Quality of Life Measurement in Neurodegenerative and Related Conditions

Quality of Life Measurement in Neurodegenerative and Related Conditions

Edited by

Crispin Jenkinson
University of Oxford

Michele Peters
University of Oxford

Mark B. Bromberg
University of Utah

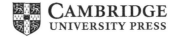
CAMBRIDGE
UNIVERSITY PRESS

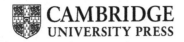

CAMBRIDGE
UNIVERSITY PRESS

Shaftesbury Road, Cambridge CB2 8EA, United Kingdom

One Liberty Plaza, 20th Floor, New York, NY 10006, USA

477 Williamstown Road, Port Melbourne, VIC 3207, Australia

314–321, 3rd Floor, Plot 3, Splendor Forum, Jasola District Centre, New Delhi – 110025, India

103 Penang Road, #05–06/07, Visioncrest Commercial, Singapore 238467

Cambridge University Press is part of Cambridge University Press & Assessment, a department of the University of Cambridge.

We share the University's mission to contribute to society through the pursuit of education, learning and research at the highest international levels of excellence.

www.cambridge.org
Information on this title: www.cambridge.org/9780521829014

First published 2011

A catalogue record for this publication is available from the British Library

Library of Congress Cataloging-in-Publication data
Quality of life measurement in neurodegenerative and related conditions / edited by Crispin Jenkinson, Michele Peters, and Mark B. Bromberg.
      p. ;   cm.
   Includes bibliographical references and index.
   ISBN 978-0-521-82901-4 (hardback)
      1. Nervous system – Degeneration – Patients – Rehabilitation.   2. Outcome assessment (Medical care)   3. Quality of life –Measurement.   I. Jenkinson, Crispin, 1962–   II. Peters, Michele   III. Bromberg, M. B. (Mark B.)
      [DNLM: 1. Nervous System Diseases.   2. Outcome Assessment (Health Care)
3. Quality of Life.   WL 140 Q12 2011]
   RC365.Q35 2011
   616.8´0471 – dc22

ISBN   978-0-521-82901-4   Hardback

Contents

List of contributors

James Bower, MD
Associate Professor of Neurology,
Mayo Clinic College of Medicine,
Rochester, Minnesota, USA

Mark B. Bromberg, MD, PhD
Professor of Neurology,
Department of Neurology,
University of Utah,
Salt Lake City, Utah, USA

David Burn, MD
Professor of Movement Disorder Neurology and
Honorary Consultant Neurologist,
Department of Neurology,
The Royal Victoria Infirmary,
Newcastle upon Tyne, UK

Stefan Cano, PhD, CPsychol
Associate Professor (Senior Lecturer) in Psychometrics,
Peninsula College of Medicine and Dentistry,
University of Plymouth,
Tamar Science Park, Plymouth, UK

Noelle E. Carlozzi, PhD
Assistant Professor,
Center for Rehabilitation Outcomes and
Assessment Research,
Department of Physical Medicine and Rehabilitation,
University of Michigan,
Ann Arbor, Michigan, USA

Elise Davis, PhD
Research Fellow,
McCaughey Centre, VicHealth Centre for
the Promotion of Mental Health and
Community Wellbeing,
School of Population Health,
University of Melbourne,
Melbourne, Australia

Jill Dawson, DPhil
Senior Research Scientist,
Health Services Research Unit,
Department of Public Health,
University of Oxford,
Oxford, UK

Ray Fitzpatrick, PhD, FMedSci
Professor of Public Health and Primary Care
and Head of the Department of Public Health,
University of Oxford, Old Road Campus,
Oxford, UK

Robert Harris, MSc
Research Officer,
Health Services Research Unit,
Department of Public Health,
University of Oxford,
Oxford, UK

Jeremy Hobart, FRCP, PhD
Associate Professor (Reader) in Clinical Neurosciences,
Peninsula College of Medicine and Dentistry,
University of Plymouth,
Tamar Science Park, Plymouth, UK

Crispin Jenkinson, DPhil
Professor of Health Services Research
and Director,
Health Services Research Unit,
Department of Public Health,
University of Oxford,
Oxford, UK

Anthony Lang, FRCPC, MD
Professor of Neurology
and Director,
Morton and Gloria Shulman Movement
Disorder Centre,
Toronto Western Hospital,
Ontario, Canada

Andrew J. Lees, MD, FRCP, FMedSci
Professor of Neurology, Honorary Consultant
Neurologist, and Director,
Reta Lila Weston Institute of Neurological Studies,
University College London,
London, UK

Irene Litvan, MD
Raymond Lee Lebby Professor of Parkinson
Disease Research,
and Director,
Division of Movement Disorders,
University of Louisville,
Kentucky, USA

Philip Low, MD
Professor of Neurology,
Mayo Clinic College of Medicine,
Rochester, Minnesota, USA

Christopher Mathias, DPhil, DSc, FRCP
Professor of Neurovascular Medicine,
and Consultant Physician,
Imperial College, London,
and Institute of Neurology,
University College London,
London, UK

Christopher Morris, DPhil
Senior Research Fellow,
Cerebra Research Unit and PenCLARHC,
Peninsula College of Medicine and Dentistry,
University of Exeter,
Exeter, Devon, UK

Michele Peters, PhD
Senior Research Scientist,
Health Services Research Unit,
Department of Public Health,
University of Oxford,
Oxford, UK

Niall Quinn, MD, FRCP
Emeritus Professor of Clinical Neurology,
and Honorary Consultant Neurologist,
Institute of Neurology,
University College London,
London, UK

Rebecca E. Ready, PhD
Associate Professor,
Department of Psychology,
University of Massachusetts,
Amherst, Massachusetts, USA

Anette Schrag, MD
Reader in Neurology,
and Honorary Consultant Neurologist,
Department of Clinical Neurosciences,
Royal Free and University College Medical School,
University College London,
London, UK

Caroline Selai, PhD, CPsychol
Senior Lecturer in Clinical Neuroscience,
Sobell Department for Motor Neuroscience
and Movement Disorders,
and Head of the Education Unit,
Institute of Neurology,
University College London,
London, UK

Amy Shelly, BSc
Project Officer,
Paediatric Integrated Cancer Service,
Children's Cancer Centre,
Royal Children's Hospital,
Parkville, Victoria, Australia

Elizabeth Waters, DPhil
Jack Brockhoff Chair of Child Public Health,
McCaughey Centre,
VicHealth Centre for the Promotion of Mental
Health and Community Wellbeing,
School of Population Health,
University of Melbourne,
Melbourne, Australia

Preface

Patient-reported outcome measures (PROMs) are now generally regarded as central to the evaluation of health and medical care. This represents a substantial change in opinion from that of just a few decades ago, when the systematic collection of patient reports of their health and quality of life was a relatively new area of research. Today, PROMs feature in routine data collection systems and are seen as important in the monitoring of health care provision. They are increasingly used as primary outcomes measures in trials. Thus, the measurement of quality of life, or what is sometimes referred to as health-related quality of life, has moved into the mainstream of evaluation. In part, this reflects the growth in "patient-centered care," and the importance now placed on public and patient views of health care. Thus, health care must reflect the needs of patients, and assessment of services must reflect both "consumer" views and "patient-reported outcomes." This text is evidence of this move toward patient-centered evaluation and documents the development and validation of quality-of-life measures for use in a wide variety of neurodegenerative, and related, conditions. This book is primarily concerned with the development, validation, and application of disease-specific measures. Such instruments are generally regarded as potentially more precise and sensitive to changes than more generic measures because they are intended to reflect the particular demands of specific conditions.

The first chapter documents established methods for the development and validation of instruments and introduces readers unfamiliar with the area to the fundamental concepts of measurement in quality-of-life measurement. The following chapters document the current state of the art in measurement of Parkinson's disease, multiple sclerosis, motor neuron disease, progressive supranuclear palsy, multiple system atrophy, Huntington's disease, and dementia. The particular demands of measuring the health status of children are explored in the chapter on cerebral palsy. Although cerebral palsy is not a neurodegenerative disorder in itself, the impact of the condition on growth for children, and on aging for adults, often causes, over time, profound changes in functioning and health status.

Consequently, the phenotype of cerebral palsy has been referred to as a "progressive neuromuscular" condition* – hence its inclusion here. The impact of serious illness can have substantial effects on family members and friends, and these issues are explored in a chapter on quality of life and carers. The final chapters of the book explore methodologic issues in translation and scoring of instruments, as well as the place of more individualized measures that are specifically designed to reflect the concerns of individual patients. This book is intended to give a clear idea of the range of instruments available, as well as the issues involved in their development, validation, and application.

* Graham HK. Painful hip dislocation in cerebral palsy. *Lancet* 2002; **359**: 907–908.

Aspects of methodology relevant to patient-reported outcome measures (PROMs)

Crispin Jenkinson, Jill Dawson,
and Christopher Morris

Introduction

Measuring patients' self-reported health status has become an established and credible way of assessing the effectiveness of medical interventions and health services; however, this was not always the case. Historically, medicine relied on clinical, radiologic, and laboratory tests and doctors' interpretations to assess treatment outcomes, and information from patients was not systematically collected and analyzed. The initial, slow uptake in measuring patient-reported outcomes (PROMs) was due in part to the view of some medical researchers and clinicians that measuring patient experience was either very difficult or impossible to do, and that such an undertaking could never be totally scientific. Consequently, traditional medical assessments gained themselves something of a reputation of being objective, "hard data," whereas patient-based material was considered subjective, "soft data" – the latter, rather pejorative term implying that the data were, one assumes, either redundant or simply inaccurate. In fact, objectivity is determined by the construct being assessed, and not by how it is measured (1). Therefore, patient-reported outcomes that assess observable constructs such as mobility are actually objective measures; in contrast, feelings, well-being, and satisfaction are more subjective measures.

Needless to say, anyone who has ever tried to develop a questionnaire will have found the process less straightforward than he or she anticipated. Furthermore, those of you who have attempted to complete questionnaires that do not make sense or that are repetitive or irrelevant will be aware that the superficially simple task of asking questions is an activity that often is done very badly. This is because some investigators have rather naïvely assumed that designing a health assessment measure or, indeed, any questionnaire requires little more than sense. In fact, a number of issues must be considered when designing a health status questionnaire or when assessing any given instrument for inclusion in a study. The purpose of this chapter is to introduce readers to some of the essential attributes of health status measures and the terminology used in this area. The chapter does not provide a definitive guide to questionnaire design and development. For those with an interest in developing measures, or who wish to seek further information, some excellent texts have been produced to guide people through the development, validation, and psychometrics of this process (2, 3). However, these texts do assume some knowledge of the topic, which is briefly discussed below.

Scales and measurement

Most health assessment questionnaires are based on scales. Thus, people may complete a questionnaire by rating their health in response to

Quality of Life Measurement in Neurodegenerative and Related Conditions, eds., Crispin Jenkinson, Michele Peters, and Mark B. Bromberg. Published by Cambridge University Press. © Cambridge University Press 2011.

individual questions. Responses to each question then are scored in some way, with individual ratings combined to produce an overall summary or scale score representing an underlying phenomenon or "construct." Such constructs might include "physical functioning," "perceived level of pain," or "anxiety." A scale is a graded system of categories, under which are four broad types with very different characteristics.

Ordinal scales are scales on which classes or objects are ordered on a continuum (e.g., from Best to Worst). No indication is given as to the distance between values, although a hierarchy is assumed to exist. Thus, when an illness is classified into 1 = mild, 2 = moderate, and 3 = severe, it cannot be assumed that the extent of difference between mild and moderate is similar to the difference between moderate and severe. Similarly, frequencies such as "never," "sometimes," and "always" are ordered, but the difference between these increments is not precise. Nonparametric rank order correlation is an appropriate statistical analysis for ordinal data because it does not involve such underlying assumptions. Tabular representation of ordinal data is appropriate, but even simple descriptive statistics (e.g., means and standard deviations) based on such data generally should be discouraged. However, although purists may adopt such principles, most researchers actually adopt a more pragmatic approach and consequently break these rules when individual ordinal responses are combined into multi-item scale scores. Indeed, some have argued that the errors produced by such analyses are generally small and insignificant (4) and therefore have advocated the use of parametric statistics (5). It is fair to say that a large number of health status measures in use today adopt ordinal scales on which numerous (sometimes quite inappropriate) statistics are applied. However, scaling procedures are often used to improve the numeric characteristics of response scales, and attempts are made to convert what are effectively ordinal response categories into interval level response scales. Such scaling procedures are discussed elsewhere and are beyond the scope of this text (4).

Interval scales are designed on the assumption that the scale is ordered and that the distances between values on one part of the scale are equal in distance to those between values on another part of the scale. Temperature is measured on such a scale. However, interval scales lack an absolute baseline anchor point. For example, a thermometer is an interval scale, but it is not possible to assume that 60 °F is twice as hot as 30 °F (because 0 °F is not as cold as it can get). Subtraction or addition of such data is appropriate, but ideally not division or multiplication. Pearson correlation, factor analysis, and discriminant analysis are appropriate analysis techniques. In health status measurement, it is not uncommon to see researchers converting ordinal responses to interval scales. Thus, attempts are made to weight responses rather than simply using arbitrary codes, such as 0 = no health problems, 1 = some health problems, and 2 = many health problems. However, a considerable body of evidence suggests that weighting schemes do not generally improve the accuracy and reliability of health status in most cases (6) and that often they seem to provide little more than a pseudoscientific level of accuracy that is unrealistic in this area of measurement.

Ratio scales are similar to interval scales but with an absolute zero point so that ratios between values can be meaningfully defined. Thus, time, weight, and height are all examples of ratio scales. For example, it is perfectly acceptable to assume that 48 hours is twice as long a time period as 24 hours. All forms of statistical analysis may be used with such data, although care should be taken in choosing methods, depending on the spread of the data. Ideally, data should be normally distributed (i.e., should follow the "bell" curve) if parametric statistics (i.e., statistical tests that assume normality in the distribution of data) are to be used, although in practice this rule is frequently broken. However, such rule breaking can mean that results are less than robust. It is something of a moot point whether any health status measure could truly claim to be a ratio scale, although the weighting schemes used for health economic measures may be regarded as falling into this category (see Chapter 5). However, in reality, we can never be certain if the zero points are truly accurate.

Ideally, measures should be developed that use interval or ratio scales, but this is no easy task in the social sciences. Measures of health status can never truly be regarded as fulfilling the requirements of these forms of measurement (7). Consequently, attempts are made to ensure that the results of measures fulfill at least certain criteria. It is to these important criteria (or "measurement properties") that we now turn our attention.

Validity and reliability

Validity

A valid assessment is one that measures what it claims to measure. Evaluation of the validity of a measure usually involves comparison with some standardized criterion or criteria. However, in the social sciences, this can be difficult, as "gold standards" against which measures can be compared are rare. Nonetheless, a number of standard aspects of validity are usually assessed for any properly constructed questionnaire. Essentially, validity comprises four aspects: face validity, content validity, criterion validity, and construct validity.

Face validity refers to whether items on a questionnaire appear both appropriate to the phenomenon being measured and to make sense, as well as being easily understood. This may seem a simple enough test for a questionnaire to pass, but ambiguities have been noted in some of the most respected and well utilized measures. In the next chapter, some problems with the wording of the Sickness Impact Profile and the 36-Item Short Form Health Survey (SF-36), two of the most utilized measures of health status, will be discussed.

Content validity refers to the choice of, and relative importance that is given to, items selected for a questionnaire. In a matter as fundamental as the selection of items, a number of approaches can be taken; items can be developed by suggestions from clinicians, through systematic searches of the literature, or from qualitative research with patients. Commonly, one would use a combination of these methods; if a substantial number of items are generated, then it may be helpful to ask a sample of potential respondents to rank them in order of importance and relevance. It is important that items appropriate to the phenomenon under investigation are chosen, and that if they are weighted in some way, the weights reflect the perceived level of difficulty, or the health problem.

Criterion validity refers to the ability of an instrument to correspond with other measures held up as "gold standards." In practice, few studies can truly claim to have evaluated criterion validity, as gold standards are hard to find in this area of research. Results from questionnaires have been compared with clinical criteria; for example, results from the Arthritis Impact Measurement Scales (AIMS) (8, 9) were compared with various rheumatologic measures; similarly, results from the Parkinson's Disease Questionnaire have been compared with various clinical assessments of disease progression, as well as with results on another health status measure (10). However, given that health status questionnaires are designed to measure different aspects of health than those tapped by traditional measures, such assessments really can provide only a very general impression that measures are related. It would be worrying if clinical assessments and health status measures were completely contradictory, but likewise it would be surprising if they correlated perfectly. Questionnaire results on one measure are often compared with those on another.

Construct validity usually involves a comparison with scores from instruments that are presumed to be measuring similar phenomena. A hypothesis is generated and tested to determine if it actually reflects these prior hypotheses. For *convergent validity*, one would expect results from one measure to be highly correlated with other variables and measures of the same construct. *Discriminant validity* is the mirror image of convergent validity – the assumption is that results will not be related when questionnaire data are compared with other data measuring distinct and unrelated concepts.

Typically, little more is sought than a set of predicted associations; however, when a shorter form of a measure is being compared with the original longer version, a more stringent criterion may be set. For example, results of the physical and mental health summary scales from the 36-item SF-36 have been compared with results from the 12-item version of the questionnaire and have been found to be almost identical (11). The gold standard in this instance is the longer-form measure, and perhaps, in the field of health status measurement, it is only when longer and shorter forms that proclaim to measure identical phenomena are compared that one could ever really say that one measure truly is a gold standard.

This form of criterion validity is sometimes referred to as *concurrent validity* (comparison of results from two measures administered at the same time). Another, although relatively rarely used, form of criterion validity is *predictive validity*, wherein results on one measure are expected to be predictive of some future event or outcome. Kazis and colleagues used AIMS and examined the relationship between health and mortality in a 5-year study of patients with rheumatoid arthritis. They found that patient-reported health was predictive of death with a significant linear trend for death and scores on both the general health and physical functioning dimensions of the questionnaire.

Reliability

A measure that fulfills the requirements for validity must also pass tests of reliability. As with validity, a number of methods may be used to assess reliability; three of these methods are common in health status measurement: internal consistency, test-retest reliability, and interobserver reliability.

Internal reliability, or internal consistency, involves checking whether items in a scale all are measuring the same construct (i.e., homogeneous). Classically, internal consistency is measured using Cronbach's alpha statistic (12) (where items have more than two response categories, such as "Never," "Sometimes," "Always") or the Kuder–Richardson (KR-20) test (for items with two response categories, such as "Yes," "No"). In practice, the alpha statistic, which was derived from the KR-20 test, is used for both types of response categories and produces very similar results on dichotomous data as are produced by the KR-20 formula. Cronbach's alpha statistics below 0.5 are regarded as low and would suggest that items in a scale are not all tapping the same underlying area of interest, whereas alpha statistics above 0.9 have been taken to mean that a measure has very high internal reliability and indicates item redundancy (i.e., that some items could be removed without loss of reliability). Rasch analysis can also be to used to check that items are assessing the same latent trait (13, 14), although this technique assumes a hierarchy of "item difficulty" (i.e., items can be ranked in terms of the difficulty they pose to respondents in the sense a respondent who answers a question stating he or she cannot walk at all must, logically, respond negatively to a question asking if he or she can walk a half mile). It has been suggested that questionnaires that measure quality of life do not always contain questions that can be ranked hierarchically (3).

Questionnaires must be stable to produce the same, or very similar, results on two or more administrations when there is good reason to believe that the health status of the respondents has not changed. This is referred to as *test-retest reliability*. To assess test-retest reliability, the questionnaire is administered to the same group of relevant people on two occasions separated by a short period of time (e.g., a few days or 2 weeks apart). The relevant time period between the two tests varies between circumstances; ideally, respondents' underlying situations should not have changed in any way between the two administrations of the questionnaire, but they should not be given so close together that respondents remember how they answered the first time. The difficulty with this method of assessing a questionnaire is that it is often unclear whether results that may indicate that a questionnaire is unreliable are, in fact, reflecting real change in peoples' health status. Respondents' familiarity with the questionnaire can also lead to changes in their responses between the two administrations.

A third form of reliability is when a proxy is used to measure health status as well as or instead of the patients. This is termed *interobserver* or *interrater reliability;* examples include parents and children or caregivers and adults. This method is often considered when it is thought that some individuals may not have the cognitive capacity to respond themselves, and a proxy who knows the person well is the next best alternative. As with test-retest reliability, one tests the hypothesis that scores derived from different observers should be highly correlated. Many health status measures find higher interobserver reliability for observable objective constructs such as physical functioning, and poorer reliability for subjective, emotional constructs.

Longitudinal validity and sensitivity to change

It is essential that evaluative instruments be able to detect change and that the level of this change be interpretable in some way. Sensitivity to change, or "responsiveness" of an instrument, is a very important criterion to consider when selecting measures to assess change. However, it has not, until relatively recently, received a great amount of attention. In part this is because researchers could present before and after treatment data and calculate whether any change was statistically significant (i.e., not a product of chance variation). Although this was traditionally commonplace, it is unsatisfactory. It is possible to find a statistically significant difference in scores on a questionnaire before and after treatment, but this could occur for a number of reasons, and it need not be clear that the difference means very much at all to clinicians or patients. Consequently, more sophisticated ways of assessing change and its relevance have been developed. Methods for evaluating responsiveness may be distribution-based (effect size, minimal detectable change, index of half a standard devi-

ation) or anchor-based (minimal important difference).

The effect size statistic is the most commonly cited interpretation of questionnaire change scores (15). The effect size, a standardized measure of the magnitude of change, is calculated by subtracting the mean score before treatment from that gained after treatment and dividing the result by the baseline standard deviation. The before treatment scores are used effectively as a proxy for control group scores. This approach treats the effect size as a standard measure of change in a "before and after" study context. Note that the purpose of the statistic is to give some idea of the magnitude of the change, rather than simply its level of statistical significance, and the standard deviation at baseline is used rather than the standard deviation of the differences between means (16). An effect size of 1.00 is equivalent to a change of 1 standard deviation in the sample. As a benchmark for assessing change, it has been suggested that an effect size of 0.2 is small, 0.5 is moderate, and 0.8 is large (17). However, although these cut-off points are useful, as a general rule some caution is needed in interpretation. For example, a very sensitive instrument may gain large effect sizes based on relatively modest changes. Other distribution-based approaches include the standardized response mean (SRM) (18) and the Guyatt responsiveness statistic (19). Norman and colleagues have shown that the different forms of responsiveness coefficients are mathematically related and recommend reporting effect size (20). The minimal detectable change (MDC) provides a distribution-based indication of the amount of change required to instill confidence that it is change beyond measurement error; a common standard is to use a 90% confidence level (21).

One potential problem with all the methods of assessing change outlined above is that they are primarily statistical. Other attempts have been made to make changes interpretable. The minimal important difference (MID) is the mean change in score reported by respondents who indicate that they had noticed some small change (22, 23). A single global rating of change on a five- or nine-point

Dimension (no of items)	Low scores	High scores
Physical functioning (10)	Limited a lot in performing bathing and dressing	Performs all types of physical activities without limitations due to health
Role limitations due to physical problems (4)	Problems with work or other daily activities as a result of physical health	No problems with work or other daily activities due to physical health
Role limitations due to emotional problems (3)	Problems with work or other daily activities as a result of emotional problems	No problems with work or other daily activities as a result of emotional problems
Social functioning (2)	Extreme and frequent interference with normal social activities due to physical or emotional problems	Performs normal social activities without interference due to physical or emotional problems
Mental health (5)	Feelings of nervousness and depression all of the time	Feels peaceful, happy, and calm all of the time
Energy/vitality (4)	Feels tired and worn down all the time	Feels full of energy all the time
Bodily pain (2)	Severe and limiting bodily pain	No pain or limitations due to pain
General health perceptions (5)	Believes personal health is poor and likely to get worse	Believes personal health is excellent

Figure 1.1 A guide to the interpretation of very high or very low scores on the SF-36. (Adapted from Ware and Sherbourne (27).)

ordinal scale is used to ask respondents to indicate whether their condition has changed, for better or worse, incrementally from very small but noticeable amounts or to a moderate or large degree. From these data, it is possible to calculate the amount of change perceived as minimally important to patients. However, one criticism of this approach is that it can be argued that all one need ask is whether or not changes are minimally important (24). Norman and associates demonstrated empirically that published MIDs are typically equivalent to half the standard deviation of the baseline scores (0.5SD) (25); hence this too has been added to reported indices of responsiveness. Estimates of responsiveness and minimal change vary across studies because of variability in populations, responses to treatments, and context. Therefore, Revicki et al. recommend that several indices of minimal change should be calculated and that they should triangulate toward a range of values in which confidence increases with replication (26).

Content-based interpretation lends itself to both disease-specific and generic measures, whereby scores on the questionnaire are interpreted by recourse to the content of questions. In other words, to gain insight into the meanings of scores, one simply looks to the items and response categories to see what needs to be affirmed (or not) to lead to certain scores. Figure 1.1 gives some indication of what given scores may mean in relation to the way questions have been completed on the SF-36, a widely used generic measure of health status (27). Of course, more detailed tables than the example shown here can be created and can be developed for all questionnaires. However, it is often possible to gain the same score by affirming very different questions. Consequently, content-based interpretation in this simple manner is not always possible or truly meaningful. A more sophisticated form of content analysis that involves three steps has been proposed by Ware (28). First, an item with good face validity should be chosen from a scale. Thus the question should be easy to interpret, and answers to it should give some indication of the severity of respondents' health state. Second, items on the scale should be dichotomized in a meaningful way (e.g., those who claim that they can always walk half a mile without problems and those who claim they cannot). Third, the percentage endorsing the item can be plotted against various scores on the dimension from which the item comes. An example of interpreting scores in this way is provided by Ware (27). Using an American population survey, he compared scores on the "physical functioning" scale from an established questionnaire (SF-36) with responses to a question asking if respondents can walk a block or farther. He found that, for example, an improvement from 45 to 55 would suggest an increase of approximately 18% among people able to walk one block. The problem with this method of interpreting data is that it places a great deal of weight upon a single question. Given that scales are developed because single questions are often viewed as unreliable measures, this can seem a rather odd way of calibrating a scale. Questionnaires that are scaled using Guttman scaling or Rasch analysis assume linearity in the phenomenon or construct that is being measured. Thus an answer to one question infers certain predictable responses to other questions, as a clear hierarchy is observed between them. However, measures developed using these techniques have been used relatively infrequently because of the rather strong assumptions and difficulties involved in creating such scales. Rasch analysis is covered in detail in Chapter 12 of this book, and use of this method in questionnaire construction is documented in Chapter 3. Interested readers can find excellent introductions to these techniques elsewhere (4, 29).

One final method of interpretation that can be adopted with generic measures is to compare results before and after treatment versus norms for the general population. For example, in one study (30), it was found that approximately 75% of patients with sleep apnea scored results on an emotional health outcome scale (the SF-36 Mental Health Component Summary (31, 32)) that would have placed them in the bottom 30% of the general population. After treatment (with continuous positive airway pressure therapy), 50% of patients' scores would have placed them in the top 50% of the population. This method of interpreting data gives some insight into the meaning of scores, but it does require normative data to be available and hence seems to rule out the possibility that results on disease-specific measures can be compared in this way (by definition, one cannot get normative "population-based" data for individuals with a specific disease).

Selecting health status measures

Health status questionnaires should be chosen and used with care. For instance, it is important to choose the right measure for the condition, context, and research questions to be addressed. This is because the measurement properties of a health status questionnaire are not just *of the* questionnaire; they are of the questionnaire *pertaining to the population and context in which it was developed, and tested*. This means that if a measure is designed and calibrated with one group of patients (e.g., patients with knee problems attending a hospital-based surgical outpatient clinic), its measurement properties may change if it is used with a different group of patients (e.g., patients with knee problems using a community-based rehabilitation service) that may represent different age groups or different clinical characteristics. Moreover, questionnaires need to be completed in accordance with any instructions provided, and missing information needs to be minimized. This requires good methods for following up with respondents, high levels of participant cooperation, and accurate questionnaire completion.

A set of criteria proposed for appraising the content and psychometric performance of health status measures includes appropriateness, reliability, validity, responsiveness, precision, interpretability, acceptability, and feasibility (33).

Summary

Health status questionnaires are not designed to be used as substitutes for traditional measures or clinical endpoints but are intended to complement existing measures and to provide a fuller picture of a health state than can be gained by clinical measures alone. Health status measures can provide a useful adjunct to the data traditionally obtained from mortality and morbidity statistics, or from traditional clinical and laboratory assessments, although careful consideration must be given to the appropriate choice of measures. Data on the reliability and validity of measures must be assessed, as must sensitivity to changes in measures in particular patient groups. At the present state of development, more research is required to determine the appropriateness of many measures for various clinical groups and to determine the sensitivity to change and validity of measures across community and patient samples. Such issues are of ever increasing importance, given the growing use of PROMs to evaluate medical interventions. Indeed, the U.S. Food and Drug Administration has provided guidelines for good-quality reporting of PROM data, which stress the importance of documenting clearly the characteristics of such measures when used in product development and evaluation (34). The present text indicates the state of the art in neurodegenerative diseases and the considerable efforts that have gone into creating meaningful measures of patient-reported outcomes.

REFERENCES

1. McDowell I. *Measuring Health*, Third Edition. Oxford: Oxford University Press, 2006.

2. Oppenheim AN. *Questionnaire Design, Interviewing and Attitude Measurement*, New Edition. London: Pinter, 1992.

3. Streiner D, Norman G. *Health Measurement Scales: A Practical Guide to Their Development and Use*, Fourth Edition. Oxford: Oxford University Press, 2008.

4. Nunnally J, Bernstein I. *Psychometric Theory*, Third Edition. New York: McGraw Hill, 1994.

5. Norman G. Likert scales, levels of measurement and the "laws" of statistics. Advances in Health Sciences Education: Theory and Practice, 2010; Available from: www.springerlink.com\content\102840\.

6. Jenkinson C. Why are we weighting? A critical examination of the use of item weights in a health status measure. *Social Science and Medicine* 1991; **32**: 1413–1416.

7. Bowling A. *Measuring Health: A Review of Quality of Life Measurement Scales*, Third Edition. Buckingham, UK: Open University Press, 2004.

8. Meenan RF, Gertman PM, Mason JH. Measuring health status in arthritis: the arthritis impact measurement scales. *Arthritis Rheum* 1980; **23**: 146–152.

9. Meenan RF, Mason JH, Anderson JJ, Guccione A, Kazis L. AIMS2: the content and properties of a revised and expanded Arthritis Impacts Measurement Scales health status questionnaire. *Arthritis Rheum* 1992; **35**: 1–10.

10. Jenkinson C, Peto V, Fitzpatrick R, Greenhall R, Hyman N. Self reported functioning and well being in patients with Parkinson's disease: comparison of the Short Form Health Survey (SF-36) and the Parkinson's Disease Questionnaire (PDQ-39). *Age Ageing* 1995; **24**: 505–509.

11. Jenkinson C, Layte R, Jenkinson D, Lawrence K, Petersen S, Paice C, Stradling J. A shorter form health survey: can the SF12 replicate results from the SF36 in longitudinal studies? *J Public Health Med* 1997; **19**: 179–186.

12. Cronbach LJ. Coefficient alpha and the internal structure of tests. *Psychometrika* 1951; **16**: 297–334.

13. Andrich D. *Rasch Models for Measurement*. Newbury Park: Sage Publications, 1988.

14. Tennant A, Conaghan PG. The Rasch measurement model in rheumatology: what is it and why is it?: when should it be applied, and what should one look for in a Rasch paper? *Arthritis Rheum* 2007; **57**: 1358–1362.

15. Lydick E, Epstein RS. Interpretation of quality of life changes. *Qual Life Res* 1993; **2**: 221–226.

16. Kazis L, Anderson JJ, Meenan RF. Effect sizes for interpreting changes in health status. *Med Care* 1989; **27** Supplement: S178–S189.

17. Cohen J. *Statistical Power for the Behavioural Sciences.* New York: Academic Press, 1977.

18. Liang M, Fossel AH, Larson MG. Comparison of five health status instruments for orthopaedic evaluation. *Med Care* 1990; **28**: 632–642.

19. Guyatt G, Walter S, Norman TG. Measuring change over time: assessing the usefulness of evaluative instruments. *J Chron Dis* 1987; **40**: 171–178.

20. Norman GR, Wyrwich KW, Patrick DL. The mathematical relationship among different forms of responsiveness coefficients. *Qual Life Res* 2007; **16**: 815–822.

21. Haley SM, Fragala-Pinkham MA. Interpreting change scores of tests and measures used in physical therapy. *Phys Ther* 2006; **86**: 735–743.

22. Jaeschke R, Singer J, Guyatt GH. Measurement of health status: ascertaining the minimal clinically important difference. *Control Clin Trials* 1989; **10**: 407–415.

23. Juniper E, Guyatt G, Willan A, Griffith L. Determining a minimally important change in a disease specific questionnaire. *J Clin Epidemiol* 1994; **47**: 81–87.

24. Revicki D, Hays RD, Cella D, Sloan J. Recommended methods for determining responsiveness and minimally important differences for patient-reported outcomes. *J Clin Epidemiol* 2008; **61**: 102–109.

25. Norman GR, Sloan JA, Wyrwich KW. Interpretation of changes in health-related quality of life: the remarkable universality of half a standard deviation. *Med Care* 2003; **41**: 582–592.

26. Revicki DA, Cella D, Hays RD, Sloan JA, Lenderking WR, Aaronson NK. Responsiveness and minimal important differences for patient reported outcomes. *Health Qual Life Outcomes* 2006; **27**: 70.

27. Ware J, Sherbourne C. The MOS 36-item Short Form Health Survey 1. Conceptual framework and item selection. *Med Care* 1992; **30**: 473–483.

28. Ware J, Snow K, Kosinsnki M, Gandek B. *SF-36 Health Survey Manual and Interpretation Guide.* Boston, MA: The Health Institute, New England Medical Center, 1993.

29. Bond TG, Fox CM. *Applying the Rasch Model: Fundamental Measurement in the Human Sciences.* London: Psychology Press, 2006.

30. Jenkinson C. The SF-36 physical and mental health summary scores: a guide to interpretation. *J Health Serv Res Policy* 1998; **3**: 92–96.

31. Ware JE, Kosinski M, Keller SD. *SF-36 Physical and Mental Health Summary Scales: A User Manual.* Boston, MA: The Health Institute, New England Medical Center, 1994.

32. Jenkinson C, Layte R, Wright L, Coulter A. *The UK SF-36: An Analysis and Interpretation Manual.* Oxford: Health Services Research Unit, 1996.

33. Fitzpatrick R, Davey C, Buxon M, Jones D. Evaluating patient-based outcome measures for use in clinical trials. *Health Technol Assess* 1998; **14**: 1–72.

34. FDA Guidance for Industry. *Patient-Reported Outcome Measures: Use in Medical Product Development to Support Labelling Claims.* Silver Spring, MD: Food and Drug Administration, 2009.

2

The development and validation of the Parkinson's Disease Questionnaire and related measures

Crispin Jenkinson and Ray Fitzpatrick

Introduction

Parkinson's disease can have a wide range of impacts on individuals' lives. Although the range of problems has been documented, attempts to assess such impacts systematically and directly from the individual's perspective are relatively recent. This chapter outlines the development of a questionnaire designed to measure health-related quality of life in patients diagnosed with Parkinson's disease, as well as the subsequent development of a shorter-form measure of this instrument.

Parkinson's disease (PD) is a common, chronic neurological condition affecting just over 1 per 1000 and increasing in incidence in older ages (1). Early diagnosis can prove difficult but is usually defined by the presence of at least two of the primary physical symptoms (tremor, rigidity, bradykinesia, and postural instability), as well as a positive response to the drug levodopa. Primary symptoms can manifest themselves in many ways, including slowness, stiffness, an inability to initiate movement, a stooped posture, an impassive face, and a shuffling gait. Difficulties may be observed with walking and balance, dressing, and speech and communication, along with loss of dexterity or fatigue. As the disease progresses, the physical symptoms may affect other aspects of daily life and create additional psychological and social problems. Currently, no cure for PD is known, although pharmaceutical and surgical

treatments can be effective in managing some of the symptoms. Therefore the aim of any treatment must primarily be to improve quality of life.

Traditionally, the impact of PD upon patients' lives was largely assessed by clinical scales such as the Hoehn and Yahr Scale (2), the Columbia Rating Scale (3), and the Unified Parkinson's Disease Rating Scale (UPDRS) (4), the latter incorporating a modified Hoehn and Yahr Scale, rated in eight stages, and also measuring activities of daily living, as assessed by the clinician, by incorporating the Schwab and England Scale (5). These measures focus largely on neurological symptoms and physical impairment (indeed, the Schwab and England is more accurately a measure of physical independence than of activities of daily living). Thus, for example, evidence of effectiveness of a drug such as selegiline in relation to disability has largely tended to come from such clinical scales (6) and from assessment of the primary symptoms of the disease, notably tremor, rigidity, bradykinesia (i.e., abnormally slow body movements), and postural instability.

In the past decade, considerable growth of interest in measuring health status from the patient's perspective has been seen in the neurological community. Indeed, patient-reported outcome measures are increasingly used as primary endpoints in clinical trials (7). This chapter outlines the growing use of health-related quality of life measures in PD. Such measures are intended to assess a broader

Quality of Life Measurement in Neurodegenerative and Related Conditions, eds., Crispin Jenkinson, Michele Peters, and Mark B. Bromberg. Published by Cambridge University Press. © Cambridge University Press 2011.

range of areas of the patient's well-being than are assessed by clinical scales.

Important areas of health-related quality of life in PD

Although no consensus has been reached as to the definition of health-related quality of life in medical research, broad agreement indicates that the focus should be on areas of experience of greatest concern to individuals who have the relevant health problem, and that the concept of health-related quality of life is multidimensional (8, 9). Research has revealed some important concerns for individuals with PD. Bulpitt and colleagues (10) have shown that some symptoms such as being frozen to the spot, grimacing, and jerking arms and legs are between 20 and 40 times more frequently experienced by individuals with PD than by others of the same age, whereas a diverse range of other experiences such as loss of interest in sex, indigestion, and headache are very commonly experienced by individuals with PD, although the extent to which these problems exceed those of age-matched controls is a matter of disagreement (11). Problems of sleep are frequently reported; an inability to turn over in bed and nocturnal cramps have been reported by more than 50% of one sample of individuals with PD (12).

Several epidemiologic surveys have demonstrated the importance of physical disability in PD, particularly in terms of walking, moving around in bed and around the house, and having mobility in public areas (1, 13). Falls are a common hazard for individuals with PD; in one study, 13% reported falls occurring more than once a week (14). As a result, hip fractures can be a common health problem in this group of patients. Individuals with PD report more work-related problems than matched controls and also more limitations in relation to household management (15). The potential social consequences of PD are diverse. Individuals may experience social isolation and limited leisure activities; in one study, 50% of individuals with PD compared with 27% of age-matched controls

reported restricted social activities (16). More than two thirds of individuals attending a specialist clinic for PD reported giving up a hobby because of their PD (17). The same series of patients commonly reported difficulties in taking holidays. Within the household, individuals with PD rated their home or family life as being far more adversely affected by health problems than did the controls.

Financial difficulties may be an important consequence of PD. Oxtoby estimated that 19% of individuals with PD experience such problems (18). Premature retirement from work, resulting in reduced income, was reported by 29% of individuals with PD in a study of quality of life of patients with PD attending a specialist clinic. Rubenstein and colleagues report a case-control study of individuals with PD identified from the U.S. population–based National Medical Expenditure Survey (19). Individuals with PD experienced significantly more health-related economic costs than did the matched controls, arising from costs of prescriptions, home care, and hospitalization. They also were significantly more likely to report that their health kept them from working or limited the kind of paid work that they could do.

Emotional well-being is a central aspect of health-related quality of life. Up to 30% of individuals with PD experience depression (20, 21). Less severe but important effects include a sense of loss of control over life, loss of confidence, embarrassment, and stigma arising from symptoms of PD (22). Also distressing are the consequences of cognitive impairment. Bulpitt and colleagues found 33% concerned about problems of concentration (9). Severe cognitive decline and dementia pose additional stresses. PD can involve particular problems with communication. Approximately a third of individuals with PD experience difficulties with speech that cause them concern (1, 12).

Patient-reported outcome measures

Patient-reported outcome measures (PROMs) are intended to assess salient aspects of disease from the patient's perspective in a way that produces standardized and valid information. It is equally important that such information be collected in a feasible and acceptable fashion, so that data collection in clinical trials does not jeopardize the care of participating patients. Two main types of PROM are used: generic and disease-specific instruments. Both types have been used in relation to PD. The two types differ in their form, content, and intended purpose.

Generic measures

Generic PROMs, as implied by the name, are intended to be relevant to a wide spectrum of health problems rather than to one specific disease alone. The main advantage of such an instrument is that it allows comparisons of health status across diverse patient groups. Generic PROMs tend to be worded in such a way that questionnaire items are relevant to the vast majority of people. This has the advantage that estimates of the health status of a population as a whole can be made as a baseline or norm against which the scores of a specific patient group or intervention can be evaluated. Four of the most widely used generic measures are the Sickness Impact Profile (SIP) (23) (Anglicized for use in the UK as the Functional Limitations Profile (24)), the Nottingham Health Profile (NHP) (25), the EuroQol EQ-5D (26), and the 36-Item Short Form Health Survey (SF-36) (27).

Reasonable evidence of the use of such generic measures in PD is now available. The SIP was administered by Longstreth and colleagues to patients with PD attending a neurological clinic and to matched controls (15). SIP scale scores correlated significantly with Hoehn and Yahr and Columbia Scale scores as assessed by the neurologist, providing evidence of construct validity. Correlations with the clinical scales were somewhat stronger for physical than for psychosocial dimensions of the SIP, and investigators concluded that the SIP assesses important impacts of PD not captured by conventional neurological scales. The problem most commonly reported by patients (75%)

was difficulty in writing. Areas of greatest difference from controls included various items regarding housework, sexual interest, problems of speech, and social activities, in all of which patients with PD had poorer scores. Another study used the SIP to demonstrate greater problems for individuals with PD in relation to physical function than were observed in a general population survey of individuals identified as disabled (14). Finally, dimensions of the SIP have been found to be sensitive to change and able to differentiate between treatment with standard carbidopa-levodopa and sustained-release carbidopa-levodopa (28).

The NHP has also been used to demonstrate higher levels of problems across all six dimensions for individuals with PD compared with a control group of the same age (29). In the same way, the membership of PD societies reported poorer scores on all dimensions of the SF-36 than were obtained by controls (30).

The SF-36 has been found to provide consistently strong associations between Hoehn and Yahr stage and SF-36 dimensions (31). Furthermore, the Mental Health dimension of the SF-36 has been found to be responsive to intervention. Mercer reports the use of a simple subset of items taken from the SF-36 to evaluate the impact of a health management program, PROPATH, on the well-being of patients with PD (32). The PROPATH program was intended to provide advice and information to assist patients in coping with the physical and psychosocial consequences of PD. Although no impact on patient satisfaction measures was apparent, significant improvement was detected in the five-item measure of mental health (the Mental Health dimension of the SF-36) 1 year after the intervention.

Some criticisms of the use of generic measures have been raised, notably that the SIP is too long a questionnaire to be useful in all situations where quality of life measures might profitably be included, that the NHP is insensitive to lower levels of ill health, and that the terminology of the SF-36 does not make it suitable for older adults, as many of the questions ask about work-related behavior

(33). However, despite such concerns, the measures appear reliable and seem to provide meaningful and useful insight into the demands of the illness upon patients.

Generic measures of quality of life are not designed for a particular disease and consequently have some limitations. For example, although they include questions about physical, social, and psychological factors, they often omit questions specifically relevant to particular disease groups, such as issues concerning the social embarrassment that individuals with PD may experience. Thus a PD-specific questionnaire is intended to give a more accurate picture of the impact of PD than is provided by a generic measure. It is also more likely to be able to detect the small but important changes anticipated with many of the modern drug therapies.

A number of disease-specific measures assess quality of life in PD: the Parkinson's Impact Scale (PIMS) (34); the Parkinson's Disease Quality of Life Questionnaire (PDQL) (35); PDQUALIF (36); the 39-item Parkinson's Disease Questionnaire (PDQ-39); and the shorter-form Parkinson's Disease Questionnaire, the PDQ-8 (37, 38).

The Parkinson's Impact Scale (PIMS)

The PIMS is a short measure that was developed on the basis of clinical judgment, with its 10 items designed by nurses from PD specialty clinics. Data collected by the developers on 149 PD patients suggest that the measure has acceptable levels of reliability and validity. Because of its brevity, Calne and followers (34) suggest that the PIMS is of potential use in clinical settings and may be applicable to other chronic illnesses.

However, longer-form measures can provide greater accuracy and validity. Consequently, we will describe the PDQL and the PDQ-39 in greater detail. Both these measures have been developed in accordance with widely accepted criteria for the construction of disease-specific, quality of life mea-

sures (39). The criteria are that questions included in the measure should reflect areas of quality of life that are of importance to the specific patient group under study and should measure aspects of physical, social, and psychological well-being. In addition, the scores generated from the measure should be amenable to statistical analysis, and the questionnaire should fulfill tests for validity and should be as short as possible and simple to complete. A review of health status quality of life measures found that both the PDQL and the PDQ-39 fulfilled most of these criteria (40).

PDQUALIF

The PDQUALIF was based on responses gathered to an open-ended question: How does PD change or affect one's quality of life? (35) Fifty-two patients, 28 spouses or significant others, and 6 PD professionals answered the question, and 73 indicators of quality of life were abstracted from the responses through content analysis. Three movement disorder professionals then rated each statement for clarity, conciseness, and relevance. The 32 highest-scoring items were then selected for inclusion in the instrument, with one additional global quality of life statement added to the list. Factor analytic techniques were then used to assign the 32 original items into subscales. The questionnaire was designed to place an emphasis on nonmotor impairments and disabilities and places greater stress on social aspects of living with the disease. At the time of this writing, the instrument has not been widely used and has not been validated for use outside of the United States.

The Parkinson's Disease Quality of Life Questionnaire (PDQL)

The PDQL was developed in two phases. In the first phase, potential questions were generated by a combination of in-depth interviews with four patients, suggestions from neurologists, who were members of the Dutch PD Society, and a literature review. Then 13 patients were asked to rate the relative importance of 73 candidate questionnaire items, the result of which task produced 37 most important items. In the second phase, completed answers to the PDQL of 384 members of the Dutch PD Society were analyzed in conjunction with demographic variables and answers to other quality of life measures. Answers from the larger survey were factor analyzed to produce the four scales of the PDQL. Moreover, the PDQL had expected patterns of correlation with the other quality of life measures. The developers made several important observations that are relevant to any assessment of quality of life in this group of patients. First, they noted that patients with PD took twice as long as a comparison group of patients with inflammatory bowel disease to complete a questionnaire. This suggests the advantages of brevity and simplicity in assessing quality of life in PD. Second, they noted that those with substantial cognitive impairment have problems completing such assessments. Although they estimated that only 1% of their sample had such impairment, this may be a greater problem in other studies and could result in bias in trials if nonresponse is not taken into consideration.

In an assessment of the PDQL on a PD sample derived from a community-based register, Hobson and colleagues found it to be a valid instrument that could be an important additional measure reflecting the impact of PD from the patient perspective (41). However, they reported that the responsiveness of this measure still needs to be determined.

The Parkinson's Disease Questionnaire (PDQ-39)

To ensure that the questionnaire captured aspects of health status important to patients with PD, in-depth interviews were conducted with 20 people with PD attending a neurology outpatient clinic. People were asked to describe the areas of their lives

The Parkinson's Disease Questionnaire (PDQ-39)

8 dimensions: 39 items
- Mobility
- Activities of daily living
- Emotional well-being
- Bodily discomfort
- Stigma
- Social support
- Cognitions
- Communication

Associated measures
- PDQ-39SI: single index derived from the PDQ-39
- PDQ-8SI: single index derived from the PDQ-8
- PDQ-8: an 8-item measure containing the most highly correlated item from each PDQ-39 dimension, designed solely to provide the PDQ-8SI

Figure 2.1 Features of the PDQ-39 and related measures.

that had been adversely affected by their PD. This generated a large number of possible questionnaire items, which could be included in the final questionnaire. These items were scrutinized for ambiguity and repetition. A 65-item questionnaire was developed and piloted to test basic acceptability and comprehension.

The next stage was to reduce the number of questionnaire items and generate scales for the different dimensions of health-related quality of life. Three hundred fifty-nine individuals completed the 65-item questionnaire. Factor analyses produced a 39-item questionnaire with eight dimensions. Reliability in terms of internal consistency of each dimension was assessed using Cronbach's alpha statistic (42), where values above 0.5 are acceptable, although ideally scores should be in excess of 0.7 (43, 44). Internal consistency was found to be good for all dimensions of the PDQ-39 and comparable with other established health status measures (28). The result was the PDQ-39, a questionnaire with 39 items covering eight discrete dimensions (Figure 2.1). The scores from each dimension are computed into a scale ranging from 0 (best, i.e., no problem at all) through to 100 (worst, i.e., maximum level of problem).

The measurement properties of the PDQ-39 – reliability, validity, and sensitivity to change – were assessed by using data from a second postal survey and an outpatient clinic sample (45). For the second postal survey, all members with PD from five different PDS branches were sent a booklet containing the PDQ-39, the SF-36, and questions about the severity of their PD symptoms. In addition, a second copy of the PDQ-39 was included in a sealed envelope. Respondents were asked to complete the second copy 3 to 6 days after the first and were asked to report any important changes in their health during that time.

In the clinic sample, individuals with PD attending neurology outpatient clinics were surveyed with the PDQ-39 and the SF-36 and were clinically assessed using the Hoehn and Yahr Index and the Columbia Rating Scale; they were reassessed with the same measures 4 months later.

Reliability

The two sets of PDQ-39 data from the second postal survey were available to examine reliability in terms of internal consistency of the eight PDQ-39 dimensions. Cronbach's alpha was satisfactory for all scales on both occasions, with the exception of social support (0.66) at time 1, which was only slightly below the accepted criterion. Test-retest reliability (reproducibility) was examined by means of correlation coefficients between scale scores at time 1 and time 2. Correlations were all significant (p < 0.001), and a *t*-test to test for changes in the distribution of scores between the two assessments produced no significant differences.

Validity

Construct validity was examined by correlating scale scores with relevant SF-36 scores. Correlations were all significant for PDQ-39 scales with matching scales of SF-36. Questionnaire items asked respondents to assess the severity of their tremor, stiffness, and slowness. A consistent pattern of worse scores on all PDQ-39 scales was obtained from patients with more severe self-assessed symptoms. Further evidence of construct validity has been established in a Spanish study, which compared the UPRDS with

the PDQ-39. All PDQ-39 scales were significantly correlated with UPRDS scores (46).

Validity of the PDQ-39 was also examined in terms of agreement with clinical assessments performed by neurologists in the clinic study: the Hoehn and Yahr Index and the Columbia Rating Scale. Significant correlations were found between both clinical scales and PDQ-39 dimensions (p < 0.05) for all dimensions except social support.

Sensitivity to change

Sensitivity to change of the PDQ-39 was evaluated in a postal survey of randomly selected members of 13 local branches of the Parkinson's Disease Society. Questionnaires were completed on two occasions, 6 months apart. At time 1, the survey contained PDQ-39 demographic questions; in addition, members were asked to provide their name and address if they were willing to take part in the 6-month follow-up. A thank you/reminder letter was sent out to all members after 3 weeks. At follow-up, the survey was sent to all respondents who had provided their name and address for this purpose. In this second survey, the questionnaire contained the PDQ-39 and nine transition questions. Eight transition questions asked respondents to judge change since the previous survey on each of the specific dimensions of the PDQ-39, and one asked about overall health. For each of the transition questions, respondents were asked if they were "a lot better," "a little better," "the same," "a little worse," or "a lot worse" than 6 months ago. A reminder letter and a questionnaire were sent to nonresponders after 3 weeks.

Mean change scores were calculated for the summary index and each dimension of the PDQ-39. The mean change for each dimension, and for the summary score, was compared with responses to its relevant transition question. A minimally important difference (MID) was defined as the mean change score of individuals reporting a little change over the 6 months since completing the first questionnaire. In principle, this could be for the better or the worse. However, the proportion of this sample reporting any change for the better within any dimension was considered too small (3.7%–13.0%) to estimate MIDs. Over a quarter of the sample reported they felt "a little worse" for all dimensions, with the exception of Stigma and Social Support. Thus minimally important differences were calculated on data from this group. Evidence suggests that a small positive or negative change from baseline can be treated as equivalent (47). Effect sizes were also calculated for each dimension and the summary score. An effect size is defined as the difference between two mean scores expressed in standard deviation units (i.e., the mean difference divided by the standard deviation at baseline) (48). One thousand three hundred seventy-two PDS members were surveyed at baseline. A total of 851 (62.0%) questionnaires were returned, of which 800 (58.3%) had been completed and included name and address details for follow-up. In all, 39 (2.8%) had been completed but with no address details, and 12 (0.9%) were returned blank with notice that the person was unable to participate in the survey. At time 2, 800 respondents who had provided their name and address for this purpose were surveyed. Of these, 735 (91.9%) questionnaires were returned, of which 728 (91.0%) had been completed, and 9 (1.1%) were returned blank with notice that the person was unable to participate.

The final analysis was carried out on 728 people (53.1% of the original sample), who completed the questionnaires at both times. The mean age of the sample was 70.4 years (range, 32.9–90.9); 58.9% were male and 41.1% female. The mean number of years with PD was 8.6 (range, 0–40 years); 75.6% were married, and 80.3% lived with at least one other adult; 3.5% lived in residential care, and 4.7% were currently employed; 29.4% needed help to complete the questionnaire.

Table 2.1 shows the mean change scores on the eight dimensions and the index score for those who indicated "no change" at follow-up as well as for those who indicated "a little change for the worse." No significant differences were found between the two administrations of the questionnaire on any dimension for those who claimed that no change had occurred. However, significant differences were

Table 2.1 Mean (SD) change scores in PDQ-39 scores of respondents reporting that their health was "About the same" or "A little worse" at follow-up (i.e., time 2)

	"About the same" Mean Change (SD) [n]	"A little worse" Mean Change (SD) [n]
Mobility	−1.5 (14.09) [249]	−3.2 (13.26) [254]∗
ADL	−0.7 (15.91) [317]	−4.4 (16.56) [242]∗
Emotional well-being	0.3 (14.18) [388]	−4.2 (17.09) [182]∗
Stigma	0.8 (18.45) [477]	−5.6 (22.98) [91]∗∗∗
Social support	−1.2 (15.66) [547]	−11.4 (23.28) [33]∗∗
Cognitions	0.4 (15.80) [360]	−1.8 (15.56) [245]
Communication	−0.8 (16.36) [419]	−4.2 (18.74) [197]∗∗
Pain	1.3 (17.72) [436]	−2.1 (18.68) [174]
Overall (PDQ-39SI)	−0.6 (9.51) [243]	−1.6 (8.89) [192]∗∗∗

t–tests (difference between time 1 and time 2): ∗ p < =0.001; ∗∗ p < =0.01; ∗∗∗ p < =0.05.

found on the index score and on six of the eight dimensions of the questionnaire for those who reported at follow-up that their health had changed for the worse. Minimally important differences for each dimension varied, with large changes required in before and after scores to indicate a meaningful alteration in perceived social support, whereas smaller numeric changes were required on all other dimensions. Such results can also be analyzed in terms of effect size, with relatively small effect sizes indicating subjectively important changes (see Table 2.2).

Cross-cultural validation

The PDQ-39 instrument is the most widely used disease-specific instrument employed in studies of PD patients. Reviews have suggested that it is the most widely validated instrument, and in most instances where quality of life of PD patients is being measured, it is likely to be the most appropriate (49, 50). Indeed, the measure has been, and is being, applied in trials that include a number of countries. For any measure to be of value in a clinical

Table 2.2 Mean (SD) PDQ–39 scores at baseline and follow-up for patients who reported at follow-up that they felt "a little worse" for each dimension of the PDQ–39

	Mean (SD) at Time 1	Mean (SD) at Time 2	Effect Size
Mobility (n=254)	63.07 (27.82)	66.23 (25.47)	.11
ADL (n=242)	52.93 (24.95)	57.37 (24.10)	.18
Emotional well–being (n=182)	46.20 (21.86)	50.39 (19.86)	.19
Stigma (n=91)	42.17 (26.88)	47.73 (24.99)	.21
Social support (n=33)	37.63 (26.69)	48.99 (21.32)	.43
Cognitions (n=245)	51.86 (21.40)	53.62 (20.00)	.08
Communication (n=197)	47.04 (24.61)	51.27 (21.21)	.17
Pain (n=174)	61.16 (23.13)	63.27 (31.35)	.10
Overall (PDQ–39SI) (n=192)	44.00 (15.85)	45.60 (15.57)	.10

trial, evidence must indicate that it is reliable, valid, and practicable (51). Manifestly, measures that fulfill such requirements in one country, but not in others, are going to be of limited use. A number of published studies have indicated that the measure is valid and reliable in countries other than the United Kingdom. The measure has been translated into more than seventy languages, and extensive validation studies have been undertaken for the American (52), Brazilian (53), Bulgarian (54), Chinese (55, 56, 57, 58), Dutch (59), Ecuadorian (60), French (61), Greek (62), Japanese (63), Spanish (64), and Iranian (65) versions of the instrument. Thus, data quality, response rates, reliability, and scaling assumptions of the measure have been supported in a large number of countries.

Discussion and conclusion

Patient-reported outcome measures, such as the PDQ-39 and related measures, are increasingly used to assess the impact of treatment regimens upon patients. Typically, traditional clinical assessments do not measure important components of well-being, and improvements in quality of life are perhaps the most important outcome variables in treatment trials (66, 67). As this chapter has indicated, a range of instruments have been shown to be of value in assessing a broader range of aspects of health-related quality of life in PD. Generic instruments have an important role in showing the range of impacts of PD because results can be compared with scores on the same instrument for the general population and for other illness groups. Consequently, it is possible to "norm" the data and interpret scores from specific patient groups with the health of the population at large. Disease-specific questionnaires are more likely to be sensitive to the specific concerns of individuals with PD and to be particularly appropriate for use in clinical trials. It is important to note that thresholds for sensitivity of the dimensions of PDQ-39 are available (see Tables 2.1 and 2.2), and thus standard "rules of thumb" need not be used. It is clear that information gained by such instruments directly complements the evidence obtained by conventional clinical scales, and it has been suggested that they be used to evaluate treatment and long-term care regimens (68) when clinical measures provide only a limited view of the impact on the subjective experience of patients. Such a view may once have been controversial, but given the widespread use of the PDQ-39 throughout the world, it would appear this is no longer the case: patient views are now truly at the center of health care evaluation.

REFERENCES

1. Sutcliffe R, Prior R, Mawby B, McQuillan W. Parkinson's disease in the district of Northampton Health Authority, UK. A study of prevalence and disability. *Acta Neurologica Scand* 1985; **72**: 363–379.

2. Hoehn M, Yahr M. Parkinsonism: onset, progression and mortality. *Neurology* 1967; **17**: 427–442.

3. Hely M, Chey T, Wilson A, Williamson PM, O'Sullivan DJ, Rail D, Morris JGL. Reliability of the Columbia Scale for assessing signs of Parkinson's Disease. *Movement Disord* 1993; **8**: 466–472.

4. Fahn S, Elton RL, and members of the UPDRS development committee. Unified Parkinson's Disease Rating Scale. In: Fahn S, Marsden M, Goldstein M, Calne DB, eds. *Recent Developments in Parkinson's Disease*, Volume 2. New York: MacMillan, 1987.

5. Schwab RS, England AC. Projection technique for evaluating surgery in Parkinson's disease. In: Gillingham FJ, Donaldson MC, eds. *Third Symposium of Parkinson's Disease*. Edinburgh: Livingstone, 1969.

6. Bryson H, Milne R, Chrisp P. Selegiline: An appraisal of the basis of its pharmacoeconomic and quality-of-life benefits in Parkinson's Disease. *ParmacoEconomics* 1992; **2**: 118–136.

7. Williams A, Patel S, Ives N, Rick C, Daniels J, Jenkinson C, Gill S, Varma T, Wheatley K. (2008) PD SURG: A large, randomised trial to assess the impact of surgery in Parkinson's disease. *Movement Disord* 2008; **23** (Suppl 1): 360.

8. Guyatt G, Cook D. Health status, quality of life, and the individual. *JAMA* 1994; **272**: 630–631.

9. Bowling A, What things are important in people's lives? A survey of the public's judgements to inform scales of health-related quality of life. *Soc Sci Med* 1995; **41**: 1447–1462.

10. Bulpitt C, Shaw K, Clifton P, Stern G, Davies J, Reid J. The symptoms of patients treated for Parkinson's disease. *Clin Neuropharmacol* 1985; **8**: 175–183.

11. Quinn W, Oertel N. Parkinson's disease drug therapy. *Ballieres Clin Neurology* 1997; **97**: 89–108.

12. Lees A, Blackburn N, Campbell V. The night-time problems of Parkinson's disease. *Clin Neuropharmacol* 1988; **11**: 512–519.

13. Mutch W, Strudwick A, Roy S, Downie A. Parkinson's disease: disability, review, and management. *BMJ* 1986; **293**: 675–677.

14. Koller W, Vetere-Overfield B. Abstract: Falls and Parkinson's disease. *Ann Neurol* 1988; **24**: 153–154.

15. Welburn P, Walker S. Assessment of quality of life in Parkinson's disease. In: Teeling Smith G, ed. *Measuring Health: A Practical Approach*. Chichester: John Wiley, 1988.

16. Longstreth W, Nelson L, Linde M, Munoz D. Utility of the Sickness Impact Profile in Parkinson's disease. *J Geriatr Psychiatry Neurol* 1992; **5**: 142–148.

17. Clarke C, Zobkiw R, Gullaksen E. Quality of life and care in Parkinson's disease. *Br J Clin Pract* 1995; **49**: 288–293.

18. Oxtoby M. *Parkinson's Disease Patients and Their Social Needs*. London: Parkinson's Disease Society, 1982.

19. Rubenstein L, Chrischilles E, Voelker M. The impact of Parkinson's disease on health status, health expenditures, and productivity. *Pharmacoeconomics* 1997; **12**: 486–498.

20. Shindler J, Brown R, Welburn P, Parkes J. Measuring the quality of life of patients with Parkinson's disease. In: S Walker, R Rosser, eds. *Quality of Life Assessment: Key Issues in the 1990s*. Dordrecht: Kluwer Academic Publishers, 1993.

21. Gotham A, Brown R, Marsden C. Depression in Parkinson's disease: a quantitative and qualitative analysis. *J Neurol Neurosurg Psychiatry* 1986; **49**: 381–389.

22. Nijhof G. Parkinson's disease as a problem of shame in public appearance. *Sociol Health Illn* 1995; **17**: 193–205.

23. Bergner M, Bobbitt RA, Carter WB, Gilson B. The Sickness Impact Profile: development and final revision of a health status measure. *Med Care* 1981; **19**: 787–805.

24. Patrick D, Peach H. *Disablement in the Community*. Oxford: Oxford University Press, 1989.

25. Hunt S, McEwen J, McKenna S. *Measuring Health Status*. London: Croom Helm, 1986.

26. Greiner W, Weijnen T, Nieuwenhuizen M, Oppe S, Badia X, Busschbach J, Buxton M, Dolan P, Kind P, Krabbe P, Ohinmaa A, Parkin D, Roset M, Sintonen H, Tsuchiya A, de Charro F. A single European currency for EQ-5D health states. Results from a six-country study. *Eur J Health Econ* 2003; Sep **4**(3): 222–231.

27. Ware J, Sherbourne C. The MOS 36-Item Short-Form Health Survey 1: Conceptual framework and item selection. *Med Care* 1992; **30**: 473–483.

28. Pahwa R, Lyons K, McGuire D, Silverstein P, Zwiebel F, Robischon M, Koller W. Comparison of standard Carbidopa-Levodopa and sustained release Carbidopa-Levodopa in Parkinson's disease: pharmackinetic and quality of life measures. *Movement Disord* 1997; **12**: 677–681.

29. Karlsen KH, Larsen PJ, Tandberg E, Maeland JG. Influence of clinical and demographic variables on quality of life in patients with Parkinson's disease. *J Neurol Neurosurg Psychiatry* 1999; **66**: 431–435.

30. Jenkinson C, Peto V, Fitzpatrick R, Greenhall R, Hyman N. Self-reported functioning and well-being in patients with Parkinson's disease: a comparison of the Short-Form Health Survey (SF-36) and the Parkinson's Disease Questionnaire (PDQ-39). *Age Ageing* 1995; **24**: 505–509.

31. Chrischilles EA, Rubenstein LM, Voelker MD, Wallace RB, Rodnitzky RL. The health burdens of Parkinson's disease. *Movement Disord* 1998; **13**: 406–413.

32. Mercer B. A randomized study of the efficacy of the PROPATH program for patients with Parkinson's disease. *Arch Neurol* 1996; **53**: 881–884.

33. Hobson P, Meara J. Letter to the Editor. Self-reported functioning and well being in patients with Parkinson's Disease. *Age Ageing* 1997; **25**: 334–335.

34. Calne S, Schulzer M, Mak E, Guyette C, Rohs G, Hatchard S, Murphy D, Hodder J, Gagnon C, Weatherby S, Beaudet L, Duff J, Pegler S. Validating a quality of life rating scale for Idiopathic Parkinsonism: Parkinson's Impact Scale (PIMS). *Parkinsonism Relat Disord* 1996; **2**: 55–61.

35. De Boer AGEM, Wijker W, Speelman JD de Haes J. Quality of life in patients with Parkinson's disease: development of a questionnaire. *J Neurol Neurosurg Psychiatry* 1996; **61**: 70–74.

36. Welsh M, McDermott MP, Holloway RG, Plumb S, Pfeiffer R, Hubble J; Parkinson Study Group. Development and testing of the Parkinson's disease quality of life scale. *Movement Disord* 2003 Jun; **18**(6): 637–645.

37. Peto V, Jenkinson C, Fitzpatrick R, Greenhall R. The development and validation of a short measure of functioning and well being for individuals with Parkinson's disease. *Qual Life Res* 1995; **4**: 241–248.

38. Jenkinson C, Fitzpatrick R, Peto V. *The Parkinson's Disease Questionnaire. User Manual for the PDQ-39, PDQ-8 and PDQ Summary Index*, 2nd ed. Oxford: Health Services Research Unit, 2008.

39. McDowell I, Jenkinson C. Development standards for health measures. *J Health Serv Res Policy* 1996; **1**: 238–246.

40. Damiano AM, Snyder C, Strausser B, Willian MK. A review of health-related quality-of-life concepts and measures for Parkinson's disease. *Qual Life Res* 1999; **8**: 235–243.

41. Hobson P, Holden A, Meara J. Measuring the impact of Parkinson's disease with the Parkinson's Disease Quality of Life questionnaire. *Age Ageing* 1999; **28**: 341–346.

42. Cronbach L. Coefficient alpha and the internal structure of tests. *Psychometrica* 1951; **16**: 297–234.

43. Carmines E, Zeller R. *Reliability and validity assessment: quantitative applications in the social sciences.* Beverly Hills: Sage, 1979.

44. Nunnally JC, Bernstein I. *Psychometric theory,* 3rd ed. New York: McGraw Hill, 1994.

45. Fitzpartick R, Peto V, Jenkinson C, Greenhall R, Hyman N. Health-related quality of life in Parkinson's disease: a study of out-patient clinic attenders. *Movement Disord* 1997; **6**: 916–922.

46. Martinez-Martin P, Frades Payo B, and the Grupo Centro for Movement Disorders. Quality of life in Parkinson's disease: validation study of the PDQ-39 Spanish version. *J Neurol* 1998; **245** (Supp 1): S34–S38.

47. Jaeschke R, Singer J, Guyatt GH. (1989) Measurements of health status: ascertaining the minimal clinically important difference. *Control Clin Trials* 1989; **10**: 407–415.

48. Cohen J. *Statistical Power Analysis for the Behavioural Sciences*, 2nd ed. Hillsdale, NJ: Lawrence Erlbaum, 1988.

49. Marinus J, Ramaker C, van-Hilten JJ, Stiggelbout AM. Health related quality of life in Parkinson's disease: a systematic review of disease specific instruments. *J Neurol Neurosurg Psychiatry* 2002; **72**: 241–248.

50. Damiano AM, Snyder C, Strausser B, Willian M. A review of health-related quality-of-life concepts and measures for Parkinson's disease. *Qual Life Res* 1999; **8**: 235–243.

51. Loge JH, Kaasa S, Hjermstad M, Kvien T. Translation and performance of the Norwegian SF-36 Health Survey in patients with rheumatoid arthritis. 1: Data quality, scaling asumptions reliability and construct validity. *J Clin Epidemiol* 1998; **51**: 1069–1076.

52. Bushnell DM, Martin ML. Quality of life and Parkinson's disease: translation and validation of the US Parkinson's Disease Questionnaire (PDQ-39). *Qual Life Res* 1999; **8**: 345–350.

53. Carod-Artal FJ, Martinez-Martin P, Vargas AP. Independent validation of SCOPA-psychosocial and metric properties of the PDQ-39 Brazilian version. *Mov Disord* 2007; **22**(1): 91–98.

54. Hristova DR, Hristov JI, Mateva NG, Papathanasiou JV. Quality of life in patients with Parkinson's disease. *Folia Med (Plovdiv)* 2009; **51**: 58–64.

55. Tsang KL, Chi I, Shu-Leong H, Lou VW, Lee TMC, Chu LW. Translation and validation of the standard Chinese version of the PDQ-39: A quality-of-life measure for patients with Parkinson's disease. *Movement Disord* 2002; **17**: 1036–1040.

56. Tan LC, Lau PN, Au WL, Luo N. Validation of PDQ-8 as an independent instrument in English and Chinese. *J Neurol Sci* 2007; **255**(1–2):77–80.

57. Luo N, Tan LC, Li SC, Soh LK, Thumboo J. Validity and reliability of the Chinese (Singapore) version of the

Parkinson's Disease Questionnaire (PDQ-39). *Qual Life Res* 2005; **14**: 273–279.

58. Ma HI, Hwang WJ, Chen-Sea MJ. Reliability and validity of a Chinese-translated version of the 39-item Parkinson's Disease Questionnaire (PDQ-39). *Qual Life Res* 2005; **14**: 565–569.

59. Marinus J, Visser M, Jenkinson C, A Stiggelbout. Evaluation of the of the Dutch version of the Parkinson's Disease Questionnaire 39. *Parkinsonism Relat Disord* 2008; **14**: 24–27.

60. Martinez-Martin P, Sarrano-Duena M, Vaca-Baquuero V. Psychometric charecteristics of the Parkinson's disease questionnaire (PDQ-39) – Ecuadorian version. *Parkinsonism Relat D* 2005; **11**: 297–304.

61. Auquier P, Sapin C, Ziegler M, Tison F, Destée A, Dubois B, Allicar MP, Thibault JL, Jenkinson C, Peto V. (2002) Validation en Française d'un questionnaire de qualité de vie dans le maladie de Parkinson: le Parkinson's Disease Questionnaire – PDQ-39. *Rev Neurol (Paris)* 2002; **158**: 41–50.

62. Katsarou Z, Bostantjopoulou S, Peto V, Alevriadou A, Kiosseoglou G. Quality of life in Parkinson's disease: Greek translation and validation of the Parkinson's disease questionnaire (PDQ-39). *Qual Life Res* 2001; **10**: 159–163.

63. Kohmoto J, Ohbu S, Nagaoka M, Suzukamo Y, Kihira T, Mizuno Y, Ito YM, Hith M., Yamaguchi T, Ohashi Y, Fukuhara S, d Kondo T. Validity of the Japanese version of the Parkinson's Disease Questionnaire. *Clin Neurol* 2003; **43**: 71–76.

64. Martinez-Martin P, Frades Payo B, and the Grupo Centro for Movement Disorders. Quality of life in Parkinson's disease: validation study of the PDQ-39 Spanish version. *J Neurol* 1998; **245** (Supp 1): S34–S38.

65. Nojomi M, Mostafavian Z, Ali Shahidi G, Jenkinson C. Quality of life in patients with Parkinson's disease: Translation and psychometric evaluation of the Iranian version of PDQ-39. *J Res Med Sci* 2010; **15**: 63–69.

66. Ives NJ, Jenkinson C, Fitzpatrick R, Wheatley K, Clarke CE. The PDQ-39 is a sensitive measure of change in quality of life in early Parkinson's disease. *Movement Disord* 2004; **19** (Supplement 9): S208.

67. Martinez-Martin P, Frades Payo B, Fontan-Tirado C, Martinez Sarries FJ, Guerrero M, del Ser Quijano T. Valoracion de la calidad de vida en la enfermedad de Parkinson mediante el PDQ-39. Estudio piloto. *Neurolagia* 1997; **12**: 56–60.

68. Fukunaga H, Kasai T, Yoshidome H. Clinical findings, status of care, comprehensive quality of life, daily life therapy and treatment at home in patients with Parkinson's disease. *Eur Neurol* 1997; **38** Suppl 2: 64–69.

Parkinson's Disease Quality of Life Questionnaire

DUE TO HAVING PARKINSON'S DISEASE, how often have you experienced the following, <u>during the last month?</u>

Due to having Parkinson's disease, how often <u>during the last month</u> have you. ...

*Please tick **one box** for each question.*

	Never	Occasionally	Sometimes	Often	Always or cannot do at all
1. Had difficulty doing the leisure activities which you would like to do?	☐	☐	☐	☐	☐
2. Had difficulty looking after your home, e.g. DIY, housework, cooking?	☐	☐	☐	☐	☐
3. Had difficulty carrying bags of shopping?	☐	☐	☐	☐	☐
4. Had problems walking half a mile?	☐	☐	☐	☐	☐
5. Had problems walking 100 yards?	☐	☐	☐	☐	☐
6. Had problems getting around the house as easily as you would like?	☐	☐	☐	☐	☐
7. Had difficulty getting around in public?	☐	☐	☐	☐	☐
8. Needed someone else to accompany you when you went out?	☐	☐	☐	☐	☐
9. Felt frightened or worried about falling over in public?	☐	☐	☐	☐	☐
10. Been confined to the house more than you would like?	☐	☐	☐	☐	☐
11. Had difficulty washing yourself?	☐	☐	☐	☐	☐
12. Had difficulty dressing yourself?	☐	☐	☐	☐	☐
13. Had problems doing up buttons or shoe laces?	☐	☐	☐	☐	☐

Please check that you have ticked <u>one box for each question</u> before going on to the next page.

Parkinson's Disease Quality of Life Questionnaire (*cont.*)

	Never	Occasionally	Sometimes	Often	Always or cannot do at all
14. Had problems writing clearly?	☐	☐	☐	☐	☐
15. Had difficulty cutting up your food?	☐	☐	☐	☐	☐
16. Had difficulty holding a drink without spilling it?	☐	☐	☐	☐	☐
17. Felt depressed?	☐	☐	☐	☐	☐
18. Felt isolated and lonely?	☐	☐	☐	☐	☐
19. Felt weepy or tearful?	☐	☐	☐	☐	☐
20. Felt angry or bitter?	☐	☐	☐	☐	☐
21. Felt anxious?	☐	☐	☐	☐	☐
22. Felt worried about your future?	☐	☐	☐	☐	☐
23. Felt you had to conceal your Parkinson's from people?	☐	☐	☐	☐	☐
24. Avoided situations which involve eating or drinking in public?	☐	☐	☐	☐	☐
25. Felt embarrassed in public due to having Parkinson's disease?	☐	☐	☐	☐	☐
26. Felt worried by other people's reaction to you?	☐	☐	☐	☐	☐
27. Had problems with your close personal relationships?	☐	☐	☐	☐	☐
28. Lacked support in the ways you need from your spouse or partner? *If you do not have a spouse or partner, please tick here* ☐	☐	☐	☐	☐	☐
29. Lacked support in the ways you need from your family or close friends?	☐	☐	☐	☐	☐
30. Unexpectedly fallen asleep during the day?	☐	☐	☐	☐	☐
31. Had problems with your concentration, e.g. when reading or watching TV?	☐	☐	☐	☐	☐

Please check that you have ticked <u>one box for each question</u> before going on to the next page.

Parkinson's Disease Quality of Life Questionnaire (*cont.*)

	Never	Occasionally	Sometimes	Often	Always or cannot do at all
32. Felt your memory was bad?	☐	☐	☐	☐	☐
33. Had distressing dreams or hallucinations?	☐	☐	☐	☐	☐
34. Had difficulty with your speech?	☐	☐	☐	☐	☐
35. Felt unable to communicate with people properly?	☐	☐	☐	☐	☐
36. Felt ignored by people?	☐	☐	☐	☐	☐
37. Had painful muscle cramps or spasms?	☐	☐	☐	☐	☐
38. Had aches and pains in your joints or body?	☐	☐	☐	☐	☐
39. Felt unpleasantly hot or cold?	☐	☐	☐	☐	☐

Please check that you have ticked <u>one box for each question</u>.

Thank you for completing this questionnaire.

3

The Multiple Sclerosis Impact Scale (MSIS-29)

Initial development, subsequent revision, lessons learned

Jeremy Hobart

Chapter overview

The Multiple Sclerosis Impact Scale (MSIS-29) is a 29-item self-report rating scale for measuring the physical and psychological impact of multiple sclerosis (MS). The aim of this chapter is to document its development and subsequent revision, and the lessons learned.

Development of the MSIS-29 was prompted by the perceived lack of suitable rating scales for measuring outcomes in clinical trials of MS. Development began in 1997 following a grant application to the U.K. National Health Service Health Technology Assessment Board. The scale was developed using traditional psychometric methods. These methods of scale development and evaluation remain the dominant psychometric paradigm, and we would like to think that we applied them rigorously. The resultant MSIS-29 Scale comfortably satisfied traditional psychometric criteria as a reliable and valid measurement instrument scale and provided preliminary evidence of responsiveness. This was confirmed in a large subsequent study. Consequently, the MSIS-29 has been used in clinical trials of MS and has been officially translated into 29 languages by MAPI (available on request).

At the time of publication in 2001, we acknowledged the increasingly recognized role of the modern psychometric methods, Rasch measurement and item response theory, in rating scale research.

Thus we recommended that these methods should be used to evaluate the scale. From late 1999, our group took an interest in modern psychometric methods and, over a period of time, became educated in their theory and practice. The Rasch analysis of our existing MSIS-29 data led to the revision of the scale, MSIS-29v2. Although the revision might appear small, with reduction of the number of item response categories from five to four, it is very important in terms of the measurement performance of the scale. Thus, since 2005, we have recommended the use of version 2 rather than the original (Appendix 1). One beauty of using Rasch analysis is that it allows MSIS-29v1 and MSIS-29v2 data to be equated on the same metric (details available on request).

Rasch analysis of our MSIS-29 data also raised other issues in relation to the measurement of physical and psychological health in MS and the development of rating scales in general. These have led to continued developments in our thinking and practice. Essentially, we have learned two key lessons from the MSIS-29 experience: first, that Rasch analysis is far superior to traditional methods in the development of new rating scales and the evaluation and modification of existing rating scales; and second, that the way most rating scales are developed ought to change.

The MSIS-29 is a useful measure of the physical and psychological impact of MS. It serves

Quality of Life Measurement in Neurodegenerative and Related Conditions, eds., Crispin Jenkinson, Michele Peters, and Mark B. Bromberg. Published by Cambridge University Press. © Cambridge University Press 2011.

as an important milestone in the history of maximizing rating scale measurement in MS. We would, of course, do things differently given our time again.

Background to the development of the MSIS-29

Multiple sclerosis is an incurable, progressive neurological disorder that has a profound impact on individuals and their families. Although the incidence in the United Kingdom is relatively low (2,500 new cases/year), the prevalence is much higher (85,000). This is because MS tends to begin in young age groups, is incurable, and in the majority of people is progressive over many decades. Although MS has little effect on longevity, it has a major impact on physical function, employment, and quality of life. It is a complex disorder with diverse effects, an unpredictable course, and variable manifestations that pose unique problems to patients and their families. Moreover, the cost of MS in the United Kingdom is estimated to be 1.2 billion per year (1) and is expected to increase (2). Costs due to MS have been shown to increase as disability progresses (3, 4). Psychosocial costs are less easily quantified, but no less real.

Because MS is a major public health concern in Britain, beneficial interventions are to be welcomed. However, the outcomes of therapeutic interventions must be rigorously evaluated if policy decisions and clinical practice are to be evidence based. The need for more rigorous evaluation of treatments for MS has recently become critically important for several reasons. First, an increasing number of therapeutic pharmaceutical agents aimed at altering the course of MS are being introduced, and their effectiveness needs to be determined (5). Second, because the relative benefits of different interventions are likely to be marginal, analyses of comparative effectiveness are necessary (6). Third, because treatments are expensive and may be required on a long-term basis, decisions about interventions based on short-term evaluation may have long-term economic implications. Fourth, because resources

for the treatment of MS are required for other aspects of service provision, including rehabilitation and community support, resource allocation must be equitable. Finally, it is important that the current limited resources are allocated appropriately.

Evidence-based policy and clinical decision making require rigorous measurement of outcomes. This information is of value when the outcomes that are evaluated are appropriate to patients and the instruments that are used are clinically useful and scientifically sound. Outcome measures in MS have traditionally focused on physiologic parameters of disease and simple, easy to measure entities such as mortality, morbidity, and duration of survival. Although these assessments are important, they only partly address patients' concerns (7), offer little information about diverse clinical consequences, fail to address the personal impact of disease (8), and are of limited relevance in conditions that do not affect longevity. Because new treatments for MS are aimed at altering its natural history or modifying its impact, traditional outcomes are inadequate in a comprehensive evaluation of therapeutic effectiveness.

Historically, outcome measurement in MS has relied heavily on the Expanded Disability Status Scale (EDSS) (9). This is an observer (neurologist)-rated scale that grades "disability" due to MS in 20 steps on a continuum from 0 (normal neurological examination) to 10 (death due to MS). The EDSS was developed on the basis of the extensive clinical experience of a neurologist specializing in MS. It addresses impairment [symptoms and signs] at the lower levels (0–3.5), mobility at the middle range (4.0–7.5), and upper limb (8.0–8.5) and bulbar function (9.0–9.5) at higher levels. Although the EDSS evaluates disability, it was developed before psychometric methods became familiar to clinicians, was not based on recognized techniques of scale construction (10), and did not directly involve people with MS. More important, the EDSS is rated by neurologists rather than by patients themselves and has limited measurement properties (11, 12).

The lack of validated MS-specific measures has led to the use of generic measures, such as the

Medical Outcomes Study 36-Item Short Form Health Survey (SF-36) (13), the Sickness Impact Profile (SIP) (14), and the EuroQoL (15). Although generic measures have the advantage of enabling comparisons across diseases, it is increasingly recognized that they do not cover some areas of outcome that are highly relevant in specific diseases (16), and they may have limited responsiveness (17). Psychometric limitations of the SF-36 in MS include significant floor and ceiling effects (18), limited responsiveness (18), underestimation of mental health problems (19), and failure to satisfy assumptions for generating summary scores (20). Disease-specific instruments, consisting of items and domains of health that are specific to a particular disease, are more relevant and important to patients and clinicians and consequently are more likely to be responsive to subtle changes in outcome (7, 17, 21).

A number of MS-specific measures have been developed over the past 5 years. These include the Functional Assessment of MS (FAMS (22)), the MSQoL-54 [23]), the MS Functional Composite (24), the Leeds MSQoL scale (25), the Guy's (now U.K.) Neurological Disability Scale (GNDS/UKNDS (26)), the MS Quality of Life Inventory (MSQLI (27)), and the health-related quality of life questionnaire for MS (HRQoL-MS (28)). Although all are encouraging, one limitation of these measures is that none was developed using the standard psychometric approach of reducing a large item pool generated *de novo* from people with MS. The FAMS and MSQoL-54 were developed by adding MS-specific items to existing measures – an approach that has been demonstrated to have some limitations (29). The HRQoL-MS was developed through factor analysis of items from two generic and one MS-specific measure, and the MSQLI combines a large number of existing disease-specific and generic instruments. Items for the GNDS were developed through expert clinical opinion rather than on the basis of interviews with people with MS. Consequently, an outcome measure that is MS-specific and combines patient perspective with rigorous psychometric methods will complement existing instruments.

The facts indicated that clinical trials of MS needed a new rating scale that was derived from people with MS and was rigorously developed.

The MSIS-29: initial development

The MSIS-29 was developed using traditional psychometric methods for scale development. Three stages occurred. In stage 1 (item generation), a 141-item questionnaire was generated from patient interviews, expert opinion, and a literature review. In stage 2 (item reduction and scale generation), the 141-item questionnaire was administered by postal survey to a large sample of people with MS, and the MSIS-29 was generated by the selection of items on their psychometric performance. In stage 3 (psychometric evaluation), a comprehensive traditional psychometric evaluation of the measurement properties of the MSIS-29 was undertaken in a large sample of people with MS.

Full details of the development and evaluation are described elsewhere (30, 48). Briefly, some 3,000 statements concerning the impact of MS were generated from 30 tape-recorded one-on-one patient interviews, literature review, and expert opinion. These statements were examined for their content, overlap, and redundancy. From the statements, 141 potential scale items were written. These items were administered as a questionnaire to a large, randomly selected, geographically stratified sample of people with MS (n = 1,532) drawn from the membership database of the MS Society of Great Britain and Northern Ireland.

Data analysis focused on 129 items because 12 items concerning walking were excluded, as they were appropriate only to a limited number of people with MS. These 12 items formed the MS Walking Scale (MSWS-12) (31), which has since been generalized for neurological conditions (32, 33) and revised to the MSWS-12v2 (submitted for publication, details on request).

Full details of the item reduction process, which comprises the methods used to select the final 29 items from the original 129, are provided elsewhere (30). First, 36 items were removed because of high item-item correlations and thus presumed redundancy. Next, 51 items were removed on the basis of psychometric performance (that is, high item level floor/ceiling effects and poor endorsement profiles). The remaining 42 items were entered into an exploratory factor analysis. A number of possible factor solutions were examined. The two-factor solution was the most clinically and statistically appropriate, but three items were removed because they loaded similarly on both factors. The other 39 items were grouped into two scales (26 items; 13 items) whose content concerned the physical and psychological impact of MS. Refinement of the two scales using tests of item convergence and discriminate validity identified items that might confound measurement, which were thus removed. The final instrument had two scales: a 20-item physical impact scale and a 9-item psychological impact scale.

The reliability and validity of the MSIS-29 were examined in a second large independent survey of 1,250 members of the MS Society. A nested test-retest reliability substudy was conducted (n = 150). Participants were sent booklets containing the MSIS-29 and other health measurement scales. The return rate was 81.8%, and the response rate 69.1%. In the test-retest subsample, 90.6% (n = 136) of people returned both questionnaires.

We examined data quality, scaling assumptions, targeting, reliability (internal consistency and test-retest reliability), and validity (convergent and discriminate construct validity, group differences, and hypothesis testing), and undertook a provisional responsiveness study. Table 3.1 summarizes the results. Data quality was high. Item-level missing data were low (range, 1.1%–3.6%). Complete data were provided for 84%. Item test-retest reproducibility was high. Scaling assumptions were satisfied, targeting criteria were met, and reliability was high (for both internal consistency and test-retest reproducibility). Evidence for validity was based on correlations with multiple other scales, analysis of group differences, and relative validity testing.

Preliminary evidence for responsiveness and relative responsiveness was found in pretreatment and posttreatment data from 55 people with MS admitted for inpatient rehabilitation and for intravenous steroids for treatment of relapse. Change scores for both MSIS-29 scales were similar in magnitude and statistically significant. Effect sizes were large to moderate. Subsequently, we have reported a large (n = 245) comprehensive responsiveness study examining the relative responsiveness of the MSIS-29 in different clinical circumstances and have compared it with a range of other scales measuring similar constructs. The MSIS-29 physical scale was the most responsive of the scales tested. Although the General Health Questionnaire (GHQ)-12 was the most responsive of the psychological scales tested, the MSIS-29 psychological scale performs better than other measures of psychological impact. We also studied the differential responsiveness of the MSIS-29 across different clinical circumstances (rehabilitation, steroid treatment, primary progressive MS) and found this to be good.

Across the range of health outcomes measurement literature, it is extremely rare to find examples that include the extent of scale evaluation in all the areas we have examined in the case of the MSIS-29. Subsequent evaluations (34, 35, 36, 37), also using traditional psychometric methods, have supported the reliability, validity, and responsiveness of the scale.

Results from initial testing showed that the MSIS-29 satisfied traditional psychometric criteria as a summed rating scale. Therefore, it could be considered an acceptable, reliable, and valid measure of the physical and psychological impact of MS. We adopted stringent criteria for item selection in an attempt to develop an instrument with strong psychometric properties. In an effort to create a responsive scale, items were selected that discriminated well between individuals, and items with maximum endorsement frequencies over 40% were eliminated. Similarly, to reduce overlap, MSIS-29 physical and psychological scale items that did not show good evidence of item convergence and discriminant validity were eliminated. Subsequently,

Table 3.1 Psychometric properties of MSIS-29v1 (n = 713 unless stated otherwise)

	MSIS-29 subscale physical impact	Psychological impact
Number of items	20	9
Number of item response categories	5	5
Data quality		
% missing item data	3.6	1.8
% computable scores	98.0	98.7
Scaling assumptions		
Range of item mean scores	2.54–3.83	2.57–3.28
Range of item SD	1.20–1.56	1.27–1.37
Corrected item total correlations	0.60–0.86	0.49–0.77
Item other scale correlations	0.41–0.57	0.34–0.56
Definite scaling success rate	100%	100%
Targeting		
Scale range (mid point)*	0–100	0–100
Observed score range	0–100	0–100
Mean (SD)	56.0 (26.6)	45.5 (25.2)
% floor effect	0.9	1.7
% ceiling effect	3.9	1.9
Score distribution skewness	−0.285	0.172
Reliability		
Test-retest reproducibility (n = 128)	0.94	0.97
Scale score ICC	0.65–0.90	0.72–0.82
Range of item score ICCs		
Internal consistency	0.96	0.91
Scale score alpha	0.58	0.52
Mean item-item correlation		
Validity (correlations with other scales)		
SF-36 PF	−0.79	−0.41
SF-36 MH	−0.41	−0.76
FAMS mobility	−0.88	−0.50
EQ5D usual activities	0.69	0.42
EQ5D anxiety depression	0.36	0.68
GHQ-12	0.46	0.68
Postal Barthel index	−0.71	−0.35
Responsiveness ES(SRM)		
Primary progressive MS: n = 104	0.01 (0.02)	−0.15 (−0.16)
Inpatient rehabilitation: n = 64	0.61 (0.64)	0.44 (0.54)
IV steroid treatment for relapse: n = 77	1.01 (1.11)	0.72 0.90)

* For ease of interpretation, the scale ranges of the physical (20−100) and psychological (9−45) impact scales have been rescaled to a range of 0−100.

Abbreviations: MSIS = Multiple Sclerosis Impact Scale; SD = standard deviation; ICC = intraclass correlation coefficient; SF-36PF = Medical Outcome Study 36-item short-form health survey physical functioning dimension; SF-36MH = Medical Outcome Study 36-item short-form health survey mental health dimension functioning scale; FAMS mobility = Functional Assessment of MS Mobility Scale; EQ5D = Euroqol; GHQ-12 = 12-item version of the General Health Questionnaire; ES = effect size; SRM = standardized response mean.

others have studied the psychometric properties of the MSIS-29 using traditional psychometric methods and have provided further evidence of its reliability, validity, and responsiveness. A firm approach to the development and validation of health outcome measures is important because the results of studies are dependent on the quality of the measures used for data collection. Furthermore, the limitations of measures cannot be overcome easily by improvements in study design and powerful statistical methods (38).

Subsequent revision of MSIS-29 to form MSIS-29 version 2

When we published the MSIS-29, we highlighted the increasing importance of the modern psychometric methods, Rasch measurement and item response theory, in health rating scale research. We recommended that they be used to evaluate the MSIS-29.

New psychometric methods are by no means new. The seminal texts were published in 1960 (39) and 1968 (40). However, they have been slow to transfer to psychometric practice. The reasons for this are covered to some extent in Chapter 12 on the Rasch analysis of health rating scale data and include their inherent complexity, inaccessible literature, misunderstandings and misconceptions, confrontation between proponents of Rasch measurement and of item response theory, and the skepticism of psychometricians trained in traditional psychometric methods who are often not willing to invest effort in understanding what they have to offer.

Since 1999, our group has invested heavily in these methods. This was prompted by an increasing understanding of the limitations of traditional psychometric methods. Our existing MSIS-29 dataset gave us the opportunity to evaluate the scale using Rasch measurement and to compare and contrast Rasch measurement and traditional psychometric methods.

Both traditional psychometric methods and Rasch analysis have the same goal: to determine if it

is legitimate to generate a total score by combining the integer scores from a group of items, and if that total score is reliable and valid. The two approaches differ in the evidence used to achieve that goal. Traditional psychometric analyses are based on Classical Test Theory and are embodied in the work of Likert (41, 42) and others. Their evidence comes mainly from the analysis of descriptive statistics and correlations. New psychometric methods stem from the work of Thurstone (43), Lord and Novick (40), and Rasch (39). Their evidence comes from checking the observed data against *a priori* explicit mathematical models of how a set of items must behave to permit the summation of items to generate a reliable and valid total score (44).

New psychometric methods offer potential scientific and clinical advantages over traditional methods. From a scientific perspective, they enable more conceptually grounded and sophisticated evaluations of scales. From a clinical perspective, they offer, among other things, the ability to transform ordinal scores into interval measures and legitimate individual person measurement. However, comparisons in the literature to determine the added value of using the new psychometric methods are limited.

Different psychometric methods use a different range of evidence to achieve that goal. As we have seen, in traditional psychometric methods, the range of evidence comes, predominantly, from correlation-based analyses. In a Rasch analysis, the range of evidence stems from a mathematical conceptualization of the conditions of measurement that permit the summation of integer scores. Essentially then, the observed data should fit, within reason, for measurement to be considered achieved. In circumstances where the data fit the model, two fundamental inferences can be made. First, measurement of the persons can be considered to be on a linear scale. Second, these measurements are invariant across designated groups for *which the fit has been confirmed*.

Like all psychometric analyses, the Rasch analysis of an existing scale consists of gathering and integrating the evidence from a series of analyses.

Typically, these analyses are not reported in the literature under the subheadings in the same way that we and others have used for traditional methods. Although some have compared and contrasted the reliability and validity evidence from traditional and Rasch analyses (45), it might be more clinically meaningful to build on the approach documented by Wright and Masters (46). This is because a Rasch analysis gives us explicit and separate information about the scale and the sample. It seems to us clinically meaningful then to think separately about scale and sample after first considering, in general terms, the suitability of the sample for evaluating the scale, and the suitability of the scale for measuring the sample. With this in mind we recommend considering reporting Rasch analyses under three main questions:

1) Is the scale-to-sample targeting adequate for making judgments about the performance of the scale and the measurement of people?

2) Has a measurement ruler been constructed successfully?

3) Have the people been measured successfully?

A detailed explanation of how each of these three questions is addressed is given in Chapter 12 of this book (Rasch analysis), and in a recent Health Technology Assessment (HTA) report on the role of new psychometric methods (47).

MSIS-29 data from a total of 1,725 people with MS were Rasch analyzed. These data were generated by the two field tests of the MS Society membership databases (n = 768 and n = 712) undertaken during development of the MSIS-29 (30, 48) and a study of its responsiveness (n = 245) (49).

Rasch analysis highlighted the strengths and limitations of the MSIS-29. Evidence in support of the measurement properties of the MSIS-29 came from a demonstration that: both scales are well targeted to the study samples (Figure 3.1); the items of both subscales map out continua of increasing intensity; are located along those continua in a clinically sensible order; work reasonably well together to define single variables; consist of items that are locally independent; and do not exhibit differential item functioning. Further support for the use of the subscales came from the finding that both subscales were able to separate the sample reliably, and people's patterns of responses were consistent with expectations.

However, Rasch analysis detected important limitations of the MSIS-29 that were not identified by traditional psychometric methods. It detected that the five-category item scoring function did not work as intended for nine items in the physical subscale and for one item in the psychological subscale (Figure 3.2). This implied that these items had too many response options. In fact, good evidence from the analyses indicated that all items would benefit from having fewer response categories. Because of this finding, we undertook a *post hoc* rescoring of the items by collapsing adjacent categories (so that all items had four response categories), as suggested by each category probability curve. Reanalysis of the data demonstrated that all thresholds were now correctly ordered. The rest of the analyses were similar. Clearly, this needed to be tested prospectively because collapsing categories make assumptions about how people would respond.

A second limitation of the MSIS-29 detected by Rasch analysis, and applicable to both subscales but especially the psychological subscale, was the range and spread of the item locations and thresholds. Neither scale mapped a very wide variable. Both scales demonstrated bunching of item thresholds at the center of the scale range (Figure 3.1) and gaps in their continua. The implication of these findings is that measurement could be improved further. It is also important to note that these findings are a function of traditional psychometric methods. Correlation-based analyses (e.g., item-total correlations, item-item correlations, alphas), which are the mainstay underpinning item selection, tend to identify items in the middle of the scale range as superior. A number of problems arise from packing items in the central region of the scale range. One problem is that the scale is a precise measure only over a limited range. A second problem is that scales could become overly precise in the center relative to the extremes. Thus, the relationship between raw scores and interval measures becomes increasingly

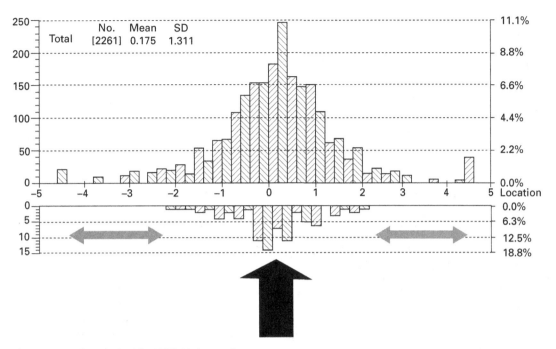

Figure 3.1 Rasch analysis of the MSIS-29v1: targeting.

This figure produced by the Rasch analysis software program RUMM2020 shows the targeting. This is the relationship between the physical impact scales and the sample. More specifically, it is the relationship between the "ruler" of physical functioning measured by the 20 items of the MSIS-29v1 physical impact subscale items (lower histogram) and the distribution of physical impact measurements in the sample (upper histogram).

This simple plot gives vast information. First, it tells us about the suitability of the study sample for evaluating the performance of the scale and the suitability of the scale for measuring physical impact in the study sample. This plot shows good targeting as the distributions are pretty well matched. However, it is clear that the physical functioning of people toward the extremes (i.e., < -2.25 logits and $> +2.0$ logits) is suboptimal.

The plot also tells us much about the continuum mapped out by the items. Here we can see that there is bunching of items toward the center of the scale range (large vertical arrow), implying some degree of item redundancy. It also shows how and where the scale might be improved (horizontal arrows).

Finally, the plot shows us the distributions of person measurements. Here they have a near "normal" distribution. This is not a requirement. The distribution can be of any type. It is an empirical finding of the sample.

S-shaped, and therefore increasingly nonlinear, so that the "real" implications of raw score changes and differences become increasingly distorted (Figure 3.3). For the MSIS-29, the change in interval level measurement implied by a fixed change in raw score varies up to 27-fold.

A third limitation of the MSIS-29, detected by Rasch analysis, relates to the extent to which the items work together to define a single variable. Both subscales, but especially the physical scale,

demonstrated misfit on the two numeric indicators of fit of the data to the Rasch model (item-person fit residuals; item-trait chi-square values). The third graphic indicator of fit implied that this misfit was less of a concern. These findings could be interpreted in two ways. On the one hand, we could favor the graphic indicator, play down the numeric values, and argue that the items in each subscale scale work well together to define a single variable. On the other hand, we could be more

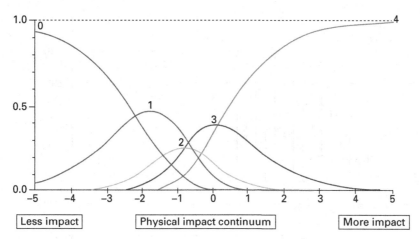

Figure 3.2 Rasch analysis of the MSIS-29v1: performance of item response options.

This RUMM plot is called a category probability curve (CPC). It shows the probability (y-axis) of endorsing each of the five item response categories (lines numbered 0-4 rather than 1-5) for each level of physical impact (x-axis). This is the CPC for item 1. It has been selected because it typifies the CPCs for most of the 29 items.

It is logical to expect that as people become more disabled, that is, move from left to right along the physical impact continuum measured by the 20-item set, they would move sequentially through the five-item response options for each item in the sequence they are written (0 = not at all, 1 = a little, 2 = moderately, 3 = quite a bit, 4 = extremely). This plot shows the test of that requirement.

Note curve line 2 in the above plot. It is the CPC for the third response option (2 = moderately) for this item. Nowhere along the continuum does the green curve have the highest probability of endorsement. This means that nowhere along the continuum is the option "moderately" most likely to be chosen. Put another way, "moderately" is NEVER the most likely item response category to be endorsed at ANY level of physical impact. Thus, the sequential ordering of the five response categories is not working as intended for item 1 within the frame of reference of the 20-item set.

Further evaluation, beyond the scope of this chapter, showed that the problem lay in people's ability to distinguish "moderately" from "quite a bit." We explored the empirical benefit of combining these two categories. This worked both retrospectively and prospectively (details from author).

This is an important plot. When the item response categories are working as intended, the plot tells us the best estimate of the measurement range associated with ANY response to ANY item. For example, in the above example, a response of "a little" to item 1 (that is, represented by curve line 1) is associated with a best estimate of physical impact of −2.25 to −0.75 logits because this is the range of the physical impact continnum over which this is the most likely response to be endorsed. However, a response of "moderately" (curve line 2) is not associated with a clear estimate of measurement. Thus, the validity of this item response option is questioned.

This "problem" with the "moderately" category was a consistency finding for many MSIS-29 items. Even when the categories were working correctly, the area of the continuum represented by the "moderately" category was small. This implies that there were too many item response categories for people with MS for reliable distinctions to be made between them.

circumspect and try to diagnose why an instrument that passes all traditional tests of validity demonstrates notable misfit on some – but not all – tests of fit. The second approach is that favored by leading Rasch analysts (50, 51, 52) and in line with Kuhnian theory, which argues that the role of measurement is to highlight anomalies for further investigation (53, 54).

In keeping with this approach, the results of the test of fit provoked a careful examination of the items, a consideration of the scale development process, and an explanation for the findings. For

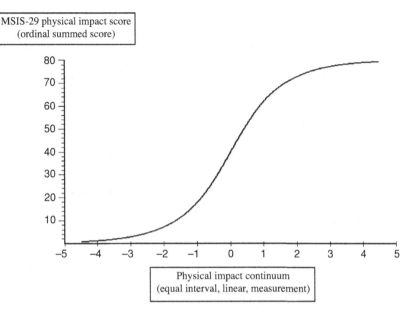

Figure 3.3 Rasch analysis of the MSIS-29v1: relationship between scores and measurements.

This plot shows the relationship between the physical impact scores, which are by definition ordinal data, and the interval-level measurements that can be derived from those data (provided the data fit the Rasch model adequately). The relationship is S-shaped. Thus, the rate of change of interval measurements changes across the range of the raw score. At low raw scores (e.g., 0–20) and high raw scores (e.g., 60–80), a change of 1 MSIS point on the y-axis is associated with a large change in linear physical impact measurement (x-axis). In the middle of the scale range (e.g., 30–50), a 1-point change in MSIS score (y-axis) is associated with a small change in linear measurement (x-axis). Thus, the "meaning" (i.e., change in linear measurement) of a 1-point change in MSIS SCORE varies, depending where the person is on the range.

example, the 20 items of the physical impact sub-scale can be grouped into three themes: activity limitations, symptoms causing physical limitations, and limitations in social functioning. The amalgamation of these related but different subconstructs into a single set operationalizes a broad physical functioning variable and would explain why the data are less cohesive statistically. Why did this happen? Because the scale development process used a factor analysis that groups items that are related but distinct from other groups of items. Moreover, because factor analysis is based on correlations, it will tend to bring together items that measure at a similar point on the scale, irrespective of their content.

The findings of this Rasch analysis have led us to revise the MSIS-29 to produce version 2. Prospec-tive evaluation of MSIS-29v2 data confirms that it is a superior measurement instrument (unpublished data).

Lessons learned

Two key lessons have been learned from our experience developing, evaluating, and revising the MSIS-29. The first lesson concerns the choice of psychometric method to guide scale construction and evaluation. The second lesson concerns the basic approach taken to scale development. These lessons are related but different.

The first key lesson is that Rasch analysis is vastly superior to traditional psychometric methods as a vehicle for developing and evaluating rating scales.

We have provided a clear example of this. The MSIS-29 was developed using traditional psychometric methods. Those of us involved in its development would like to think that we applied those methods rigorously. Others think so (55). We followed the well-established three-stage approach of item generation, item reduction and scale formation, and scale validation. People with MS were intimately involved at all stages, and the study was done in collaboration with the MS Society of Great Britain and Northern Ireland. To generate a pool of items, we interviewed people with MS, representing the full range of the condition, until redundancy; canvassed expert opinion from a range of health professionals; and undertook a comprehensive literature review. This process generated in the region of 3,000 statements concerning the health impact of MS. A preliminary questionnaire was prepared from these statements and was pretested in a sample of people with MS before it was sent to a large sample of people with MS across the United Kingdom. The final instrument was comprehensively evaluated for six psychometric properties: data quality, targeting, scaling assumptions, reliability, validity, and responsiveness. All traditional psychometric criteria were comfortably satisfied. Yet Rasch analysis identified anomalies and avenues for improvement. This is because it is conceptually and scientifically stronger, provides a more comprehensive and sophisticated evaluation of scales, and enables clear visualization of scale performance; it therefore acts as a helpful vehicle for scale construction and improvement.

The ability to formally examine item scoring functions means that this can be built into scale development, so that the number of item response categories is determined empirically rather than by assumption. At the moment, item response categories are typically chosen because they seem to be sensible. Our own research, as well as that of others, demonstrates that the numbers of response options that "work" vary from scale to scale. In addition, traditional psychometric method has tended to impose the same number and wording of item response categories for each item in a scale. We

think that this can affect the clinical meaningfulness of items to patients. It would be far more appropriate for the number and type of response options to be item specific and empirically determined. Rasch analysis enables this, but traditional psychometric methods do not.

The fact that Rasch analysis enables investigators to visualize the relative locations of items and their thresholds, and the knowledge that these locations are independent of the distributional properties of the study sample, have implications for scale development, evaluation, and refinement. This means that the variable mapped out by a set of items can be constructed to cover a suitable range. Gaps in the measurement continuum can be identified early and appropriate items identified and tested. Item bunching and redundancy can be minimized. Application of these methods is likely to produce more responsive scales. Traditional methods do not allow this to be done, and the fact that items are highly correlated does not mean that they are redundant.

Rasch analysis enables investigators to understand better the relationship between raw ordinal scale scores (achieved by summing item scores) and interval-level measurements that can be derived from those item response data. Although the nonlinear (S-shaped) relationship between ordinal raw scores and interval measures is well known, the implications of this relationship for the measurement of change are underestimated. Rasch analysis shows that a fixed 1-point change in raw scores implies a variable change in interval-level (that is, equal-interval) measurements. The variability is scale dependent and is 27-fold for the MSIS physical subscale. The direct implication is that studies using raw scores have almost certainly underestimated change in the samples; the problem is that we do not know to what extent, nor the circumstances in which different inferences would have been made. However, if clinical trials strive to deliver truthful inferences, then it seems hard to argue against methods that enable interval-level measurement of patient-reported outcomes.

Rasch analysis enables legitimate measurement at the individual person level. Traditional methods are not recommended for this (56). This is because Rasch analysis generates a standard error for every person, determined by the items they answer, their location on the continuum, and the targeting of the items to their location. In contrast, traditional methods generate one standard error for all locations on the scale that is determined by the reliability of the scale and the standard deviation of the sample. Thus, even when the reliability is very high, the error is wide (unless the sample SD is low, in which case the reliability is unlikely to be high). Moreover, the standard error associated with measurements of people is logical and empirically dependent on their location on the continuum. This makes the concept of a single standard error scientifically weak as well as illogical.

Rasch analysis, therefore, allows clinical trialists to evaluate their data at both the group level and the individual person level. This is important in that the treatment effect is typically variable: different people benefit different amounts. Ideally, clinical trials should have the facility to differentiate responders from nonresponders, as well as the overall group effect. In addition, group-based statistical tests do not account for the differing measurement precision of rating scales (see (47)).

Rasch analysis demonstrates that rating scales are really good measures only over a limited range. Typically, the samples used in clinical trials are variable in the construct of interest. This implies that we need scales with good precision over a wide range. By definition, this means scales with large numbers of items well spread over the range of the continuum. Such scales would almost certainly be unsuitable for use in clinical trials. The alternative is targeted measurement – that is, present each individual with a selection of items whose locations are similar to those of the person being measured. This process requires a large pool of calibrated items – known as an item bank – and a method of administering those items to individuals.

Targeted measurement represents a "sea change" from our current thinking about rating scales. Typically, trials use scales with fixed numbers of items (e.g., MSIS-29, SF-36, PDQ-39). These scales are inflexible in that they are good measures over a limited range that does not change. Essentially, therefore, when we use a fixed-length rating scale, we hope the sample will fit the scale. This situation needs to be reversed: scales need to be tailored to fit samples and the individuals within them. This process is achievable with item banking and computer adaptive testing.

Rasch analysis is a more sophisticated psychometric method. It has been regarded as a refinement or advance on traditional psychometric methods (44). Therefore, we expect it to identify limitations not identified using traditional methods. But there is a trade-off. Investment is required to understand the underpinning concepts, to read and understand an initially inaccessible literature, then to use and interpret the software programs. Do the advantages outweigh the investment? We think that moral, theoretical, and empirical arguments in favor can be presented.

The moral argument is that no compromise can be accepted in the efforts made to improve the quality of measurement in clinical studies. Rating scales are increasingly the primary outcome measures in clinical trials. In this role, they are the central dependent variables on which decisions are made about the treatment of people, prescribing habits, the expenditure of public funds, and future research. Moreover, vast amounts of public money are spent on clinical trials. It seems hard to argue against state-of-the-art clinical trials using state-of-the-art measurement methods.

The theoretical scientific arguments in favor of Rasch analysis are many. These include the use of an explicit mathematical model that realizes the requirements for measurement; the use of a mathematical model that enables construction of stable (invariant) linear measurements and sophisticated checks on the internal validity and consistency of scores; the ability to generate interval-level measurements from ordinal data; the ability to undertake legitimate individual person measurements; the ability to facilitate the development of item banks from which any subset of items can be taken; and scientific handling of missing data.

The information presented in this chapter goes some way toward providing empirical scientific arguments for the advantages of Rasch analysis over traditional psychometric methods. We have demonstrated that a scale developed using traditional psychometric methods has important limitations that went undetected by traditional methods. In addition, we have been able to estimate measurements of the physical and psychological impact of MS from the ordinal response to the 29 MSIS items. Finally, we have demonstrated how Rasch analysis could lead to improvement in scale development and could guide modification of existing scales.

It is sometimes difficult to demonstrate the advantages of one method over another. Head-to-head comparisons of scales are uncommon. Similarly, and for this reason, some people argue that there is still no "proof" that new psychometric methods provide meaningful advances on traditional methods because no evidence suggests that the results of a clinical trial are changed by using "Rasch scoring rather than Likert scoring." We think this argument misses the point.

The second lesson we have learned from the MSIS-29 experience concerns the basic approach to scale development. Typically, scales are developed "top down," that is, a pool of items is generated and items are grouped into subscales on the basis of statistical tests, such as factor analysis, or thematic similarity. This has two potential limitations. First, grouping items statistically does not ensure that they measure the same construct. Second, grouping items thematically does not ensure that they map out a variable in a clinically meaningful fashion.

It seems clear to us that the scale development process has to be underpinned by a clear definition, and conceptualization, of the variable to be measured. Without this foundation, it is impossible to map out a variable (referred to as "operationalize") in a clinically meaningful and measurable fashion. It then follows that the purpose of a psychometric evaluation is to establish the extent to which a pro-posed quantitative conceptualization has been successfully operationalized (44).

Taking a "top-down" approach to scale development may mean that scale developers might not invest fully in the process of defining, conceptualizing, and operationalizing variables that we now (6, 57) and others (58, 59) believe are central to valid measurement. Indeed, a critical look at our development of the MSIS-29 and most other published rating scales indicates that those processes were not formally undertaken. Many scales consist of items of mix-related constructs, and the variables they purport to measure may not be clear from the scale content. This is not helped by the fact that psychometric evaluations of scales can produce apparently excellent results in the face of limited content/clinical validity. This is because there is a difference, perhaps subtle, between a set of items being related and a set of items mapping out a variable. In both situations, it is highly likely that responses to the items will be correlated (the basis of traditional analyses) and related probabilistically (the basis of Rasch analysis). It is also because statistical evaluations of any set of items cannot be expected to tell us directly *what* a scale measures. Conversely, the fact that a set of items appears clinically meaningful does not tell us *how* they will perform as a measurement instrument.

Rasch analysis and more correctly the underpinning Rasch approach can assist in this process. In a Rasch analysis, the investigator is testing the fit of the data to a model, the Rasch model. The model is a mathematical articulation of a theory of how items should perform for measurements to be constructed from the ordinal responses to a set of items. Thus we are testing the data against a theory. Departures from that theory are anomalies for investigation.

Summary

Evidence suggests that the MSIS-29 is a useful scale for measuring the physical and psychological impact of MS. It was developed using traditional psychometric methods, and according to that paradigm, the evidence for psychometric soundness is very strong. Rasch analysis, however, identified limitations that led to revisions and the availability of MSIS-29v2. This version also has strong psychometric properties. Moreover, it enables linear estimates of physical and psychological health to be derived from MSIS-29v2 data. And, it enables legitimate analysis of study data at the individual person level.

The development, evaluation, and revision of the MSIS-29 taught us that modern psychometric methods are vastly superior to traditional ones and that the basic process of scale development needs to change. Thus we expect to see the MSIS29v2 replaced in the future by better instruments, by which I mean scales that generate better measurements of more clinically explicit variables. The MSIS-29v1 and v2 are stepping stones in the history of MS measurement.

REFERENCES

1. Holmes J, Madgwick T, Bates D. The cost of multiple sclerosis. *Br J Med Econ* 1995; **8**: 181–193.
2. Hatch J. The economic impact of multiple sclerosis. *MS Manag* 1996; **3**(1): 40.
3. Harvey C. Economic costs of multiple sclerosis: how much and who pays? Health Services Research Report: *National Multiple Sclerosis Society*, 1995 January. Report No.: ER-6005.
4. Prouse P, Ross-Smith K, Brill M, Singh M, Brennan P, Frank A. Community support for young physically handicapped people. *Health Trends* 1991; **23**: 105–109.
5. Thompson AJ, Noseworthy JH. New treatments for multiple sclerosis: a clinical perspective. *Curr Opin Neurol* 1996; **9**: 187–198.
6. Hobart JC, Thompson AJ. Clinical trials of multiple sclerosis. In: Reder AT, ed. *Interferon therapy of multiple sclerosis*. New York: Marcel Dekker, 1996; 398–407.
7. Guyatt GH, Freeny DH, Patrick DL. Measuring health-related quality of life. *Ann Int Med* 1993; **118**(8): 622–629.
8. Jenkinson C, Peto V, Fitzpatrick R, Greenhall R, Hyman N. Self-reported functioning and well-being in patients with Parkinson's disease: comparison of the Short-Form Health Survey (SF-36) and the Parkinson's Disease Questionnaire (PDQ-39). *Age Ageing* 1995; **24**: 505–509.
9. Kurtzke JF. Rating neurological impairment in multiple sclerosis: an expanded disability status scale (EDSS). *Neurology* 1983; **33**: 1444–1452.
10. Nunnally JC Jr. *Tests and measurements: assessment and prediction*. New York: McGraw-Hill; 1959.
11. Sharrack B, Hughes RAC, Soudain S, Dunn G. The psychometric properties of clinical rating scales used in multiple sclerosis. *Brain* 1999; **122**: 141–159.
12. Hobart JC, Freeman JA, Thompson AJ. Kurtzke scales revisited: the application of psychometric methods to clinical intuition. *Brain* 2000; **123**: 1027–1040.
13. Ware JE Jr, Snow KK, Kosinski M, Gandek B. *SF-36 Health Survey manual and interpretation guide*. Boston, Massachusetts: Nimrod Press; 1993.
14. Bergner M, Bobbitt RA, Pollard WE, Martin DP, Gibson BS. The Sickness Impact Profile: validation of a health status measure. *Med Care* 1976; **14**: 57–67.
15. EuroQol Group. EuroQoL: a new facility for the measurement of health-related quality of life. *Health Policy* 1990; **16**: 199–208.
16. Peto V, Jenkinson C, Fitzpatrick R, Greenhall R. The development and validation of a short measure of functioning and well-being for individuals with Parkinson's disease. *Qual Life Res* 1995; **4**: 241–248.
17. Patrick D, Deyo R. Generic and disease-specific measures in assessing health status and quality of life. *Med Care* 1989; **27**(3 Suppl): S217–S232.
18. Freeman JA, Hobart JC, Langdon DW, Thompson AJ. Clinical appropriateness: a key factor in outcome measure selection. The 36-item Short Form Health Survey in multiple sclerosis. *J Neurol Neurosurg Psychiatry* 2000; **68**: 150–156.
19. Norvedt MW, Riise T, Myer K-M, Nyland HI. Performance of the SF-36, SF-12 and RAND-36 summary scales in a multiple sclerosis population. *Med Care* 2000; **38**: 1022–1028.
20. Hobart JC, Freeman JA, Lamping DL, Fitzpatrick R, Thompson AJ. The SF-36 in multiple sclerosis: why assumptions must be tested. *J Neurol Neurosurg Psychiatry* 2001; **71**: 363–370.
21. Fitzpatrick R, Ziebland S, Jenkinson C, Mowat A, Mowat A. Importance of sensitivity to change as a criterion for selecting health status measures. *Qual in Health Care* 1992; **1**: 89–93.
22. Cella DF, Dineen K, Arnason B, Reder A, Webster KA, Karabatsos G, et al. Validation of the Functional

Assessment of Multiple Sclerosis quality of life instrument. *Neurology* 1996; **47**: 129–139.

23. Vickrey BG, Hays RD, Harooni R, Myers LW, Ellison GW. A health-related quality of life measure for multiple sclerosis. *Qual Life Res* 1995; **4**: 187–206.

24. Rudick R, Antel J, Confavreux C, Cutter G, Ellison G, Fischer J, et al. Recommendations from the National Multiple Sclerosis Society Clinical Outcomes Assessment Task Force. *Ann Neurol* 1997; **42**: 379–382.

25. Ford HL, Tennant A, Johnson MH. Developing a disease-specific quality of life measure for people with multiple sclerosis. *Clin Rehabil* 2001; **15**: 247–258.

26. Sharrack B, Hughes RAC. The Guy's Neurological Disability Scale (GNDS): a new disability measure for multiple sclerosis. *Mult Scler* 1999; **5**: 223–233.

27. Fischer JS, Rocca NL, Miller DM, Ritvo, PG, Andrews, H, Paty, D. Recent developments in the assessment of quality of life in multiple sclerosis. *Mult Scler* 1999; **5**: 251–259.

28. Pfennings LE, Cohen L, Van Der Ploeg HM, Bramsen I, Polman CH, Lankhorst GJ, et al. A health-related quality of life questionnaire for multiple sclerosis patients. *Acta Neurol Scand* 1999; **100**: 148–155.

29. Freeman JA, Hobart JC, Thompson AJ. Does adding MS-specific items to a generic measure (SF-36) improve measurement. *Neurology* 2001; **57**: 68–74.

30. Hobart JC, Riazi A, Lamping DL, Fitzpatrick R, Thompson AJ. Improving the evaluation of therapeutic interventions in multiple sclerosis: development of a patient-based measure of outcome. *Health Technol Asses* 2004; **8**(9): 1–48.

31. Hobart JC, Riazi A, Lamping DL, Fitzpatrick R, Thompson AJ. Measuring the impact of MS on walking ability: the 12-item MS Walking Scale (MSWS-12). *Neurology* 2003; **60**: 31–36.

32. Holland A, O'Connor RJ, Thompson AJ, Playford ED, Hobart JC. Talking the talk on walking the walk: a 12-item generic walking scale for neurological conditions. *J Neurol* 2006; **253**(12): 1594–1602.

33. Graham RC, Hughes RA. Clinimetric properties of a walking scale in peripheral neuropathy. *J Neurol Neurosurg Ps* 2006; **77**(8): 977–979.

34. Riazi A, Hobart J, Lamping D, Fitzpatrick R, Thompson A. Multiple Sclerosis Impact Scale (MSIS-29): reliability and validity in hospital-based samples. *J Neurol Neurosurg Psychiatry* 2002; **73**: 701–704.

35. Riazi A, Hobart J, Lamping D, Fitzpatrick R, Thompson A. Evidence-based measurement in multiple sclerosis: the psychometric properties of the physical and psychological dimensions of three quality of life rating scales. *Mult Scler* 2003; **9**(4): 411–419.

36. Hoogervorst EL, Zwemmer JN, Jelles B, Polman CH, Uitdehaag BM. Multiple Sclerosis Impact Scale (MSIS-29): relation to established measures of impairment and disability. *Mult Scler* 2004; **10**(5): 569–574.

37. McGuigan C, Hutchinson M. The multiple sclerosis impact scale (MSIS-29) is a reliable and sensitive measure. *J Neurol Neurosurg Psychiatry* 2004; **75**(275): 266–269.

38. McHorney CA, Haley SM, Ware JE Jr. Evaluation of the MOS SF-36 Physical Functioning Scale (PF-10): II. comparison of relative precision using Likert and Rasch scoring methods. *J Clin Epidemiol* 1997; **50**(4): 451–461.

39. Rasch G. *Probabilistic models for some intelligence and attainment tests.* Copenhagen, Chicago: Danish Institute for Education Research, 1960.

40. Lord FM, Novick MR. *Statistical theories of mental test scores.* Reading, MA: Addison-Wesley, 1968.

41. Likert RA. A technique for the measurement of attitudes. *Arch Psychol* 1932; **140**: 5–55.

42. Likert RA, Roslow S, Murphy G. A simple and reliable method of scoring the Thurstone attitude scales. *J Soc Psychol* 1934; **5**: 228–238.

43. Thurstone LL. A method for scaling psychological and educational tests. *J Educ Psychol* 1925; **16**(7): 433–451.

44. Andrich D, Styles IM. *Report on the psychometric analysis of the early development instrument (EDI) using the Rasch model.* Perth, WA: Murdoch University, 2004.

45. Smith EV Jr. Evidence for the reliability of measures and validity of measure interpretation: a Rasch measurement perspective. *J Appl Meas* 2001; **2**: 281–311.

46. Wright BD, Masters G. *Rating scale analysis: Rasch measurement.* Chicago: MESA, 1982.

47. Hobart JC, Cano SJ. Improving the evaluation of therapeutic interventions in multiple sclerosis: the role of new psychometric methods. *Health Technol Assess* 2009; **13**(12): 1–200.

48. Hobart JC, Lamping DL, Fitzpatrick R, Riazi A, Thompson AJ. The Multiple Sclerosis Impact Scale (MSIS-29): a new patient-based outcome measure. *Brain* 2001; **124**: 962–973.

49. Hobart JC, Riazi A, Lamping DL, Fitzpatrick R, Thompson AJ. How responsive is the MSIS-29? A comparison with other self-report scales. *J Neurol Neurosurg Psychiatry* 2005; **76**(11): 1539–1543.

50. Andrich D. Controversy and the Rasch model: a characteristic of incompatible paradigms? *Med Care* 2004; **42**(1): I7–I16.

51. Andrich D, de Jong JHAL, Sheridan BE. Diagnostic opportunities with the Rasch model for ordered response categories. In: Rost J, Langeheine R, editors. *Applications of latent trait and latent class models in the social sciences*. Münster, Germany: Waxmann Verlag GmbH, 1997;59–70.

52. Wright BD. Misunderstanding the Rasch model. *J Educ Meas* 1977; **14**: 219–225.

53. Kuhn TS. *The structure of scientific revolutions*. Chicago: University of Chicago Press, 1962.

54. Kuhn TS. *The essential tension*. Chicago: University of Chicago Press, 1977.

55. Herndon R. *Handbook of Neurologic Rating Scales*. New York: Demos Medical Publishing, 2006.

56. McHorney CA, Tarlov AR. Individual-patient monitoring in clinical practice: are available health status surveys adequate? *Qual Life Res* 1995; **4**: 293–307.

57. Nicholl L, Hobart JC, Cramp AFL, Lowe-Strong AS. Measuring quality of life in multiple sclerosis: not as simple as it sounds. *Mult Scler* 2005; **11**: 708–712.

58. Andrich D. A framework relating outcomes based education and the taxonomy of educational objectives. *Stud Educ Eval* 2002a; **28**: 35–59.

59. Andrich D. Implication and applications of modern test theory in the context of outcomes based research. *Stud Educ Eval* 2002b; **28**: 103–121.

Multiple Sclerosis Impact Scale, version 2 (MSIS-29v2)

- The following questions ask for your views about the impact of MS on your day-to-day life during **the past 2 weeks**.
- For each statement, please circle the one number that best describes your situation.
- Please answer all questions.

In the past 2 weeks, how much has your MS limited your ability to …	Not at all	A little	Moderately	Extremely
1. Do physically demanding tasks?	1	2	3	4
2. Grip things tightly (e.g., turning on taps)?	1	2	3	4
3. Carry things?	1	2	3	4

In the past 2 weeks, how much have you been bothered by …	Not at all	A little	Moderately	Extremely
4. Problems with your balance?	1	2	3	4
5. Difficulties moving about indoors?	1	2	3	4
6. Being clumsy?	1	2	3	4
7. Stiffness?	1	2	3	4
8. Heavy arms and/or legs?	1	2	3	4
9. Tremor of your arms or legs?	1	2	3	4
10. Spasms in your limbs?	1	2	3	4
11. Your body not doing what you want it to do?	1	2	3	4
12. Having to depend on others to do things for you?	1	2	3	4

In the past 2 weeks, how much have you been bothered by …	Not at all	A little	Moderate	Extremely
13. Limitations in your social and leisure activities at home?	1	2	3	4
14. Being stuck at home more than you would like to be?	1	2	3	4
15. Difficulties using your hands in everyday tasks?	1	2	3	4
16. Having to cut down the amount of time you spent on work or other daily activities?	1	2	3	4
17. Problems using transport (e.g., car, bus, train, taxi)?	1	2	3	4
18. Taking longer to do things?	1	2	3	4
19. Difficulty doing things spontaneously (e.g., going out on the spur of the moment)?	1	2	3	4
20. Needing to go to the toilet urgently?	1	2	3	4
21. Feeling unwell?	1	2	3	4
22. Problems sleeping?	1	2	3	4
23. Feeling mentally fatigued?	1	2		4
24. Worries related to your MS?	1	2	3	4
25. Feeling anxious or tense?	1	2	3	4
26. Feeling irritable, impatient, or short-tempered?	1	2	3	4
27. Problems concentrating?	1	2	3	4
28. Lack of confidence?	1	2	3	4
29. Feeling depressed?	1	2	3	4

4

Patient-reported outcome measurement in motor neuron disease/amyotrophic lateral sclerosis – the ALSAQ-40 and ALSAQ-5

Crispin Jenkinson

Introduction

Motor neuron disease (MND) refers to a family of related progressive disorders in which upper and lower motor neurons cease to function, thus causing increasing disability. A French neurologist, Jean-Martin Charcot, first suggested grouping together disparate conditions that affect the lateral horn of the spinal cord as MND in 1869. The disease came to public awareness in 1939, when the New York Yankees baseball icon Lou Gehrig was diagnosed with the disease and died a few years later at the age of 37. Despite the relative rarity of the disease, a number of high-profile cases, including the actor David Niven and Cambridge Professor of Mathematics Stephen Hawking, have kept the disease in the public arena.

Although the symptoms of the various forms of MND vary at the outset, they overlap in later stages. Amyotrophic lateral sclerosis (ALS) is the most common type, accounting for approximately 8 of 10 cases. Initial symptoms are typically stiffness and weakness in the hands and feet. ALS is a fatal condition, with people living between 2 and 5 years from initial symptoms. Almost all other cases of MND are progressive bulbar palsy (PBP), with initial bulbar involvement, causing difficulties with speech, chewing, and swallowing. Once again, this disease is fatal with the majority of people with the condition dying within 3 years from presentation of the first symptoms. Two other forms of MND have been documented but are very rare. Progressive muscular atrophy begins with weakness, but not stiffness, in the hands and feet. The disease progresses relatively slowly, with most people with the condition living longer than 5 years from first symptoms. Finally, primary lateral sclerosis typically begins with weakness in the legs and some patients reporting clumsiness with the hands and difficulty with speech. Progression of the disease is very slow and may not lead to death. However, it is believed that the disease can develop into ALS, which is fatal.

The incidence of all types of MND is approximately 2/100,000/year, with a prevalence of about 6/100,000 (1). Progressive weakness of limb, trunk, and ventilatory and bulbar muscles causes increasing dependency on family and other caregivers (2). In the longer term, this will lead to a state of physical dependency and immobility. Intellectual capacity is unaffected. This chapter outlines the use of generic health status measures in the assessment of amyotrophic lateral sclerosis/motor neuron disease (3), and outlines the development and validation of the first measure designed specifically for patients diagnosed with these conditions.

Clinical assessment of MND

The most common primary outcome points in trials of treatment regimens for ALS/MND are muscle

Quality of Life Measurement in Neurodegenerative and Related Conditions, eds., Crispin Jenkinson, Michele Peters, and Mark B. Bromberg. Published by Cambridge University Press. © Cambridge University Press 2011.

strength, pulmonary function, and mortality. Perhaps the most widely known measure is the Norris ALS Scale (4), which was designed to track clinical changes in ALS patients after treatment. This scale measures both impairments and disabilities. The scale provides scores for bulbar, respiratory, arm, trunk, and leg domains, as well as a general domain, measuring, among other things, fatigue and emotional health. The measure assigns weights of equal value to different aspects of patient functioning, which does not seem appropriate given that it also assesses areas of health state seldom influenced by ALS, such as bladder and bowel function (5). The Appel Scale is a widely used measure that consists of assessments of bulbar involvement (speech and swallowing), respiratory involvement, muscle strength in arms and legs, lower extremity function, and upper extremity function. Assessments are determined by clinical evaluation. The disparate scores gained from the assessment are used to obtain a single total scale score. Although the construct validity of the measure has been supported by evidence of increasing scores on the overall index as the disease progresses (6), such addition of the various assessments has been criticized as having limited meaning (7). The most recent attempt to develop a clinimetric scale, which is simple to use and can provide meaningful data, is the ALS Functional Rating Scale (ALSFRS) (7). The ALSFRS is a 10-item functional inventory that was devised for use in therapeutic trials in ALS and covers the areas of speech, salivation, swallowing, handwriting, cutting food, dressing and hygiene, turning in bed, walking, climbing stairs, and breathing. Each item is rated on a 0 to 4 scale by the patient, caregiver, or both, yielding a maximum score of 40 points. The ALSFRS assesses patients' levels of self-sufficiency in areas of feeding, grooming, ambulation, and communication. The ALSFRS has been validated both cross-sectionally and longitudinally against muscle strength testing, the Schwab and England Activities of Daily Living rating scale, the Clinical Global Impression of Change (CGIC) scale, and independent assessments of patients' functional status. Evidence has also been provided in

a large, multicenter clinical trial for ALS test-retest reliability and consistency of the ALSFRS (8). One weakness of the ALSFRS is that it grants disproportionate weighting to limb and bulbar, as compared with respiratory, dysfunction. A revised version of the ALSFRS has been developed that incorporates additional assessments of dyspnea, orthopnea, and the need for ventilatory support (9). The Revised ALSFRS (ALSFRS-R) retains the properties of the original scale and shows strong internal consistency and construct validity. More recently, on the basis of a survey of an on-line community for people with ALS, three new items were selected that conform to the existing factor structure of the ALFRS-R. These relate to ability to use fingers to manipulate devices, ability to show emotional expression in the face, and ability to get around inside the home (10). This measure (ALSFRS-EX) has not yet been fully validated.

However, despite the excellent qualities of the ALSFRS, the impact of newly developed therapies increasingly requires a broader assessment of outcome in terms of subjective health status. For example, the ALSFRS does not attempt to assess the impact of ill health on emotional functioning or social functioning. Thus, measures of health status that provide a more subjective and, hence, of a more complete impact of the disease upon functioning and well-being are needed.

Generic measures of health status

The 36-item Short Form Health Survey questionnaire (SF-36) (11) is perhaps, at present, the most widely used measure of general health status, and it has recently been evaluated for use in ALS/MND patients. In one study, the progression of disability and the patients' perception of their health were assessed in a small group of MND patients (n = 14) 6 months from the point of diagnosis or very soon after and were compared with a group of patients of similar age with Parkinson's disease (PD). MND patients showed a far more rapid deterioration in health status on a number of clinical measures.

However, for both groups, perception of their physical health on the SF-36 was very poor at recruitment compared with age- and sex-matched population norms. In both groups, the SF-36 could not be used to monitor changes in perception of health because of floor effects on a number of domains (12). However, these results are at odds with those gained from an American study that compared results from the SF-36 with those gained on the Tufts Quantitative Neuromuscular Exam (TQNE). This study examined the reliability and responsiveness of each measure and contrasted the health status between individuals with ALS and the general population. Subjects (n = 31) completed the SF-36 and TQNE at two time points within 1 week to determine reliability. Furthermore, 17 subjects also completed both the TQNE and the SF-36 each month for 1 year after diagnosis of ALS to establish the relationship between the two assessment tools. The authors claim that both measures were highly reliable and responsive. This paper argued that both the TQNE and the SF-36 were reliable and responsive and appeared important in the characterization of patient status after ALS is diagnosed (13).

The SF-36 was used in the European ALS-Health Profile Study (14). This large-scale study was undertaken throughout Europe to evaluate the health status of patients with ALS/MND. Evidence indicated floor effects, particularly in the "role physical" dimension of the instrument. However, more recently, the SF-36 was modified to overcome this problem, and the subsequent SF-36 version 2 is likely to be a more appropriate instrument for use in evaluation of the consequences of ALS/MND (15). A subset of items from the SF-36 has been used to construct the 12-item Health Survey Questionnaire (SF-12) (16). Evidence suggests that it provides a picture of health status similar to that of the SF-36 (17).

Recent trials of ALS therapies have included the Sickness Impact Profile (SIP) to evaluate health-related quality of life; the feasibility, psychometric properties, and interpretation of the SIP have been evaluated in this setting. The SIP is a questionnaire containing 136 items; it can provide an overall scale score, scores for 12 subdimensions, or both, as well as physical and psychosocial summary scores. In one study, the SIP was administered at baseline and at 3, 6, and 9 months during a double-blind, placebo-controlled study of recombinant human insulin-like growth factor I. The frequency of missing SIP data and administration time were recorded. Patients' scores on the Appel ALS Rating Scale were used to identify a stable subgroup for reliability testing and clinically distinct groups for validity testing. Internal consistency, reliability, and reproducibility were evaluated using Cronbach's alpha and intraclass correlation coefficients, respectively. Analysis of variance (ANOVA) models and t-tests were used to assess validity. Effect sizes and the responsiveness index were used to assess responsiveness. At baseline, 259 (97%) patients completed a 30-minute interview, which included the SIP. At subsequent assessments, response rates ranged from 92% to 97% and mean administration times ranged from 25 to 27 minutes. The overall SIP score demonstrated high internal reliability and stability coefficients. Baseline overall SIP scores discriminated between patients in the two Appel ALS score defined groups. Similarly, mean overall SIP change scores discriminated patients progressing at different rates. With few exceptions, dimension scores met similar criteria. Responsiveness statistics for the physical and overall SIP scores were lower at 3 months and higher at 6 and 9 months as the disease progressed. The authors concluded that these findings support the validity of the SIP for assessing outcomes of ALS and its treatment in future clinical trials (18). However, they themselves claim that the study design they adopted had limitations in assessing the usefulness of the SIP as a measure of psychosocial well-being because the primary end points of the trial were measures of physical function. Indeed, this limitation is present in other assessments of the SIP in ALS. For example, the TQNE is a standardized tool used for measuring muscle strength and pulmonary function in patients with amyotrophic lateral sclerosis; in a study of 524 ALS patients, a significant relationship was found between TQNE and SIP scores, both in cross section and over time (19). Again, this provides evidence for the ability of the SIP to measure physical functioning in ALS but offers limited evidence for its appropriateness to assess psychosocial aspects of health state. Nonetheless, available evidence seems to suggest that the SIP is an appropriate tool for this patient group.

One obvious criticism of the SIP is that it takes considerable time to complete, and this can be demanding for patients with serious conditions such as ALS/MND. Consequently, a shorter version has been developed specifically for use with ALS/MND patients (20). The authors examined SIP subscales and clinically derived item sets in relation to the TQNE combination megascore (CM) in an effort to define a briefer measure of quality of life for use in clinical trials. Two "Mini-SIP" indices performed as well as the overall SIP in reflecting the impact of muscle weakness on ALS patients' quality of life: a combination of two SIP subscales (SIP-33) and a 19-item set of questions independently chosen by a panel of ALS specialists (SIP/ALS-19). The developers suggest that either index could potentially be useful in ALS clinical trials, but more extensive evaluation of the measures is required. The SIP/ALS-19 is currently being used in a national ALS database (the ALS CARE program), providing an opportunity to evaluate its utility prospectively against other quality of life measures in ALS patients (15). To date, only limited data have been available on this shortened, disease-specific version of the SIP.

A more individualized quality of life measure has been proposed, which asks patients to nominate their own areas of health adversely affected by their health status and to score these areas: the Schedule for Individual Quality of Life (Direct Weighted version) (SEIQoL-DW) (21). In a study of 120 patients with ALS, results of the SEIQoL-DW were not highly correlated with fixed-format quality of life measures. The authors argue that the study demonstrates that the SEIQoL-DW is of great value in identifying those factors that contribute to the psychosocial well-being of an individual with ALS. However, SEIQoL index scores may not reflect aggregate QoL

of groups of patients with ALS and may be measuring a construct other than QoL. Caution should be exercised in using the SEIQoL index score to measure QoL of groups, such as would be needed in interventional trials (22).

Ideally, however, disease-specific measures are not adapted from existing measures but are designed from "the ground up"; at present, only one such measure exists: the 40-item ALS Assessment Questionnaire and its shorter form – the five-item ALSAQ-5 (23). The development and validation of this measure are outlined below.

The ALSAQ-40 disease-specific health status measure

To develop a disease-specific health status measure for ALS/MND, a three-stage development process was followed. In the first stage, in-depth semistructured interviews with 18 patients presenting with ALS were tape-recorded. The sample size for this stage of the study was determined by the point at which no new significant themes appeared to emerge from the interviews. Patients presented with ALS across the breadth of the disease process, and at different ages. They were asked to describe the areas of their lives that had been influenced by their ALS/MND. A list of aspects of life adversely affected by the disease was extracted from the transcribed interviews. Four researchers then independently devised questionnaire items from this list. These were then discussed jointly and scrutinized for repetition and ambiguity, and a final set of items was agreed on. This led to a final pool of 78 items, which were drafted to ask about the influence of ALS on a specific area of life over the last 2 weeks. For each question, respondents could select from a range of answers: Never (0); Occasionally (1); Rarely (2); Often (3); and Always (or cannot do at all) (4). The face validity of the questionnaire was assessed at this stage by two patients, a regional care advisor, and two neurologists. No alterations were suggested. Consequently, 75 copies of the form were sent to patients with MND with a request to complete the questionnaire and indicate any alterations that they would suggest. A telephone number was provided to enable patients to call in with comments. Few comments on the measure were made, and no one issue was consistently raised. Consequently, it was decided to make no alterations to the measure.

In the second stage of development of the measure, the 78-item questionnaire, developed in the first stage, was administered, by postal survey, to a sample of individuals with ALS. Care advisors for regions of the Motor Neurone Disease Association Society in England, Wales, and Northern Ireland were approached for help in recruiting. A small number of patients (n = 25) were not contacted in this way but volunteered to take part in the study, which had been outlined in a copy of *Thumbprint*, the U.K. MND Association newsletter. In total, the measure was mailed to 208, of whom 29 people did not respond, and 6 blank questionnaires were returned. Thus a response rate of 173 (83.2%) was achieved. The mean age of the sample was 62.6 years (min = 31, max = 92, n = 168). Sixty-six (38.2%) of the sample were female and 104 (60.1%) male. The mean period since diagnosis was 37.9 months (min = 2, max = 211, n = 165). Statistical analysis of these data suggested that the measure contained five dimensions and 40 items. The statistical procedures employed at this stage are documented in full elsewhere (14). Areas measured by the instrument include the following:

- *Eating and Drinking* (3 items): addresses problems eating solid foods, swallowing, and drinking liquids.
- *Communication* (7 items): addresses a variety of problems communicating with others, for example, difficulties with speech such as talking slowly, stuttering while speaking, and feeling self-conscious about speech.
- *Activities of daily living/Independence* (10 items): addresses a variety of limitations in activities of daily living (ADLs), for example, difficulties in washing oneself, dressing oneself, and doing tasks around the house, as well as difficulties in writing and getting dressed.

- *Mobility* (10 items): addresses problems of mobility, for example, difficulties of walking, standing up, going up and down stairs, and falling.
- *Emotional well-being* (10 items): addresses various emotional problems, for example, feeling lonely, bored, or depressed, feelings of embarrassment in social situations, and feeling worried that the disease will progress in the future.

The purpose of the measure is to indicate the extent of ill health up to each domain measured. Consequently, each scale is transformed to have a range from 0 (the best health status as measured on the questionnaire) through 100 (the worst health status measured on the questionnaire), with each scale calculated as follows: scale score = the total of the raw scores of each item in the scale divided by the maximum possible raw score of all items in the scale multiplied by 100.

The correlations of items with their scale totals and the internal consistency reliability of scales (that is, the extent to which items in a scale tap a single underlying dimension) were evaluated to assess the psychometric soundness of the instrument. Items were found to be highly correlated with their own scale score (corrected so as not to include the item to which it was being correlated). Internal reliability was assessed using Cronbach's alpha statistic (24), and all scales were found to have very high internal consistency reliability by any standards but particularly high by the standard for group comparisons (25, 26).

Construct validity was assessed in two small-scale studies. In the first, it was examined by means of correlations of scales for ALSAQ-40 with relevant scales for SF-36. The Mobility scale of the ALSAQ-40 correlated with the Physical Function scale of the SF-36. The Activities of Daily Living/Independence scale of the ALSAQ-40 correlated with both the Physical Function scale and the Role Limitations due to Physical Problems scale of the SF-36. The Emotional Well-being of the ALSAQ-40 was found to be correlated with both the Mental Health and Role Limitations due to Emotional Problems scales of the SF-36. These associations were previously hypothesized and provide further evidence that the

ALSAQ-40 is providing a meaningful picture of health status.

The acceptability and construct validity of the ALSAQ were also assessed in a pilot study undertaken in a neurology clinic in the United States. Patients completed the forms without trouble. Internal reliability of the measure was found to be comparable with that gained in the U.K. samples. High correlations were found between conceptually similar domains on a clinician-completed form (the ALS-FRS) and domains of the ALSAQ. The eating and drinking domain (ALSAQ-40) correlated with speech, swallowing, and breathing (ALS-FRS); communication (ALSAQ-40) correlated with the ALS-FRS dimensions of speech, salivation, swallowing, and breathing. ALSAQ-40 ADL/independence domain scores correlated with ALS-FRS domains of writing, cutting food, dressing and hygiene, turning in bed, walking, and climbing stairs. Physical mobility (ALSAQ-40) correlated with turning in bed, walking, and climbing stairs. The only unexpected association was that found between emotional reactions (ALSAQ-40) and the turning in bed dimension of the ALS-FRS. However, this may be accounted for by the fact that discomfort in bed is likely to lead to poor sleep, causing in turn tiredness and fatigue, which evidence suggests are associated with adverse mental health (27).

The ALSAQ-40 has been translated and validated in Dutch (28), Italian (29), Spanish (30), and Japanese (31). Domains were found to have high levels of internal consistency. Construct validity was assessed by comparing scores on ALSAQ with both clinical measures and generic patient-reported outcome measures, and was supported in all validation studies.

The ALSAQ-5

Despite the relative brevity of the ALSAQ-40, there are situations in which an even shorter instrument is desirable. Certainly in the case of large-scale trials, it has been suggested the chance of patient and physician participation is greater when the data required are simple to collect and relatively brief. Indeed, the quality of recorded data in trials often suffers when too many data are collected on each patient (32). Furthermore, it is evidently desirable to reduce patient burden in data collection, especially when the demands of the illness can be considerable, as in neurological disorders such as ALS. The purpose of this chapter, therefore, is to report on the development of a short-form ALSAQ, which may be used in large-scale studies when the ALSAQ-40 is believed to be impracticable. Many attempts to reduce the length of instruments ignore, or at least do not report, appropriate methodologic and statistical procedures (33). Most important, the choice of instrument for item reduction is usually inappropriate because little or no evidence confirms the reliability and validity of the original measure. Manifestly reducing the length of an instrument that is unreliable is not a worthwhile exercise. In this instance, the ALSAQ-40 has proven validity and reliability and is used as the "gold standard" for consequent item reduction. Results on any short form should produce results that are as close as possible to those of the long form. This section documents the methods used to select items for a shorter version of the ALSAQ-40 and compares results between the two versions of the instrument.

A survey of members of the MND Association (Northampton, United Kingdom) was used to determine which items should be included in a shortened version of the ALSAQ. Scores were calculated for the five dimensions of the ALSAQ-40 on a standardized scale of 0 (best possible health state measured by the ALSAQ) to 100 (worst possible health state measured by the ALSAQ). Furthermore, all 40 items on the questionnaire were transformed onto a scale from 0 to 100, and each item was compared with its dimension total. Items whose mean scores were not found to be statistically significantly different from their scale total, and that most closely reflected the distribution of the scale, were selected for inclusion in the short-form measure. Ninety-five percent confidence intervals were calculated for each scale item representing the scale in the short-form, five-item ALSAQ (referred to here as the ALSAQ-5).

Each selected item was then correlated with the five scale scores to ensure that it was highly associated with the (uncorrected) scale score to which it contributes, and, further, was less well correlated with the other four scales.

The operating characteristics of the two measures were then assessed on another dataset – the MND Regional Survey. First, correlations of items to scale scores was undertaken again on this dataset to corroborate the results obtained from the MND Association survey. The ALSAQ-40 and ALSAQ-5 scores were then correlated with the Physical and Mental Summary Scores (PCS and MCS) of the SF-36 to determine whether a similar pattern of associations was observed. It was hypothesized that if the operating characteristics of the two versions of the instrument were similar, then the pattern of correlations between ALSAQ-5 items and the PCS and MCS should closely resemble the pattern of correlations between dimensions of the ALSAQ-40 and the PCS and MCS. Analyses supported these hypotheses, and a five-item questionnaire was created. The instrument addresses the following areas: difficulty standing up (question 9 on the original instrument), difficulty using arms and hands (question 11), difficulty eating solid food (question 22), speech not easy to understand (question 25), and feeling hopeless about the future (question 34) (34).

Discussion

Research into patient-based outcome and quality of life takes a wider perspective than the purely medical model of disease that has hitherto dominated clinical trials and other assessments of the value of treatments. The future of treatment for ALS is beginning to show promise, and simply assessing functional ability or length of life will not give full insight into the impact of new treatment regimens. Subjective reports of patients will provide a far more comprehensive understanding of the effects of treatment. Furthermore, a very strong case can be made for measuring caregiver burden and quality of life. The full potential of quality of life measurements

will begin to be realized only when the full social and economic effects are understood. After the development and application of new disease-specific measures for ALS, the next important task will be the creation of measures to be completed by those who care for people with the disease.

In conclusion, it is argued that in studies of future treatments for ALS, research should systematically measure quality of life and health status. Given the limited impact that medicine can have at present on the prognosis of this disease, it is essential that treatment at the very least improve well-being and quality of life. Further validation and experience with generic measures will increase their use and value to the neurological community, and the application of ALS-specific outcome measures will provide important endpoint measures for future trials and cohort studies. A User Manual and Guide are available (35).

REFERENCES

1. Brooks BR. Clinical epidemiology of amyotrophic lateral sclerosis. *Neurol Clin* 1966; **14**: 399–420.

2. Leigh PN, Swash M. Motor Neuron Disease; *Biology and Management.* London: Springer-Verlag, 1995.

3. Rosser R. A health index and output measure. In: Walker SR and Rosser R., eds. *Quality of Life Assessment: Key Issues in the 1990s.* London: Kluwer, 1993.

4. Norris FH, Calanchini PR, Fallat RJ, Pantry S, Jewett B. The administration of guanidine in amyotrophic lateral sclerosis. *Neurology* 1974; **34**: 721–728.

5. Brooks B, Sufit R, DePaul R, Tan Y, Senjak M, Robbins J. Design of clinical therapeutic trials in amyotrophic later sclerosis. *Adv Neurol* 1991; **56**: 521–546.

6. Appel V, Stewart SS, Smith G, Appel SH. A rating scale for amyotrophic lateral sclerosis: description and preliminary experience. *Ann Neurol* 1987; **22**: 328–333.

7. The ALS CNTF Treatment Study Phase I-II Study Group. The Amyotrophic Lateral Sclerosis Functional Rating Scale. Assessment of Activities of Daily Living in Patients with Amyotrophic Lateral Sclerosis. *Arch Neurol* 1996; **53**: 141–147.

8. Cedarbaum JM, Stambler N. Performance of the Amyotrophic Lateral Sclerosis Functional Rating Scale (ALSFRS) in multicenter clinical trials. *J Neurol Sci* 1997; **152** Supp: S1–S9.

9. Cedarbaum JM, Stambler M, Malta E. The ALSFRS-R: A revised ALS functional rating scale that incorporates assessment of respiratory function. *J Neurol Sci* 1999; **169**: 13–21.

10. Wicks P, Massagli MP, Wolf C, Heywood J. Measuring function in advanced ALS: validation of ALSFRS-EX extension items. *Eur J Neurol* 2009; **16**: 353–359.

11. Ware J, Sherbourne C. The MOS 36-Item Short Form Health Survey 1: Conceptual Framework and Item Selection. *Med Care* 1992; **30**: 473–483.

12. Young CA, Tedman BM, Williams IR. Disease progression and perceptions of health in patients with motor neurone disease. *J Neurol Sci* 1995; **129** Supp: 50–53.

13. Shields RK, Ruhland JL, Ross MA, Saehler MM, Smith KB, Heffner ML. Analysis of health-related quality of life and muscle impairment in individuals with amyotrophic lateral sclerosis using the medical outcome survey and the Tufts Quantitative Neuromuscular Exam. *Arch Phys Med Rehab* 1998; **79**: 855–856.

14. Jenkinson C, Fitzpatrick R, Brennan C, Bromberg M, Swash M. Development and validation of a short measure of health status for individuals with amyotrophic lateral sclerosis (motor nerone disease): the ALSAQ-40. *J Neurol* 1999; **246**, Supp 3: 16–21.

15. Jenkinson C, Stewart-Brown S, Petersen S, Paice C. Evaluation of the SF-36 Version II in the United Kingdom. *J Epidemiol Community Health* 1999; **53**: 46–50.

16. Ware J, Kosinski M, Keller SD. A 12-Item Short-Form Health Survey: construction of scales and preliminary tests of reliability and validity. *Med Care* 1996; **3**: 220–223.

17. Miller RG, Anderson F, the ALS CARE Group. Assessing Quality of Life in ALS. Comparison of the Short-Form 12 Survey with the ALS Functional Rating Scale, Forced Vital Capacity and ALS Quality of Life Index. Poster presented at the Eighth International Symposium on ALS MND, Chicago, 1998.

18. Damiano AM, Patrick DL, Guzman G, Gawel MJ, Gelinas DF, Natter HM, Ingalls KK. Measurement of health-related quality of life in patients with amyotrophic lateral sclerosis in clinical trials of new therapies. *Med Care* 1999; **37**: 15–26.

19. McGuire D, Garrison L, Armon C, Barohn R, Bryan W, Miller R, Parry G, Petajan J, Ross M. Relationship of the Tufts Quantitative Neuromuscular Exam (TQNE) and the Sickness Impact Profile (SIP) in measuring progression of ALS. SSNJV (CNTF ALS) Study Group. *Neurology* 1996; **46**: 1442–1444.

20. McGuire D, Garrison L, Armon C, Barohn RJ, Bryan WW, Miller R, Parry GJ, Petajan JH, Ross MA. A brief quality-of-life measure for ALS clinical trials based on a subset of items from the sickness impact profile. The Syntex-Synergen ALS (CNTF) Study Group. *J Neurol Sci* 1997; **152** (Suppl 1): S18–S22.

21. Hickey A, Bury G, O'Boyle C, Bradley F, O'Kelly F, Shannon W. A new short form individual quality of life measure (SEIQoL-DW): application in a cohort of individuals with HIV (AIDS). *BMJ* 1996; **313**: 29–33.

22. Felgoise SH, Stewart JL, Bremer BA, Walsh SM, Bromberg MB, Simmons Z. The SEIQoL-DW for assessing quality of life in ALS: strengths and limitations. *Amyotroph Lateral Scler* 2009; **10**: 456–462.

23. Epton J, Harris R, Jenkinson C. Quality of life in amyotrophic lateral sclerosis (motor neuron disease): a structured review. *Amyotroph Lateral Scler* 2009; **10**: 15–26.

24. Cronbach LJ. Coefficient alpha and the internal structure of tests. *Psychometrika* 1951; **16**: 297–334.

25. Nunnally JC, Bernstein IH. *Psychometric Theory: The Third Edition.* New York: McGraw Hill, 1994.

26. Ware JE, Kosinski M, Keller SD. SF-36 Physical and Mental Health Summary Scales. *A User's Manual.* Boston, Massachusetts: The Health Institute, New England Medical Center, 1994.

27. Walker EA, Katon WJ, Jemalka RP. Psychiatric disorders and medical care utilisation among people in the general population who report fatigue. *J Gen Int Med* 1993; **8**: 436–440.

28. Maessen M, Post MW, Maillé R, Lindeman E, Mooij R, Veldink JH, Van Den Berg LH. Validity of the Dutch version of the Amyotrophic Lateral Sclerosis Assessment Questionnaire, ALSAQ-40, ALSAQ-5. *Amyotroph Lateral Scler* 2007; **8**: 96–100.

29. Palmieri A, Sorarù G, Lombardi L, D'Ascenzo C, Baggio L, Ermani M, Pegoraro E, Angelini C. Quality of life and motor impairment in ALS: Italian validation of ALSAQ. *Neurol Res* 2010; **32**: 32–40.

30. Salas T, Mora J, Esteban J, Rodríguez F, Díaz-Lobato S, Fajardo M. Spanish adaptation of the Amyotrophic Lateral Sclerosis Questionnaire ALSAQ-40 for ALS patients. *Amyotroph Lateral Scler* 2008; **9**: 168–172.

31. Yamaguchi T, Ohbu S, Saito M, Ito Y, Moriwaka F, Tashiro K, Ohashi Y, Fukuhara S. Validity and clinical applicability of the Japanese version of amyotrophic

lateral sclerosis–assessment questionnaire 40 (ALSAQ-40). *No To Shinkei* 2004 Jun; **6**: 483–494. (Japanese).

32. Pocock SJ. *Clinical Trials: A Practical Approach.* Chichester: John Wiley and Sons, 1983.

33. Coste J, Guillemin F, Pouchot J, Fermanian J. Methodological approaches to shortening composite measurement scales. *J Clin Epidemiol* 1997; **50**: 247–252.

34. Jenkinson C, Fitzpatrick R. A reduced item set for the Amyotrophic Lateral Sclerosis Assessment Questionnaire: Development and validation of the ALSAQ-5. *J Neurol Neurosurg Psychiatry* 2001; **70**: 70–73.

35. Jenkinson C, Swash M, Fitzpatrick R, Swash M, Levvy G. *ALSAQ User Manual.* Oxford: Health Services Research Unit, 2001.

ALSAQ-40

The following statements all refer to certain difficulties that you may have had <u>during the last 2 weeks</u>. Please indicate, by ticking the appropriate box, how often the following statements have been true for you.

If you cannot walk at all please tick *Always/cannot do at all*, for questions 1 to 9.

How often <u>during the last 2 weeks</u> have the following been true?

*Please tick **one box** for each question.*

	Never	Rarely	Sometimes	Often	Always or cannot do at all
1. I have found it difficult to walk short distances, (e.g., around the house).	☐	☐	☐	☐	☐
2. I have fallen over while walking.	☐	☐	☐	☐	☐
3. I have stumbled or tripped while walking.	☐	☐	☐	☐	☐
4. I have lost my balance while walking.	☐	☐	☐	☐	☐
5. I have had to concentrate while walking.	☐	☐	☐	☐	☐
6. Walking has tired me out.	☐	☐	☐	☐	☐
7. I have had pains in my legs while walking.	☐	☐	☐	☐	☐
8. I have found it difficult to go up and down the stairs.	☐	☐	☐	☐	☐
9. I have found it difficult to stand up.	☐	☐	☐	☐	☐
10. I have found it difficult to get myself up out of chairs.	☐	☐	☐	☐	☐
11. I have had difficulty using my arms and hands.	☐	☐	☐	☐	☐
12. I have found turning and moving in bed difficult.	☐	☐	☐	☐	☐
13. I have found picking things up difficult.	☐	☐	☐	☐	☐
14. I have found holding books or newspapers, or turning pages, difficult.	☐	☐	☐	☐	☐
15. I have had difficulty writing clearly.	☐	☐	☐	☐	☐
16. I have found it difficult to do jobs around the house.	☐	☐	☐	☐	☐

*Please make sure that you have ticked **one box for each question** before going on to the next page.*

ALSAQ-40 (*cont.*)

	Never	Rarely	Sometimes	Often	Always or cannot do at all
17. I have found it difficult to feed myself.	☐	☐	☐	☐	☐
18. I have had difficulty combing my hair or cleaning my teeth.	☐	☐	☐	☐	☐
19. I have had difficulty getting dressed.	☐	☐	☐	☐	☐
20. I have had difficulty washing at the hand basin.	☐	☐	☐	☐	☐
21. I have had difficulty swallowing.	☐	☐	☐	☐	☐
22. I have had difficulty eating solid food.	☐	☐	☐	☐	☐
23. I have found it difficult to drink liquids.	☐	☐	☐	☐	☐
24. I have found it difficult to participate in conversations.	☐	☐	☐	☐	☐
25. I have felt that my speech has not been easy to understand.	☐	☐	☐	☐	☐
26. I have slurred or stuttered while speaking.	☐	☐	☐	☐	☐
27. I have had to talk very slowly.	☐	☐	☐	☐	☐
28. I have talked less than I used to do.	☐	☐	☐	☐	☐
29. I have been frustrated by my speech.	☐	☐	☐	☐	☐
30. I have felt self-conscious about my speech.	☐	☐	☐	☐	☐
31. I have felt lonely.	☐	☐	☐	☐	☐
32. I have been bored.	☐	☐	☐	☐	☐
33. I have felt embarrassed in social situations.	☐	☐	☐	☐	☐
34. I have felt hopeless about the future.	☐	☐	☐	☐	☐
35. I have worried that I am a burden to other people.	☐	☐	☐	☐	☐
36. I have wondered why I keep going.	☐	☐	☐	☐	☐
37. I have felt angry because of the disease.	☐	☐	☐	☐	☐
38. I have felt depressed.	☐	☐	☐	☐	☐
39. I have worried about how the disease will affect me in the future.	☐	☐	☐	☐	☐
40. I have felt as if I have no freedom.	☐	☐	☐	☐	☐

*Please make sure that you have ticked **one box for each question**. Thank you for completing this questionnaire.*

5

Measuring quality of life in progressive supranuclear palsy

The PSP-QoL

Anette Schrag, Caroline Selai, Niall Quinn, Jeremy Hobart, Andrew J. Lees, Irene Litvan, Anthony Lang, James Bower, and David Burn

Introduction

Progressive supranuclear palsy (PSP) is a neurodegenerative disorder causing parkinsonism, visual dysfunction, and balance impairment, as well as cognitive impairment and psychiatric complications. These problems, together with the emotional and social consequences of having a progressively disabling disease with shortened life expectancy, have an enormous impact on patients' health-related quality of life (HRQoL) (1, 2, 3). PSP was first delineated as a distinct disorder, separate from Parkinson's disease, in 1962. It is sometimes referred to as Steele–Richardson–Olszewski syndrome after the scientists who originally described the condition (4). It is estimated that the disease has a prevalence of 6 per 100,000, similar to that of motor neuron disease, with the average age of onset being in the seventh decade. Mean survival from the onset of symptoms is approximately 6 years (5, 6, 7, 8, 9, 10).

To date, there has been little validation of any HR-QoL generic instruments in this patient group. In one small-scale study, some limited evidence for the appropriateness of the European Quality of Life Five Dimensions (EQ-5D) in this patient group was found, but less support was found for the

36-Item Short-Form Health Survey (SF-36), which some patients indicated did not cover areas of relevance to them (3). The Parkinson's Disease Questionnaire (PDQ-39) has been assessed for its suitability in this patient group, but it was found to lack some aspects of quality of life that are important to patients with PSP (3). Disease severity is typically assessed using a clinically based rating scale – the PSP Rating Scale (PSPRS) (11, 12). However, the PSPRS does not cover many aspects of a patient's HRQoL and was not designed for patient completion. Given the importance attributed to patient-reported outcome measures, a PSP-specific patient-reported outcome measure (PROM) has recently been developed – the PSP QoL (13, 14, 15, 16). This chapter summarizes the development and validation of this instrument.

Development of the PSP-QoL

The PSP-QoL was developed and tested in three stages (17). First, a pool of items was generated from in-depth patient interviews, expert opinion, and literature review. Second, people with PSP completed these items, formatted as a questionnaire, and

Quality of Life Measurement in Neurodegenerative and Related Conditions, eds., Crispin Jenkinson, Michele Peters, and Mark B. Bromberg. Published by Cambridge University Press. © Cambridge University Press 2011.

standard item reduction methods were used to develop a 45-item instrument measuring the physical and mental health impact of PSP. Third, five psychometric properties of the PSP-QoL (data quality, scaling assumptions, acceptability, reliability, and validity) were evaluated in a further sample of people with PSP.

An item pool was generated from semistructured interviews of 27 people with PSP and their caregivers (3), a review of the literature, and consultation with five experts in PSP. Interviewees were selected from movement disorder clinics to represent the full spectrum of the disorder, and new interviews were conducted until no new themes emerged. The problems most frequently reported by patients and caregivers were related to physical limitations and associated problems (e.g., pain, slowness of movement, difficulty swallowing), psychological difficulties (e.g., anxiety, depression, sexual problems), social impairment (e.g., family difficulties, problems meeting people), activities of daily living (e.g., difficulties going out and pursuing hobbies, needing help with self-care), and cognitions (e.g., memory impairment, poor concentration, loss of motivation). The issues rated as most severe were similar to those reported most commonly, although drooling and having to stop driving were also rated as severe problems among those reporting them. Less important QoL issues, which were infrequently reported by patients with PSP or were rated as of relatively low importance, included tremor, emotional lability, weight loss, hallucinations, irritability, personality change, and financial issues. Issues in the domain of cognitive dysfunction were less commonly or severely rated than those in the domains of physical dysfunction, psychological impact, social impairment, or activities of daily living. The interviews indicate that, although many issues relevant to patients with PD are also relevant to patients with PSP, some issues less frequently experienced by patients with PD are among the most relevant to patients with PSP. These include difficulties related to balance and falls, to visual disturbances, and to dysarthria and dysphagia. Other reported issues not

common in PD were those of muddled thinking, confusion, and apathy, which are not addressed in the PD-specific QoL questionnaires. On the other hand, the consequences of PSP for activities of daily living and social and emotional functioning were similar to those of PD, although they were more severe because of the often acute parkinsonism in PSP. Overall, caregivers and patients reported similar problems and rated them at similar severity. Items generated were given a five-response option format (0 = no problem to 4 = extreme problem) (18). A "not applicable" response option was also included to account for people unable to answer any of the items, but this was not assigned a score. A time frame of 4 weeks was used, as this was considered to be clinically meaningful. The items were formatted as a questionnaire, reviewed by movement disorder experts, and adjusted after pretesting in a small sample of patients with PSP (n = 8) for readability, ambiguity, and clarity.

The preliminary questionnaire, containing 87 items, was distributed by the PSP (Europe) Association to all eligible patient members (n = 302), and 192 (64%) usable responses were gained. The questionnaire included instructions requesting that the questions should be completed according to the patients' answers, even if help was provided by a caregiver. It also included questions on demographic variables, time of onset, the PSP staging system modified for self-completion, and a visual analogue scale (VAS) of how satisfied the patient felt overall with his or her life (10). The questionnaire was also administered to patients who fulfilled NINDS-SPSP (National Institute for Neurological Disorders and Society for PSP) diagnostic criteria for probable or possible PSP and who were attending movement disorders clinics in London (n = 16) and North America (n = 48) (19). Patient characteristics on the analyzed 225 questionnaires were similar across all patient groups (17). Twenty-five percent of questionnaires were completed by the patients themselves and 75% by a caregiver, with no difference in age or gender between these, but those requiring help had a more severe self-reported disease severity (p < 0.001) (10).

The initial analysis involved examining the percent of missing data for each item; those items with values exceeding 10% were removed (20). An exploratory factor analysis (principal components analysis, varimax rotation) was performed on the remaining items to determine the potential measurement dimensions, and item groups derived from factor analysis were refined to generate scales that satisfied standard psychometric criteria (17).

The instrument developed as a result of the analyses above contained 45 items measuring the physical (22-items) and mental (23-items) impact of PSP. Scores for the two subscales were generated by summation of items and transformation to a range of 0 to 100 (100 × [(observed score – min possible score) / (max possible score – min possible score)]). The psychometric properties of this questionnaire were examined in a second field test. The questionnaire was sent to 275 members of the PSP Association approximately 2.5 years after the first field test; 173 completed it (response rate, 63%) and 15 consecutive patients attended movement disorder clinics in North America.

Convergent and discriminant validity were tested using the PSP staging system (10); the 39-item Parkinson's Disease Questionnaire (PDQ-39) (21); the EuroQoL (EQ-5D, a generic HRQoL measure) (22); the Hospital Anxiety and Depression Scale (HADS) (23); and a VAS of how satisfied the person felt with his or her life. A subset of 30 patients was sent a second identical questionnaire 2 weeks later to examine test-retest reliability. The content validity of the final subscales was assessed by the expert panel and was considered to be good. Internal construct validity was supported by the moderate interscale correlation between the physical and mental subscales, implying that the two PSP-QoL subscales measure related but different health constructs. Convergent and discriminant construct validity was supported by finding correlations with other scales and variables that were consistent with *a priori* predictions (17). Group differences validity

was supported by finding that the PSP-QoL physical subscale was better at detecting group differences in mobility, self-care, and usual activities, but the PSP-QoL mental health scale was better at detecting differences in anxiety/depression. Results also indicated high levels of data completion, and scaling assumptions were met. Internal consistency reliability was good with Cronbach's alpha of 0.93 and 0.95 for the two subscales. For both scales, corrected item–total correlations exceeded the recommended criterion of 0.40, and all reliability estimates exceeded 0.90 (23). The standard error of measurement (SEM) for each of the subscores was approximately 5.5, giving 95% CIs for individual patient scores of approximately +/−10 scale points.

Conclusion

Previous evidence has suggested that the generic EQ-5D and the disease-specific PDQ-39 have limited validity in patients with PSP because they do not incorporate many of the aspects of PSP and thus underestimate health problems in PSP (3). On the other hand, assessments of disease severity using clinical rating scales omit patient views about issues of importance to their health, particularly those of cognitive and emotional functioning and the impact of dysfunction on activities of daily living. Hence, the decision was made to create a new instrument to assess patients with PSP, developed on the basis of patient and clinician views together with psychometric analysis of data from a large field test in patients with PSP. The development techniques sought to ensure that the scale was derived from patient report and had a low number of missing values; applicability of the scale to patients at all stages of disease; no undue skewness; homogeneity of items with the scales, allowing for replacement of missing values and robustness of the scale; high reliability and clinical significance; good discriminative power between different patient groups; and low ceiling or floor effects. Results of psychometric testing of the instrument suggest that it satisfies standard criteria as a summed rating scale, is highly reliable, and has good face and construct validity. The validity of the scale has to be tested further in other populations and other clinic and community populations. Further work is needed to evaluate the responsiveness of the PSP-QoL; however, item discrimination was used as a criterion for item selection, and an evaluation of scale discriminant validity was included. This would suggest that the instrument should prove sensitive to subjectively important changes.

REFERENCES

1. Schrag A, Ben Shlomo Y, Quinn NP. Prevalence of progressive supranuclear palsy and multiple system atrophy: a cross-sectional study. *Lancet* 1999; **354**: 1771–1775.

2. Nath U, Ben Shlomo Y, Thomson RG, et al. The prevalence of progressive supranuclear palsy (Steele-Richardson-Olszewski syndrome) in the UK. *Brain* 2001; **124**: 1438–1449.

3. Schrag A, Selai C, Davis J, Lees AJ, Jahanshahi M, Quinn N. Health-related quality of life in patients with progressive supranuclear palsy. *Movement Disord* 2003; **18**: 1464–1469.

4. Richardson JC, Steele J, Olszewski J. Supranuclear ophthalmoplegia, pseudobulbar palsy, nuchal dystonia and dementia. A clinical report on eight cases of 'heterogeneous system degeneration'. *Trans Am Neurol Assoc* 1963; **88**: 25–29.

5. Wakabayashi K, Takahashi H. Pathological heterogeneity in progressive supranuclear palsy and corticobasal degeneration. *Neuropathology* 2004; **24**: 79–86.

6. Papapetropoulos S, Gonzalez J, Mash DC. Natural history of progressive supranuclear palsy: a clinicopathologic study from a population of brain donors. *Eur Neurol* 2005; **54**: 1–9.

7. Litvan I, Mangone CA, McKee A, et al. Natural history of progressive supranuclear palsy (Steele-Richardson-Olszewski syndrome) and clinical predictors of survival: a clinicopathological study. *J Neurol Neurosurg Psychiatry* 1996; **60**: 615–620.

8. Brusa A, Mancardi GL, Bugiani O. Progressive supranuclear palsy 1979: an overview. *Ital J Neurol Sci* 1980; **1**: 205–222.

9. Maher ER, Lees AJ. The clinical features and natural history of the Steele-Richardson-Olszewski syndrome (progressive supranuclear palsy). *Neurology* 1986; **36**: 1005–1008.

10. Williams DR, de Silva R, Paviour DC, et al. Characteristics of two distinct clinical phenotypes in pathologically proven progressive supranuclear palsy: Richardson's syndrome and PSP-parkinsonism. *Brain* 2005; **128**: 1247–1258.

11. Golbe LI, Lepore FE, Johnson WG, Belsh JM, Powell AL, Treiman DM. Inter-rater reliability of the Progressive Supranuclear Palsy Scale. *Neurology* 1999; **52**(suppl 2): A227.

12. Golbe LI, Ohman-Strickland PA. A clinical ratings scale for progressive supranuclear palsy. *Brain* 2007; **130**(Pt 6): 1552–1565.

13. Nunnally JC, Bernstein IH. *Psychometric Theory*. 3rd ed. New York: McGraw-Hill, 1994.

14. Juniper EF, Guyatt GH, Jaeschke R. How to develop and validate a new health-related quality of life instrument. In: Spilker B, ed. *Quality of Life and Pharmacoeconomics in Clinical Trials*. Philadelphia, New York: Lippincott-Raven Publishers, 1996.

15. Marx RG, Bombardier C, Hogg-Johnson S, Wright JG. Clinimetric and psychometric strategies for development of a health measurement scale. *J Clin Epidemiol* 1999; **52**: 105–111.

16. Streiner DL, Norman GR. *Health Measurement Scales: A Practical Guide to Their Development and Use. Fourth Edition*. Oxford: Oxford University Press, 2008.

17. Schrag A, Selai C, Quinn N, Litvan I, Lang A, Poon Y, Bower J, Burn D, Hobart J. Measuring quality of life in PSP. *Neurology* 2006; **67**: 39–44.

18. Nagata C, Ido M, Shimizu H, Misao A, Matsuura H. Choice of response scale for health measurement: comparison of 4, 5, and 7-point scales and visual analog scale. *J Epidemiol* 1996; **6**: 192–197.

19. Litvan I, Agid Y, Calne D, et al. Clinical research criteria for the diagnosis of progressive supranuclear palsy (Steele-Richardson-Olszewski syndrome): report of the NINDS-SPSP international workshop. *Neurology* 1996; **47**: 1–9.

20. World Health Organization. The World Health Organization Quality of Life Assessment (WHOQOL):

development and general psychometric properties. *Soc Sci Med* 1998; **46**: 1569–1585.

21. Peto V, Jenkinson C, Fitzpatrick R. PDQ-39: a review of the development, validation and application of a Parkinson's disease quality of life questionnaire and its associated measures. *J Neurol* 1998; **245**(suppl 1): S10–S14.

22. The EuroQol Group. EuroQol–a new facility for the measurement of health-related quality of life. *Health Policy* 1990; **16**: 199–208.

23. Zigmond AS, Snaith RP. The hospital anxiety and depression scale. *Acta Psychiatr Scand* 1983; **67**: 361–370.

The Health-Related Quality of Life questionnaire for Patients with Progressive Supranuclear Palsy (PSP-QoL)

Having a health problem can affect a person's quality of life in many different ways. To help us understand how your illness affects your life, we would like to know which of the following problems you have experienced, and how problematic each has been. If the problem does not apply to you, please note why. If someone helps you to fill in the questionnaire, please make sure the answers reflect <u>your own</u> answers. Should you and your helper disagree on the most correct answer, this could be noted at the end.

<u>Please note that this list includes many problems that you may never experience.</u>
There are no right or wrong answers, and we would like you to …
- Think about how you have been feeling during the past 4 weeks
- Put a cross in the box corresponding to the answer that best fits your feelings

In the last 4 weeks, have you…	No problem	Slight problem	Moderate problem	Marked problem	Extreme problem	Not appl.
1. Had difficulty moving?	☐	☐	☐	☐	☐	☐
2. Had difficulty walking?	☐	☐	☐	☐	☐	☐
3. Had difficulty climbing stairs?	☐	☐	☐	☐	☐	☐
4. Had difficulty turning in bed?	☐	☐	☐	☐	☐	☐
5. Had falls?	☐	☐	☐	☐	☐	☐
6. Had problems moving your eyes?	☐	☐	☐	☐	☐	☐
7. Had problems opening your eyes?	☐	☐	☐	☐	☐	☐
8. Had difficulty eating?	☐	☐	☐	☐	☐	☐
9. Had difficulty swallowing?	☐	☐	☐	☐	☐	☐
10. Had drooling of saliva?	☐	☐	☐	☐	☐	☐
11. Had problems communicating?	☐	☐	☐	☐	☐	☐
12. Had difficulty with your writing?	☐	☐	☐	☐	☐	☐
13. Had difficulty grooming, washing, or dressing yourself?	☐	☐	☐	☐	☐	☐
14. Had difficulty using the toilet on your own?	☐	☐	☐	☐	☐	☐

The Health-Related Quality (*cont.*)

In the last 4 weeks, have you...	No problem	Slight problem	Moderate problem	Marked problem	Extreme problem	Not appl.
15. Had difficulty holding urine?	☐	☐	☐	☐	☐	☐
16. Had difficulty reading?	☐	☐	☐	☐	☐	☐
17. Had difficulty doing your hobbies (e.g., playing chess or an instrument)?	☐	☐	☐	☐	☐	☐
18. Had problems doing things around the house (e.g., housework, DIY)?	☐	☐	☐	☐	☐	☐
19. Had difficulty enjoying sports, including gardening or walking?	☐	☐	☐	☐	☐	☐
20. Had difficulty going out to see a play or film?	☐	☐	☐	☐	☐	☐
21. Had difficulty going out for a meal?	☐	☐	☐	☐	☐	☐
22. Had difficulty using public transport?	☐	☐	☐	☐	☐	☐
23. Felt not in control of your life?	☐	☐	☐	☐	☐	☐
24. Felt frustrated?	☐	☐	☐	☐	☐	☐
25. Felt a bit down, sad, or depressed?	☐	☐	☐	☐	☐	☐
26. Felt pessimistic about the future?	☐	☐	☐	☐	☐	☐
27. Felt anxious?	☐	☐	☐	☐	☐	☐
28. Felt isolated?	☐	☐	☐	☐	☐	☐
29. Had difficulty sleeping not due to problems moving?	☐	☐	☐	☐	☐	☐
30. Found yourself crying?	☐	☐	☐	☐	☐	☐
31. Become more withdrawn?	☐	☐	☐	☐	☐	☐
32. Felt stuck at home?	☐	☐	☐	☐	☐	☐
33. Felt embarrassed in public?	☐	☐	☐	☐	☐	☐
34. Felt you cannot show your feelings?	☐	☐	☐	☐	☐	☐
35. Found your personality is different compared to before your illness?	☐	☐	☐	☐	☐	☐

The Health-Related Quality (*cont.*)

In the last 4 weeks, have you…	No problem	Slight problem	Moderate problem	Marked problem	Extreme problem	Not appl.
36. Felt the relationship with your spouse/partner has changed?	☐	☐	☐	☐	☐	☐
37. Felt your relationship with other family members has changed?	☐	☐	☐	☐	☐	☐
38. Seen family less than before you had this condition?	☐	☐	☐	☐	☐	☐
39. Had problems with your memory?	☐	☐	☐	☐	☐	☐
40. Found yourself repeating things a lot?	☐	☐	☐	☐	☐	☐
41. Found your thinking is slower than before the illness?	☐	☐	☐	☐	☐	☐
42. Found your thinking is muddled?	☐	☐	☐	☐	☐	☐
43. Felt confused?	☐	☐	☐	☐	☐	☐
44. Felt not motivated to do things?	☐	☐	☐	☐	☐	☐
45. Found it difficult to make decisions?	☐	☐	☐	☐	☐	☐

Please check that you have ticked one box for each question.

Experiencing any illness has an effect on one's life. Please indicate how satisfied you feel overall with your life at the moment by putting a cross on the line between 0 and 100.

0   100

|++++++++|++++++++|++++++++|++++++++|++++++++|++++++++|++++++++|++++++++|++++++++|++++++++|

Extremely dissatisfied   Extremely satisfied
with my life   with my life

Did you complete this questionnaire on your own?   ☐
If you filled in this questionnaire for someone else
• Did you fill in the patient's answers?   ☐
• Or did you answer on behalf of the patient according to what you thought was correct?   ☐
Do you have any other comments?

Thank you for completing the questionnaire!

6

Measuring quality of life in multiple system atrophy

Anette Schrag, Caroline Selai, Christopher Mathias, Philip Low, Jeremy Hobart, and Niall Quinn

Introduction

Multiple system atrophy (MSA) is a rare, progressive, neurodegenerative disease and a form of atypical parkinsonism. It has a prevalence of about 2 to 5 per 100,000 (1, 2, 3) and has a considerable impact on patient outcomes, including reduced life expectancy, increased disability, and lower health-related quality of life (HRQoL) (4, 5). Average age of onset is about 54 years, and mean survival from the onset of symptoms is around 5 to 9 years (6, 7, 8). MSA often presents with features similar to those of Parkinson's disease (PD) in its early stages and consequently may be difficult to diagnose correctly. As a result, many patients may not receive appropriate treatment for their condition. However, despite the intial similarities, MSA has a wider range of symptoms and a differing and more aggressive disease progression and is poorly responsive to treatments commonly associated with PD, such as levopoda. Some evidence suggests that rates of depression are high in patients diagnosed with MSA. Currently, no treatment consistently benefits patients, resulting in increasing dependency on the patient's family and other caregivers, which in turn can have consequences for their HRQoL. MSA has two different subtypes (9). MSA-P is so called because of the predominance of parkinsonism symptoms (9), whereas MSA-C is identified by a predominance of cerebellar dysfunction.

At present, few direct studies have evaluated HRQoL for patients with a diagnosis of MSA. Although Parkinson's disease has been the focus for a number of studies in the 1990s/2000s, very little research has been undertaken to study other forms of parkinsonism such as MSA. This is unfortunate because, although superficial similarities between the conditions have been noted, the more aggressive nature of MSA requires its own body of evidence to better study patients' outcomes, HRQoL, and health needs.

Few data are available on quality of life or patient-reported outcomes for MSA patients. This is not surprising because of the scarcity of the disease, the similarities to Parkinson's, and the more recent nosologic classification of MSA. The lack of an MSA-specific patient-reported outcome measure (PROM) until 2007 has had an obvious impact on the amount of evidence about health status in MSA. The purposes of this chapter are to focus on the development of PROMs in MSA research, and to provide an overview of the psychometric properties of the PROMs that have been used to assess patient outcomes in MSA. PROMs that have been used in MSA include the 39-item Parkinson's Disease Questionnaire (PDQ-39) and the MSA Quality

Quality of Life Measurement in Neurodegenerative and Related Conditions, eds., Crispin Jenkinson, Michele Peters, and Mark B. Bromberg. Published by Cambridge University Press. © Cambridge University Press 2011.

of Life questionnaire (MSA-QoL). The development of the Unified Multiple System Atrophy Rating Scale (UMSARS) will also be outlined, although it is a clinical scale rather than a PROM. The MSA-QoL is the only disease-specific PROM for MSA, and an in-depth description of its development will be given.

The Unified Multiple System Atrophy Rating Scale (UMSARS)

A clinical scale for the objective assessment of MSA has been developed for use in clinical assessment and research: the Unified Multiple System Atrophy Rating Scale (UMSARS) (10). The UMSARS was based on established clinical scales as templates, such as the Hoehn and Yahr Scale (11), the Schwab and England Scale, the Unified Parkinson's Disease Rating Scale (12), the International Ataxia Rating Scale (13), and the Composite Autonomic Symptom Scale (COMPASS) (14). The final UMSARS comprises four parts. The first part consists of a historical review and covers a patient's disease-related impairments; part two covers aspects of motor function in all areas of the body affected by MSA. For sections one and two, each question is scored from zero (no impairment) to 4 (severe impairment). The subscores of parts one and two are sometimes reported as separate findings (i. e., UMSARS-I and UMSARS-II). The third part covers an autonomic examination, and the fourth part is a global disability scale that yields a score of 1 to 5, depending on the extent of the disease.

The European MSA Study Group (4) used the UMSARS alongside generic QoL questionnaires such as the Short-Form 36 (SF-36) (15, 16) and the European Quality of Life Five Dimensions (EQ-5D) (17), and clinical measurements such as the Hoehn and Yahr Parkinson's Disease Staging Scale (11), COMPASS (14), and the Beck Depression Inventory (BDI) (18). UMSARS and COMPASS results proved a good predictor for the SF-36's PCS summary score (Physical Summary Score made up of the questions that covered any physical action), and the UMSARS and BDI were good predictors of the SF-36's MCS

summary score (Mental Summary Score derived from any questions regarding mental activities or emotional responses) (4). This suggests that the UMSARS has good construct validity with the SF-36 and provides some evidence for recommending the use of the SF-36 for MSA patients. The UMSARS has been validated for use by clinicians inasmuch as it reflects disease progression; however, because of the nature of its questions, it cannot be completed by the patient. This makes it unsuitable as a self-complete outcome measure.

PDQ-39

The Parkinson's Disease Questionnaire 39-item (PDQ-39) (19) was developed to measure HRQoL of patients with PD. The 39 items make up eight scales: mobility, activities of daily living, emotions, stigma, social support, cognitions, communication, and bodily discomfort. It was developed by researchers and clinicians on the basis of interviews with patients and has been thoroughly validated for use with PD patients. Because of similarities between MSA and PD, one study has examined the appropriateness of the PDQ-39 for MSA patients (20). Two hundred seventy-nine MSA patients completed the PDQ-39 (19), the EQ-5D (17), the Hospital Anxiety and Depression Scale (HADS) (21), and scales of life satisfaction and disease severity. The study found high internal consistency for all dimensions apart from the social support dimension (20). Factor analysis supported the 8-factor solution of the PDQ-39, and all items loaded on the same factors as previously found in PD patients. The findings of the study did not support a single PDQ-39 index in this patient group. Convergent and divergent validity with the EQ-5D and the HADS was good. However, a floor effect was found for the social support dimension and a ceiling effect for the mobility dimension. The mobility dimension was also skewed.

The mixed psychometric findings show that the PDQ-39 has limited validity in MSA patients. One reason may be that MSA is associated with a number of issues, such as severe autonomic dysfunction, that are not a problem in PD and hence are not reflected in the PDQ-39. The authors conclude that findings highlight the importance of developing a disease-specific measure for MSA (20).

The Multiple System Atrophy Quality of Life Questionnaire (MSA-QOL)

The Multiple System Atrophy Quality of Life Questionnaire (MSA-QoL) was developed because no disease-specific measure existed for MSA (22). This section will describe the development of an MSA-specific PROM based on clinician and patient involvement using standard scale development techniques (23, 24, 25, 26).

The MSA-QoL was developed and tested in three stages. First, 105 items were generated from patient interviews, the literature, and consultations with neurologists specializing in MSA. In a second stage, these items, formatted as a questionnaire, were sent to 444 MSA patients, and standard item reduction methods were used to develop a clinically meaningful and psychometrically sound 40-item instrument. Finally, the psychometric properties of the MSA-QoL were evaluated in another sample of 286 people with MSA.

Stage One: Item generation

An item pool (n = 105) was generated from semi-structured interviews of 20 people with MSA, a review of the existing literature, and consultation with five neurologists specializing in MSA. Patients were selected from neurology clinics to represent the full spectrum of the disorder, and new interviews were conducted until data saturation was reached. The median age of participants was 62 years (range 45 to 71), and 50% were female. Ten had the parkinsonian subtype of MSA (MSA-P), and 10 the cerebellar subtype (MSA-C). Items generated by this process were given a standard five-response option format (0 = no problem to 4 = extreme problem) (31). A "not applicable" response option, which

was not scored, was also included for people unable to answer an individual item. A time frame of 4 weeks was used because this was considered to be clinically relevant. Items were formatted as a questionnaire, reviewed by neurologists, and piloted in six MSA patients.

Stage Two: Scale development and item reduction

The preliminary questionnaire of 105 items was sent to all eligible patient members (n = 444) of the Sarah Matheson Trust for MSA (SMT) in the United Kingdom, and to 62 patients who fulfilled consensus criteria for probable or possible MSA (28) and who were attending clinics at the Mayo Clinic, Rochester. The questionnaire included instructions requesting that responses should reflect the patients' answers, even if the questionnaire was completed by a caregiver. Data were also collected on demographic features, time of onset, severity of MSA, and a visual analogue scale (VAS) of how satisfied the patient felt overall with his or her life.

The preliminary questionnaire was returned by 317 members of the SMT in the United Kingdom (71.4%) and 62 consecutive patients attending the neurology clinic at the Mayo clinic. In the U.K. sample, 69 questionnaires were excluded from the analysis for a variety of reasons. All questionnaires from the Mayo Clinic were eligible for inclusion, leading to a total of 310 questionnaires in the analysis. Patients had a mean age of 66.2 years, mean disease duration of 5.8 years, mean disease severity of 2.7 (range, 0 to 4), and a mean overall life satisfaction of 36.5 (range, 0 to 100). Forty-six percent of patients completed the questionnaires themselves, and 54% were completed by a caregiver. Those who completed the questionnaire themselves did not differ in age or gender from those whose caregiver had completed it, but they had a significantly more severe self-reported disease severity (p < 0.001) on the self-rated MSA staging system.

Standard item reduction methods were used to develop a clinically meaningful and psychometrically sound instrument. First, the percentage of missing data for each item was examined, and those with values exceeding 10% were removed (29). This led to exclusion of 17 items. An exploratory factor analysis (principal components analysis, varimax rotation) was performed on the remaining items, and a range of potential factor solutions were examined and compared to determine which were the most clinically sensible and statistically clear (4).

The factor analysis had not produced a pure solution; therefore, two-, three-, four-, and five-factor solutions were examined. The three-factor solution was the most statistically clear and clinically sensible. Factor one, defined as the "motor scale," included items on mobility, coordination, self-care, and activities of daily living. Factor two, labeled "nonmotor scale," covered autonomic dysfunction, energy/sleep, pain, vision, and cognition. Factor three, the "emotional social scale," included items on social and emotional aspects. All items could be referenced back to statements made by patients or caregivers.

Because of the large number of items, the potential to reduce the number of items further was assessed to produce a user-friendly PROM. Item groups derived from factor analysis were refined to generate scales that satisfied psychometric criteria.

This process of item reduction led to a final instrument with 40 items measuring the motor (14 items), nonmotor (12 items), and emotional/social impact of MSA (14 items). Scores for the three subscales were generated by summing items and, for ease of interpretation, transforming to a range of 0 to 100 ($100 \times$ [(observed score – min possible score) / (max possible score – min possible score)]).

Stage 3: Scale evaluation and validation

A second field test was conducted to test the psychometric properties of the final questionnaire. This consisted of sending the questionnaire to 505 members of the SMT approximately 2.5 years after the first field test. Convergent and discriminant validity was assessed using the self-rated MSA severity on a 5-point scale, the PDQ-39 (19), the EQ-5D (17), the HADS (31), and a VAS of how satisfied the person felt

with his or her life (17, 19, 31). To examine test-retest reliability, 100 patients were sent a second identical questionnaire 2 weeks later.

The final questionnaire was returned by 346 patients (68.5% response rate). Sixty replies were excluded for a variety of reasons. The response rate in the test-retest sample was 80%. Item level missing data were low (range, 0.3% to 2.8 %), and subscale scores could be calculated for 99% of the sample.

Corrected item-total correlations exceeded the recommended 0.30 (30, 33), and all reliability estimates exceeded 0.80 for the three scales (23). Test-retest reliability was good, with correlations around 0.9 for all subscales. The SEM of both subscores was approximately 6, yielding 95% confidence intervals for individual patient scores of approximately $+/-12$ scale points.

Different types of validity, including content validity, internal validity, and convergent and discriminant validity, were assessed. Content validity of the final subscales, as assessed by the expert panel, was considered to be good. Construct validity was supported by the moderate interscale correlation between subscales, implying that the two MSA-QoL subscales measure related but different health constructs. Convergent and discriminant construct validity was supported by finding correlations with other scales and variables as well as group differences that were consistent with *a priori* predictions such as positive correlations of the motor subscale with motor severity, mobility, ADL, and communications subscales of the PDQ-39 and EQ-5D (4).

Conclusion

A new PROM was developed on the basis of patient and clinician views and psychometric testing to assess disease-specific quality of life in MSA. Items were selected to be psychometrically sound but also to reflect patient's and clinician's views of MSA. Because one of the main aims for a PROM is to capture change, items were selected with good discriminative power between patient groups with differing severity of disease and health impairment and for low ceiling or floor effects to ensure sensitivity at both ends of the spectrum of disease.

Results of psychometric testing of the instrument indicated that the MSA-QoL satisfies standard criteria as a summed rating scale, is highly reliable, and has good face and construct validity. These data suggest that this scale could be a PROM in clinical trials.

The development of the questionnaire has some limitations. Although care was taken to include patients at all stages of MSA in development of the questionnaire, it is likely that patients in more advanced stages who could not respond accurately on their own were underrepresented in the postal surveys. A second limitation is that, as of yet, the responsiveness of the MSA-QoL has not been properly tested. A third limitation is that both postal surveys were conducted primarily in members of a patient organization, and it is not known how many of these patients had a diagnosis of probable or possible MSA.

The MSA-QoL is the first disease-specific PROM for MSA, and despite its limitations, it has been developed with patient and clinician input and rigorous psychometric testing.

Summary

To date, little research has been done to assess quality of life in MSA. This may partly be a result of the low prevalence of the condition and the lack of a disease-specific PROM until recently. Although generic instruments, such as the SF-36, have been used in patients with MSA and offer the advantage that they allow comparison between disease groups, these instruments have limited feasibility and acceptability for patients with neurodegenerative disorders (4, 5, 32, 34, 35, 36, 37, 38, 39 40). Generic instruments and instruments developed for the related but different disorder of Parkinson's disease do not address, and are unlikely to be sensitive to, specific features important to patients with MSA. One MSA-specific measure, the UMSARS, assesses disease severity using clinical rating scales, but this clinical rating scale cannot be completed by individuals with MSA and omits issues of importance to MSA patients that relate to their health and emotional and social functioning and the impact of dysfunction on activities of daily living. Thus, a patient-completed, disease-specific HRQoL scale, such as the MSA-QoL, that was developed with patient and caregiver input will provide an important complement to objective clinical rating scales and to generic PROMs.

REFERENCES

1. Schrag A, Ben-Shlomo Y, Quinn NP. Prevalence of progressive supranuclear palsy and multiple system atrophy: a cross-sectional study. *Lancet* 1999 Nov 20; **354**(9192): 1771–1775.

2. Chrysostome V, Tison F, Yekhlef F, Sourgen C, Baldi I, Dartigues JF. Epidemiology of multiple system atrophy: a prevalence and pilot risk factor study in Aquitaine, France. *Neuroepidemiology* 2004 Jul; **23**(4): 201–208.

3. Vanacore N, Bonifati V, Fabbrini G, Colosimo C, De MG, Marconi R, et al. Epidemiology of multiple system atrophy. ESGAP Consortium. European Study Group on Atypical Parkinsonisms. *Neurol Sci* 2001 Feb; **22**(1): 97–99.

4. Schrag A, Geser F, Stampfer-Kountchev M, Seppi K, Sawires M, Kollensperger M, et al. Health-related quality of life in multiple system atrophy. *Mov Disord* 2006 Jun; **21**(6): 809–815.

5. Benrud-Larson LM, Sandroni P, Schrag A, Low PA. Depressive symptoms and life satisfaction in patients with multiple system atrophy. *Mov Disord* 2005 Aug; **20**(8): 951–957.

6. Wenning GK, Tison F, Ben SY, Daniel SE, Quinn NP. Multiple system atrophy: a review of 203 pathologically proven cases. *Mov Disord* 1997 Mar; **12**(2): 133–147.

7. Jellinger KA, Seppi K, Wenning GK. Grading of neuropathology in multiple system atrophy: proposal for a novel scale. *Mov Disord* 2005 Aug; **20**(suppl 12):S29–S36.

8. Ben-Shlomo Y, Wenning GK, Tison F, Quinn NP. Survival of patients with pathologically proven multiple system atrophy: a meta-analysis. *Neurology* 1997 Feb; **48**(2): 384–393.

9. Kawai Y, Suenaga M, Takeda A, Ito M, Watanabe H, Tanaka F, et al. Cognitive impairments in multiple system atrophy: MSA-C vs MSA-P. *Neurology* 2008 Apr 15; **70**(16 Pt 2): 1390–1396.

10. Wenning GK, Tison F, Seppi K, Sampaio C, Diem A, Yekhlef F, et al. Development and validation of the Unified Multiple System Atrophy Rating Scale (UMSARS). *Mov Disord* 2004 Dec; **19**(12): 1391–1402.

11. Hoehn MM, Yahr MD. Parkinsonism: onset, progression and mortality. *Neurology* 1967 May; **17**(5): 427–442.

12. Schwab RS, England AC. Projection technique for evaluating surgery in Parkinson's disease. In: Gillingham FJ, Donaldson IML, eds. *Third Symposium on Parkinson's Disease*. Edinburgh: Livingstone, 1969; pp. 152–157.

13. Trouillas P, Takayanagi T, Hallett M, Currier RD, Subramony SH, Wessel K, et al. International Cooperative Ataxia Rating Scale for pharmacological assessment of the cerebellar syndrome. The Ataxia Neuropharmacology Committee of the World Federation of Neurology. *J Neurol Sci* 1997 Feb 12; **145**(2): 205–211.

14. Suarez GA, Opfer-Gehrking TL, Offord KP, Atkinson EJ, O'Brien PC, Low PA. The Autonomic Symptom Profile: a new instrument to assess autonomic symptoms. *Neurology* 1999 Feb; **52**(3): 523–528.

15. Ware JE, Jr., Sherbourne CD. The MOS 36-item short-form health survey (SF-36). I. Conceptual framework and item selection. *Med Care* 1992 Jun; **30**(6): 473–483.

16. McHorney CA, Ware JE, Jr., Raczek AE. The MOS 36-Item Short-Form Health Survey (SF-36): II. Psychometric and clinical tests of validity in measuring physical and mental health constructs. *Med Care* 1993 Mar; **31**(3): 247–263.

17. The Euro-Qol Group. EuroQol–a new facility for the measurement of health-related quality of life. The EuroQol Group. *Health Policy* 1990 Dec; **16**(3): 199–208.

18. Beck AT, Ward CH, Mendelson M, Mock J, Erbaugh J. An inventory for measuring depression. *Arch Gen Psychiatry* 1961 Jun; **4**: 561–571.

19. Peto V, Jenkinson C, Fitzpatrick R. PDQ-39: a review of the development, validation and application of a Parkinson's disease quality of life questionnaire and its associated measures. *J Neurol* 1998 May; **245**(suppl 1): S10–S14.

20. Schrag A, Jenkinson C, Selai C, Mathias C, Quinn N. Testing the validity of the PDQ-39 in patients with MSA. *Parkinsonism Relat Disord* 2007 Apr; **13**(3): 152–156.

21. Marinus J, Leentjens AF, Visser M, Stiggelbout AM, van Hilten JJ. Evaluation of the hospital anxiety and depression scale in patients with Parkinson's disease. *Clin Neuropharmacol* 2002 Nov; **25**(6): 318–324.

22. Schrag A, Selai C, Mathias C, Low P, Hobart J, Brady N, et al. Measuring health-related quality of life in MSA: the MSA-QoL. *Mov Disord* 2007 Dec; **22**(16): 2332–2338.

23. Nunnally JC, Bernstein IH. *Psychometric Theory*. 3rd ed. New York: McGraw-Hill, 1994.

24. Juniper EF, Guyatt GH, Jaeschke R. How to develop and validate a new health-related quality of life instrument. In: Spilker B, ed. *Quality of Life and Pharmaeconomics in Clinical Trials*. Philadelphia, New York: Lippincott-Raven, 1996.

25. Marx RG, Bombardier C, Hogg-Johnson S, Wright JG. Clinimetric and psychometric strategies for development of a health measurement scale. *J Clin Epidemiol* 1999 Feb; **52**(2): 105–111.

26. Streiner DL, Norman GR. *Health measurement scales: a practical guide to their development and use*. 2nd ed. Oxford: Oxford University Press, 1995.

27. Nagata C, Ido M, Shimizu H, Misao A, Matsuura H. Choice of response scale for health measurement: comparison of 4, 5, and 7-point scales and visual analog scale. *J Epidemiol* 1996 Dec; **6**(4): 192–197.

28. Gilman S, Low PA, Quinn N, Albanese A, Ben-Shlomo Y, Fowler CJ, et al. Consensus statement on the diagnosis of multiple system atrophy. *J Neurol Sci* 1999 Feb 1; **163**(1): 94–98.

29. World Health Organization. The World Health Organization Quality of Life Assessment (WHOQOL): development and general psychometric properties. *Soc Sci Med* 1998 Jun; **46**(12): 1569–1585.

30. Ware JE, Harris WJ, Gandek B, Rogers BW, Reese PR. *MAP-R for Windows: multitrait/multi-item analysis program, revised user's guide*. Boston: Health Assessment Laboratory, 1997.

31. Zigmond AS, Snaith RP. The hospital anxiety and depression scale. *Acta Psychiatr Scand* 1983 Jun; **67**(6): 361–370.

32. Hobart J, Freeman J, Lamping D, Fitzpatrick R, Thompson A. The SF-36 in multiple sclerosis: why basic assumptions must be tested. *J Neurol Neurosurg Psychiatry* 2001 Sep; **71**(3): 363–370.

33. Likert RA. A technique for the development of attitudes. *Arch Psych* 1932; **140**: 5–55.

34. Geser F, Wenning GK, Seppi K, Stampfer-Kountchev M, Scherfler C, Sawires M, et al. Progression of multiple system atrophy (MSA): a prospective natural history study by the European MSA Study Group (EMSA SG). *Mov Disord* 2006 Feb; **21**(2): 179–186.

35. Brazier JE, Walters SJ, Nicholl JP, Kohler B. Using the SF-36 and Euroqol on an elderly population. *Qual Life Res* 1996 Apr; **5**(2): 195–204.

36. Brazier JE, Harper R, Jones NM, O'Cathain A, Thomas KJ, Usherwood T, et al. Validating the SF-36 health survey questionnaire: new outcome measure for primary care. *BMJ* 1992 Jul 18; **305**(6846): 160–164.

37. Schrag A, Selai C, Jahanshahi M, Quinn NP. The EQ-5D– a generic quality of life measure – is a useful instrument to measure quality of life in patients with Parkinson's disease. *J Neurol Neurosurg Psychiatry* 2000 Jul; **69**(1): 67–73.

38. Freeman JA, Hobart JC, Langdon DW, Thompson AJ. Clinical appropriateness: a key factor in outcome measure selection: the 36 item short form health survey in multiple sclerosis. *J Neurol Neurosurg Psychiatry* 2000 Feb; **68**(2): 150–156.

39. Hobart JC, Williams LS, Moran K, Thompson AJ. Quality of life measurement after stroke: uses and abuses of the SF-36. *Stroke* 2002 May; **33**(5): 1348–1356.

40. Neudert C, Wasner M, Borasio GD. Patients' assessment of quality of life instruments: a randomised study of SIP, SF-36 and SEIQoL-DW in patients with amyotrophic lateral sclerosis. *J Neurol Sci* 2001 Oct 15; **191**(1–2): 103–109.

Dear Patient:

We really appreciate your taking the time to complete this questionnaire about your well-being and health-related quality of life. We hope that as a result of your answers, we will be able to help improve the quality of life of people with similar problems. We realize that this questionnaire is rather lengthy. If you find it too difficult to complete, please do not feel obliged to do so. However, any answers you can give will be helpful. If someone helps you to fill in the questionnaire, please make sure responses reflect <u>your own</u> answers.

There are no right or wrong answers, and we would like you to ...

* Think about how you have been feeling during the past four weeks
* Put a cross in the box corresponding to the answer that best fits your feelings

Date filled out _ / _ / _ (day/month/year)

MSA Quality of Life Questionnaire

Having a health problem can affect a person's quality of life in many different ways. To understand how your illness affects your life, we are interested in knowing which, if any, of the following problems you have experienced. We would also like to know how problematic each has been for you.

<u>Please note that this list includes many problems that you may never experience.</u>

In the last 4 weeks, have you ...	No Problem	Slight Problem	Moderate Problem	Marked Problem	Extreme Problem	Not appl.
1. Had difficulty moving?	☐	☐	☐	☐	☐	☐
2. Had difficulty walking?	☐	☐	☐	☐	☐	☐
3. Had problems with your balance?	☐	☐	☐	☐	☐	☐
4. Had difficulty standing up without support?	☐	☐	☐	☐	☐	☐
5. Had difficulty speaking?	☐	☐	☐	☐	☐	☐
6. Had difficulty swallowing food?	☐	☐	☐	☐	☐	☐
7. Had too much saliva or drooling?	☐	☐	☐	☐	☐	☐
8. Had difficulty with handwriting?	☐	☐	☐	☐	☐	☐
9. Had difficulty feeding yourself?	☐	☐	☐	☐	☐	☐
10. Had difficulty drinking fluids?	☐	☐	☐	☐	☐	☐

MSA Quality of Life Questionnaire (*cont.*)

In the last 4 weeks, have you…	No problem	Slight problem	Moderate problem	Marked problem	Extreme problem	Not appl.
11. Had difficulty dressing yourself?	☐	☐	☐	☐	☐	☐
12. Needed help to go to the toilet?	☐	☐	☐	☐	☐	☐
13. Had to stop doing things that you liked to do (e.g., your hobbies)?	☐	☐	☐	☐	☐	☐
14. Had difficulty doing things around the house (e.g., housework)?	☐	☐	☐	☐	☐	☐
15. Experienced bladder problems?	☐	☐	☐	☐	☐	☐
16. Experienced problems with constipation?	☐	☐	☐	☐	☐	☐
17. Experienced dizziness when standing up?	☐	☐	☐	☐	☐	☐
18. Suffered from cold hands or feet?	☐	☐	☐	☐	☐	☐
19. Experienced pain in your neck or shoulders?	☐	☐	☐	☐	☐	☐
20. Experienced pain elsewhere (e.g., in your legs or your back)?	☐	☐	☐	☐	☐	☐
21. Had difficulty getting comfortable during the night?	☐	☐	☐	☐	☐	☐
22. Had difficulty breathing during the night?	☐	☐	☐	☐	☐	☐
23. Been feeling tired very quickly (without exerting yourself)?	☐	☐	☐	☐	☐	☐
24. Experienced lack of energy?	☐	☐	☐	☐	☐	☐
25. Experienced slowness of thinking?	☐	☐	☐	☐	☐	☐
26. Had difficulty with your concentration (e.g., reading, watching TV)?	☐	☐	☐	☐	☐	☐
27. Felt frustrated?	☐	☐	☐	☐	☐	☐
28. Felt depressed?	☐	☐	☐	☐	☐	☐

MSA Quality of Life Questionnaire (*cont.*)

In the last 4 weeks, have you ...	No problem	Slight problem	Moderate problem	Marked problem	Extreme problem	Not appl.
29. Experienced a loss of motivation?	☐	☐	☐	☐	☐	☐
30. Been feeling incapable?	☐	☐	☐	☐	☐	☐
31. Worried about the future?	☐	☐	☐	☐	☐	☐
32. Worried about your family?	☐	☐	☐	☐	☐	☐
33. Felt on your own or isolated?	☐	☐	☐	☐	☐	☐
34. Experienced loss of confidence when interacting with others?	☐	☐	☐	☐	☐	☐
35. Felt that your role in your family or among friends has changed?	☐	☐	☐	☐	☐	☐
36. Experienced difficulty seeing your friends?	☐	☐	☐	☐	☐	☐
37. Had to give up social activities (e.g., going out for a meal, participating in events)?	☐	☐	☐	☐	☐	☐
38. Had difficulty talking to friends about your illness?	☐	☐	☐	☐	☐	☐
39. Been embarrassed to talk to people?	☐	☐	☐	☐	☐	☐
40. Felt that life has become boring?	☐	☐	☐	☐	☐	☐

Experiencing any illness has an effect on one's life. Please indicate how satisfied you feel overall with your life at the moment by putting a cross on the line between 0 and 100.

0   20   40   60   80   100

|++++++++|++++++++|++++++++|++++++++|++++++++|++++++++|++++++++|++++++++|++++++++|++++++++|

10   30   50   70   90

Extremely dissatisfied
with my life

Extremely satisfied
with my life

Do you have any other comments?

_____

_____

A few last questions:

This questionnaire was completed by

☐ The person with Multiple System Atrophy (MSA)

☐ Somebody else according to the patient's answers

☐ Somebody else according to what you thought was correct

	Yes	No
Would you be happy for us to contact you again?	☐	☐

If you are happy to be contacted again, please give your address here:

_____

THANK YOU VERY MUCH FOR YOUR HELP!

7

Health-related quality of life in Huntington's disease

Noelle E. Carlozzi and Rebecca E. Ready

Introduction

Huntington's disease (HD) is an autosomal dominant neurodegenerative disease, affecting approximately 1 in 10,000 individuals in North America (1). HD is caused by the expansion of a normal CAG repeat within a gene on the short arm of chromosome 4 that codes for the protein huntingtin (2, 3). Every child of a parent who carries the HD gene has a 50:50 chance of inheriting the abnormal gene; therefore, an additional 150,000 individuals are considered "at risk" for inheriting the illness. An individual who inherits the HD gene will gradually develop a host of motor, cognitive, and psychiatric disturbances characteristic of the disease (2). Eventually, individuals with the HD CAG expansion are given a clinical diagnosis of HD (typically in their mid 40's) based on findings in the neurological examination of unequivocal motor signs of chorea, bradykinesia, or both. HD is fatal; the average life span is 15 to 20 years following symptom onset (2). This insidious, progressive, neurodegenerative, and fatal disease is devastating at any age. However, it is particularly devastating given that HD affects the majority of people during the prime of their lives, thus emphasizing the need to find interventions that slow the progression of symptoms, prolong healthy living, maximize health-related quality of life (HRQoL), and ultimately provide a cure for this deadly disease.

HD is a basal ganglion disorder involving the striatum (primarily the caudate nucleus) and is characterized by a triad of symptoms: motor disturbance, cognitive dysfunction, and psychiatric symptoms (4). Symptom onset is gradual, and the clinical presentation for each individual is unique; some individuals exhibit only one set of "characteristic symptoms," but others present a myriad of clinical symptoms across the triad (5). Motor symptoms may begin before clinical onset (6), often with involuntary movements, changes in saccadic eye movements, motor impersistence, balance problems, and akisthesia (7); individuals with prodromal HD often appear to be unable to sit still and fidget in their seats. As motor symptoms worsen, symptoms often become more pronounced; chorea becomes evident (involuntary "dance-like" movements), and dystonia is common. Cognitive symptoms also begin gradually and worsen over time, including difficulties with attention, psychomotor slowing, memory retrieval difficulties, difficulty multi-tasking, trouble shifting from one task to another, difficulties in planning and organizing, problems with procedural learning, decreased verbal fluency, and poor judgment; later-stage HD is often characterized by dementia (5, 8). In addition to cognitive symptoms, psychiatric symptoms or behavioral deficits also begin gradually and worsen over time. Psychiatric symptoms include irritability, depression, anxiety, obsessions/compulsions, psychosis

Quality of Life Measurement in Neurodegenerative and Related Conditions, eds., Crispin Jenkinson, Michele Peters, and Mark B. Bromberg. Published by Cambridge University Press. © Cambridge University Press 2011.

(delusions, hallucinations, paranoia), and anasagnosia. Although many of the motor, cognitive, and psychiatric symptoms characteristic of HD overlap with other neurodegenerative disorders, their presentations are unique in HD and provide a distinct clinical picture. More specifically, although individuals with Parkinson's disease exhibit motor symptoms, their symptoms are characterized by a tremor, rigidity, and bradykinesia (9), whereas motor symptoms in HD most typically are characterized by choreiform movements. Further, although individuals with Alzheimer's disease also have memory problems, these problems are characterized by a storage deficit; in HD, memory problems are characterized by a retrieval deficit (10). Also, although depression is common in HD, it is characterized by anhedonia and lack of initiation, not simple depressed mood, which is most characteristic of clinical depression.

Despite progressive motor, cognitive, and psychiatric difficulties, some improvement in the areas of functional outcome and health-related quality of life (HRQoL) or in the perceived impact of a disease or its treatment on physical, mental, and social well-being (11) can be achieved over time. Effective treatments can also prolong the number of relatively healthy years for individuals with HD before they eventually succumb to the disease. However, the full extent of such treatments is often not detected because of (1) insensitive standardized outcome measures, and (2) lack of measures that specifically target an HD population. Given the nature of the disease, the quality of a person's life is equally as important as a person's physical status. Thus, HRQoL is a critical dependent variable in HD clinical trials, as well as in the individual's life. At present, no widely accepted instrument is available with which to obtain a comprehensive HRQoL of individuals with HD. Unfortunately, although the measurement of HRQoL is required for clinical trials, and although specific HRQoL measures are available for use with HD caregivers (12, 13, 14), no published HRQoL measures have been developed specifically for use among patients diagnosed with HD.

Without a valid HRQoL outcomes assessment, it is very difficult to determine the true impact and notable advances being made in HD research. With the advent of genetic testing for HD and the ability to track the full progression of the disease from the prodromal phases through full symptom manifestation, the need for sensitive outcomes assessment measures has become more urgent. Although a handful of studies have examined quality of life in the caregivers of HD (12) and in individuals with HD (15), no HD-specific HRQoL measures have been published. Given the importance of being able to evaluate treatment interventions designed to slow the progression of symptoms in this population, the development of a sensitive measure to assess HD-related HRQoL is long overdue.

Evaluating HRQoL in HD

Because no existing HRQoL measures are targeted specifically for HD, HD research has instead utilized other methods of evaluating HRQoL. To evaluate the HRQoL assessment measures currently being used in HD, it is important to understand the distinction between HRQoL and quality of life (QoL). Cella defines HRQoL in a multi-dimensional manner, asserting that "health-related quality of life (HRQoL) refers to the extent to which one's usual or expected physical, emotional, and social well-being are affected by a medical condition or its treatment (p. 73) (16). This can be contrasted with QoL, which refers to a less clearly defined construct that assesses general well-being (17, 18). Regardless of the differences between these constructs, both emphasize the patient's perspective. Although proxy measurement may be the only alternative for individuals who are unable to provide this information (e.g., due to mental or physical incapacity), numerous studies report discrepancies between patient and companion raters (19, 20, 21, 22, 23), making this a less than ideal approach to HRQoL or QoL assessment. In sum, assessment of HRQoL and QoL information for clinicians and individuals affected by HD becomes increasingly important for those making treatment decisions that may affect length of survival, functional status, or pain and symptom management (24, 25).

A number of different approaches have been used to assess both QoL and HRQoL in HD. Specifically, many researchers and clinicians choose to employ a targeted scale that covers a single domain of functioning assessing QoL. Still others utilize generic HRQoL or QoL measures that were designed for use in the general population. Further, some individuals choose to use specialized measures that were designed for a similar population (e.g., Alzheimer's disease, amyotrophic lateral sclerosis). Finally, single-item assessments of QoL are common. The strengths and weaknesses of these approaches are explored below.

In HD research, measures that are most commonly used for QoL assessment focus on a single, limited domain (e.g., motor functioning) and by definition are not able to capture the multidimensional construct of HRQoL. For example, a number of studies have utilized the *total functional capacity score* (26) (*TFC*) from the *Unified Huntington's Disease Rating Scale* (27) (*UHDRS*), which provides a measure of functional ability (28, 29, 30, 31). The TFC is a five-question scale covering employment, finances, domestic chores, activities of daily living, and care level. Scores can range from 0 to 13, with lower scores reflecting poorer functional abilities. Although this measure can be useful in the clinic, Nance (32) point out that it is not useful in the presymptomatic stages of the disease, because it often miscategorizes individuals with psychiatric difficulties (which are common in individuals with HD), suffers from a floor effect, and is not sensitive to progression in later stages of the disease. Similarly, other studies have focused on utilizing the *motor scale* of the UHDRS (28, 31, 33, 34). This scale includes 31 questions concerning motor decline. The questions assess for dystonia, chorea, voluntary motor impairment (tongue protrusion, finger tapping, prosupination, bradykinesia, rigidity), posture, and gait. On this measure, higher scores indicate greater impairment. This scale is most commonly utilized by a neurologist or someone with specialized training in the assessment of motor functioning and requires expertise in motor assessment to administer. Although this scale provides a measure of motor functioning in HD, it does not truly assess the multi-dimensional construct of HRQoL. Further, it does not include any self-reported questions regarding quality of life or overall functioning and, as such, is not necessarily the most appropriate HRQoL assessment measure.

In addition to weaknesses in the single-domain scales listed above, outcome measures that focus on a sole domain of functioning by design overlook the various other areas of functioning that may be affected by treatment and are characteristic of HRQoL. As noted above, many researchers/clinicians choose to focus on a single domain of functioning to represent QoL, even when the scale being used is a part of a larger multimodal assessment battery (e.g., UHDRS). Although the UHDRS still does not assess the full myriad of domains of functioning that are characteristic of HRQoL, it warrants further mention because it is the most commonly used assessment measure in HD clinical trials (28, 31). The UHDRS includes four different scales that assess functional, motor, cognitive, and behavioral symptoms. First, the *Functional Ability Scale* includes three functional capacity measures: the *TFC* (which was described above), the *Independence Subscale* (a single score rating assessing individual level of independence; scores range from 0 to 100 with higher scores indicating higher levels of independence), and a *checklist of 25 common daily tasks*. Of these three, the *TFC* is the most characteristic of a QoL measure. The *Motor Scale*, described above as well, does not capture self-reported HRQoL or QoL (as it is an objective assessment of motor functioning). The *Cognitive Scale* consists of three common neuropsychological assessment measures: a test of verbal fluency (35), the Symbol Digit Modalities test (36), and the Stroop test (37), all of which require specialized training to administer and provide an objective assessment of cognitive functioning rather than HRQoL or QoL. Finally, the *Behavioral Scale* includes severity and frequency ratings for 10 different items and four clinician-judged questions regarding mental status and mood; this scale is most appropriately administered by a psychiatrist and provides indices of mood, behavior, psychosis, and obsessiveness (higher scores suggesting more severe difficulties). Although an element of QoL assessment is inherent in some of these items, the fact that a portion of this scale is based on test administrator perception disqualifies it as a true HRQoL or QoL measure. Therefore, although the UHDRS covers multiple domains of functioning, each of which in and of itself might be construed as a domain of HRQoL, the TFC is the only measure that truly captures QoL, and without any other self-reported satisfaction with other domains of functioning, this measure is not appropriate as a proxy for HRQoL. Further, this measure has been criticized as lacking reliability (38) as well as being time consuming and difficult to use in clinical practice (39).

Other common outcome measures in HD research include generic scales, or scales that are commonly used with normative samples. The *Medical Outcomes Study Short Form-36* (40) (*SF-36*) and the *Sickness Impact Profile* (41) (*SIP*) are two common examples. A number of HD studies have utilized either the SF-36 (42, 43, 44) or the SIP (42, 45, 46, 47) as their HRQoL measure. One study, using both the SF-36 and the SIP in a sample of individuals with HD, reported that the SF-36 evidenced more robust construct validity and test-retest reliability than the SIP (42). Helder and colleagues (46) also examined HRQoL in 77 individuals with HD using the SIP and found that, although the SIP was associated with more specialized measures of motor functioning (total motor score from the UHDRS) (27) and cognition (48) (using the Mini-Mental State), only the physical subscale and total score on the SIP predicted HD-related illness variables.

Unfortunately, although these more generic measures are able to identify differences between individuals with HD and controls, they cannot necessarily detect subtle differences among individuals in the prodromal phases of the disorder. For example, one study examining memory functioning in prodromal HD reported subtle declines in memory performance but was clear in specifying that these differences were very subtle and did not indicate clinical impairment but rather a statistical decline in score (49). This suggests that changes in performance are occurring and are detectable, but that they do not necessarily have an immediate impact on functioning and would not necessarily be detectable without very sensitive measures (see Schmitz and colleagues (50) for a detailed description of clinically significant versus statistically significant change). In HD, assessment measures need to capture subtle prodromal changes in function as well as more severe clinical changes, and these measures need to capture the unique symptoms of this disorder (chorea, bradykinesia, etc). Even when they are able to identify group differences, generic measures neglect to include HD-specific questions to assess things such as the complex issues associated with disease transmission of a dominant trait and the end-of-life issues that are inherent in this disorder. Further, generic measures often contain irrelevant and offensive questions that lack validity in HD populations. For instance, one item on the SF-36 asks respondents whether they expect their health to worsen. For an individual who has an insidious, progressive genetic disorder, asking a question to which the answer is apparent can appear insensitive. In conclusion, these generic instruments lack HD-related content validity, highlighting the need for an HRQoL measure that is targeted to unique patient populations.

In addition to the HRQoL and QoL measures that are typically included in HD research and practice, some individuals might consider utilizing more specialized measures of HRQoL or QoL that are used in other, similar neurological diseases. Measures developed for other degenerative (51) and genetic diseases (52) include some "targeted" items that would likely be appropriate for HD. Unfortunately, although these disease-specific measures might include some questions that are characteristic of HD HRQoL, they likely include other questions that are not appropriate or may even be perceived as offensive by participants, and they, by design, will not be able to assess the full spectrum of HD symptoms. This is particularly problematic in HD, where the expression of clinically significant symptoms occurs only after irreversible brain degeneration requiring early detection of subtle changes in symptoms.

Finally, some studies in HD have elected to utilize a single-item rating of QoL (15, 53, 54). Although this may provide a brief snapshot of the construct of QoL, a single-question assessment of any construct is problematic. For example, a study examining individuals at risk for HD found that QoL (as was determined by a single item question) was unchanged after genetic testing (54). Unfortunately, there is no way to know if the link between QoL and genetic testing outcomes 1) does not actually exist, 2) was hindered by a small sample size, or 3) was undetectable because of the limited assessment of QoL. Although single-item assessments of QoL provide the advantages of brevity, the ability for use across multiple respondents (patients, caregivers, providers), and the ability for use across disease severity, they lack the ability to evaluate the multi-dimensional construct of HRQoL, and they do not provide a sufficient range of variability for the clinician to truly understand and detect subtle changes in this construct.

To summarize, measures that are commonly used in HD either focus solely on the construct of QoL rather than HRQoL (using a single item or a single domain of functioning) or are overly generic or overly specialized for other populations and do not capture all of the unique aspects of HD. As such, these measures are typically limited in focus and fail to account for subtle improvements in functioning or satisfaction, making it impossible to ascertain the effectiveness of clinical trials. Often these measures may also be sensitive to some stages of the disease, but not others. Without sensitive outcome measures, the positive impact of emerging interventions is difficult, if not impossible, to assess, leaving a strong need for a sensitive outcome measure to evaluate HD-related clinical trials. Fortunately, researchers have come to recognize that more multi-faceted outcome measures, such as instruments that evaluate HRQoL, which measure

the impact of physical health, level of social support, participation in the community, and level of everyday functioning on QoL, represent important variables that determine long-term satisfaction and evaluate the "effectiveness" of clinical interventions. To this end, several large-scale measurement initiatives, which are currently under development, show immense promise as leading HRQoL measures.

New HRQoL measurement initiatives

As noted above, no HRQoL measures have been developed specifically for use in HD. Fortunately, a number of large-scale initiatives have recently been funded that will address this oversight in a variety of populations, including HD. Specifically, we begin with a brief discussion of the current HRQoL measurement initiatives funded by the National Institute of Health (NIH), the National Institute of Neurological Disorders and Stroke (NINDS), the National Center for Medical Rehabilitation Research (NCMRR), the National Institute on Disability and Rehabilitation Research (NIDRR), and the VA Rehabilitation Research and Development (RR&D). These projects include the Patient-Reported Outcomes Measurement Information System (PROMIS), the Neuro-QoL Instrument, and a number of complementary development studies, including the SCI-QoL, TBI-QoL, Polytrauma-QoL, and HD-QoL. (Figure 7.1 presents a graphic of these measurement systems for use in the general population and in those with adult epilepsy, stroke, amyotrophic lateral sclerosis, multiple sclerosis, Parkinson's disease, spinal cord injury, traumatic brain injury, and HD.) This is followed by a discussion of how this development work has been extended to HD and development of the HD-QoL and the larger implications that these initiatives will have on HRQoL measurement.

The NIH has identified that a significant gap in biomedical research is the lack of uniform, dynamic outcome measures for NIH-sponsored research. The large measurement initiatives noted above are designed to utilize common data elements (CDEs)

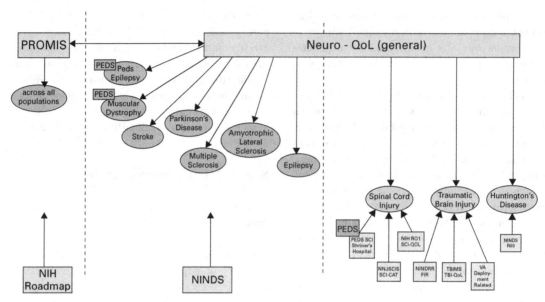

Figure 7.1 The current evolution of PROMIS and Neuro-QoL measurement systems.

This figure includes the Patient Reported Outcomes Measurement Information System (PROMIS), the Neuro-QoL Instrument, and a number of complementary development studies, including SCI-QoL, TBI-QoL, Polytrauma-QoL, and HD-QoL. The clinical population that is the focus of each project, plus the funding sources, is indicated.

in NIH-funded research across several populations. CDEs are data elements that can be used in multiple clinical studies and are required to publish primary papers reporting the results of a clinical study. The goal of CDEs is to provide investigators and study staff with a "universal language" to utilize within studies. NINDS has instituted a program to develop CDEs for clinical research in neurology to enhance the field of neurological research with the ultimate goal that data can eventually be reviewed across multiple studies. CDEs, in conjunction with item response theory and computer adaptive testing (state-of-the-art statistical techniques that will be implemented during the next phase of this study), will allow for a crosswalk between measures. Further, a movement toward utilizing computer adaptive testing (CAT) is under way, allowing the full spectrum of symptoms to be assessed while limiting the final item to a very small number of items. CAT is a method of administering individually tailored questionnaires (guided by item response the-

ory, which is a statistical framework that utilizes computational algorithms and logic to determine the specific items that a participant sees) (55). An individual who takes a CAT will be administered items that are based on his/her previous responses; the CAT uses an algorithm that estimates the participant's score (based on his/her previous response) and the score's reliability and then chooses the best next item; each individual test administration is therefore uniquely tailored to the individual. In this manner, item administration is based on predetermined specifications such as content coverage, test length, and standard error. This means that test administration can be preset on the basis of the number of domains that should be assessed, the number of items you would like each participant to see, or the minimum standard error that the examiner determines is most appropriate for the estimated response. The CAT ranks all participants on the same continuum when estimating a score, even if they have not been given any common items;

further, each participant needs to answer only a subset of items to obtain a measure that accurately estimates what would have been obtained by administering the entire set of items. CAT effectively reduces test length without loss of precision. A final advantage of this approach is that new items can be added at a later date and evaluated for consistency with the original bank, allowing for future expansion and adjustment. CAT is particularly advantageous for HD because of the wide range of disease severity that needs to be considered across respondents. Without CAT, it would be difficult to construct a measure that would be applicable from the prodromal stages to advanced HD that did not include a very large number of questions such that a large subset of questions would always be inapplicable to a portion of respondents.

The PROMIS Initiative

The Patient Reported Outcomes Measurement Information System (56) (PROMIS) is an NIH roadmap initiative designed to develop a system for dynamic assessment of patient-reported chronic disease outcomes. PROMIS is building and validating common, accessible item banks to measure key symptoms and health concepts applicable to a range of chronic conditions, enabling efficient and interpretable clinical trial research and clinical practice application of patient-reported outcomes. PROMIS utilizes patient self-report data and is expected to become a CDE in clinical trials research across populations. PROMIS measures assess several domains of functioning, including Physical Function, Pain (Behavior and Impact), Emotional Function (Depression, Anxiety, and Anger), Social Functions (Satisfaction with Social Roles and Satisfaction with Discretionary Social Activities), Fatigue, Wake Disturbance, and Sleep Disturbance. These 11 different item banks, all of which provide the option of using a short-form or a computer adaptive test, are currently available in the public domain through the following website: www.nihpromis.org.

The Neuro-QoL Initiative

Neuro-QoL is a 5-year effort funded by the NINDS to construct a psychometrically sound and clinically relevant HRQoL measurement system for people with major neurological disorders. Neuro-QoL has built upon PROMIS by including "disease targeted" scales that enhance the measurement of HRQoL in individuals with the following neurological impairments: Stroke (adult), Multiple Sclerosis (adult), Parkinson's Disease (adult), Epilepsy (adult and pediatric), Amyotrophic Lateral Sclerosis (adult), and Muscular Dystrophy (pediatric only). Neuro-QoL item banks share common items with PROMIS in several areas, including Physical, Emotional, and Social Function. This will allow for equivalency score calculations between both of these measurement systems and for cross-population comparison. In addition to the Neuro-QoL scales that overlap with PROMIS, Neuro-QoL's disease-targeted scales include Sleep Disturbance, Personality and Behavioral Changes, and Fatigue/Weakness (Cognition and Pain for children). This HRQoL scale will enable cross-disease comparisons using the generic items that are relevant to individuals across conditions as well as the evaluation of condition-specific HRQoL issues using targeted, disease-specific items. Neuro-QoL should be publicly available by September 2010; check the website for frequent updates (www.neuroqol.org). Further, additional funding has been awarded to extend Neuro-QoL to include Spinal Cord Injury (SCI) and Traumatic Brain Injury (TBI). Specifically, the NIH, NIDRR, and NCMRR, and the VA RR&D, have supported the development of SCI-QoL and TBI-QoL extensions of this study.

The HD-QoL initiative

Although HD was included in the initial pool of potential neurological disorders covered by the Neuro-QoL, it was prioritized below the aforementioned conditions (according to expert ratings), and funding was restricted to the top five conditions. The magnitude of the investments being made by NIH, NINDS, NIDRR, NCMRR, and the VA RR&D suggests that these measures will become leading, and perhaps required, outcome variables in clinical trials. Ensuring the relevance of these measures in HD research is essential given the distinct nature of HD relative to other neurological conditions (e.g., the fatality and autosomal dominant nature of the disease, the range of deficits, the particular impact on HRQoL). An HD-HRQoL measure is currently being developed (with support from NINDS) that will complement the Neuro-QoL and will include items that will allow for cross-disease comparisons. Further, the HD-QoL will include items from other HD-QoL measures that are also currently under development. For example, another is under development by the European Huntington's Disease Network (EHDN) for use in Europe that examines HRQoL in HD (57). It is hoped that the HD-QoL will be able to include items from this measure to develop a crosswalk that will allow individuals to estimate a score on the EHDN measure if the HD-QoL is administered, and vice versa. Specifically, CDEs between HD-QoL and Neuro-QoL, and between HD-QoL and measures similar to the EHDN measure, in conjunction with item response theory and CAT, will allow for a crosswalk between measures. Participants receiving the HD-QoL will also receive an estimated score on the Neuro-QoL and PROMIS, and vice versa. Further, items from other targeted scales (e.g., the EHDN measure) that are relevant to HD will be considered for the item banks that will be developed for the proposed project.

The HD-QoL will address the strong need for an outcome measure that assesses the needs of the HD community; it will evaluate areas of functioning that are unique to HD, plus include a number of items that will allow for cross-disease comparison with other neurologically based diseases. More specifically, this HRQoL HD measure will be compatible with the Neuro-QoL project that not only has NIH and NINDS support but has been expanded to include support from NIDRR, NCMRR, and the VA

RR&D. The development of a valid and meaningful instrument that measures HRQoL issues unique to the HD population is a significant step forward in HD-specific and cross-condition outcomes research. This new type of instrument will address a gap in HD outcome measurement by including the themes and domains of functioning that are relevant to this population.

The Development of the HD-QoL

The HD-QoL will utilize a community-based partnership to determine the domains and items that should be used to assess HRQoL in HD. More specifically, focus groups will be conducted with individuals with or at risk for HD, caregivers, and professionals (e.g., clinicians and researchers with more than 3 years of experience in HD) to determine domains and items relevant to HRQoL in individuals with HD. Each focus group will last approximately 90 minutes; it will begin with an open-ended question about the important issues related to HRQoL in HD and will continue with more targeted questions about specific areas of functioning. Focus groups will be transcribed and coded by two independent examiners for both thematic content and potential item identification. Kappa statistics will be examined to ensure adequate interrater agreement. Items developed on the basis of focus group content will include an adequate number of universal items to allow for cross-disease or cross-disability comparison (Neuro-QoL) and will examine a sample that spans across the stages of the disease from the earliest symptoms to the later stages of the disease process. CDEs, in conjunction with item response theory and CAT, will allow for a crosswalk between measures; participants receiving the HD-QoL will also receive an estimated score on the Neuro-QoL or PROMIS, and vice versa. Further, the HD-QoL will include items from other QoL and HRQoL measures that are under development or are in common usage. This will also allow for a crosswalk between these scales and the HD-QoL.

Summary and Recommendations

The development of a valid and meaningful instrument that measures HRQoL issues unique to the HD population will be a significant step forward in HD-specific and cross-condition outcomes research. This new type of instrument will address a gap in HD outcome measurement by including the themes and domains of functioning that are relevant to this population, such as emotional, social, cognitive, and physical functioning, end-of-life issues, and personality changes. Development of this meaningful and psychometrically sound HD-specific HRQoL scale will fulfill the need for such a scale in HD medicine and will significantly advance the understanding of outcomes of HD clinical trials. It is hoped that a final version of the HD-QoL will be available by 2013. In the meantime, utilizing the short forms that are available through the PROMIS and Neuro-QoL projects will likely provide the best alternative for HRQoL in HD. Further, after the HD-QoL has been developed, people will be able to retrospectively determine an equivalency score on the HD-QoL from these assessment measures. Overall, this advance will help people to better understand and address the needs of persons with HD to improve their HRQoL.

Acknowledgments: This chapter was supported, in part, by Grant Number R03NS065194 from the National Institute of Neurological Disorders and Stroke (NINDS). The content is solely the responsibility of the authors and does not necessarily represent the official views of NINDS or the National Institutes of Health.

REFERENCES

1. Li X. The early cellular pathology of Huntington's disease. *Molec Neurobiol* 1999; **20**[2–3]: 111–124.
2. Ho L, Carmichael J, Swartz J, Wyttenbach A, Rankin J, Rubinsztein DC. The molecular biology of Huntington's disease. *Psychol Med* 2001; **31**[1]: 3–14.
3. The Huntington's Disease Collaborative Research Group. A novel gene containing a trinucleotide repeat that is expanded and unstable on Huntington's disease chromosomes. *Cell* 1993; **72**[6]: 971–983.
4. Paulsen JS. *Understanding Behavior in Huntington's Disease.* New York, NY: Huntington's Disease Society of America, 1999.
5. Paulsen JS, Conybeare RA. Cognitive changes in Huntington's disease. *Adv Neurol* 2005; **96**: 209–225.
6. Biglan KM, Ross CA, Langbehn DR et al. Motor abnormalities in pre-manifest persons with Huntington's disease: The Predict-HD study. *Movement Disord* 2009; 24[12]: 1763–1772.
7. Siemers E, Foroud T, Bill DJ et al. Motor changes in presymptomatic Huntington disease gene carriers. *Arch Neurol* 1996; **53**[6]: 487–492.
8. Stout JC, Johnson SA. Cognitive impairment and dementia in basal ganglia disorders. *Curr Neurol Neurosci Rep* 2005; **5**: 355–363.
9. McPherson S, Cummings J. Neuropsychological aspects of Parkinson's disease and parkinsonism. Grant I, Adams KM, editors. *Neuropsychological Assessment of Neuropsychiatric and Neuromedical Disorders* 3rd ed. New York, NY: Oxford University Press, 2009:199–222.
10. Bondi MW, Salmon DP, Kaszniak AW. The neuropsychology of dementia. Grant I, Adams KM, editors. *Neuropsychological Assessment of Neuropsychiatric and Neuromedical Disorders* 3rd ed. New York, NY: Oxford University Press, 2009:159–198.
11. Cella D, Bonomi AE. Measuring quality of life: 1995 update. *Oncology* 2003; 9[11]: 47–60.
12. Aubeeluck A. Caring for the carers: Quality of life in Huntington's disease. *Brit J Nursing* 2005; **14**[8]: 452–454.
13. Aubeeluck A, Buchanan H. The Huntington's disease quality of life battery for carers: reliability and validity. *Clin Genet* 2007; **71**: 434–445.
14. Aubeeluck A, Buchanan H. A measure to assess the impact of Huntington's disease on the quality of life of spousal carers. *Brit J Neurosci Nurs* 2006; **2**[2]: 88–95.
15. Ready R, Mathews M, Leserman A, Paulsen J. Patient and caregiver quality of life in Huntington's disease. *Movement Disord* 2008; 23[5]: 721–726.
16. Cella DF. Measuring quality of life in palliative care. *Seminal Oncol* 1995; **22**: 73–81.
17. Campbell A, Converse PE, Rodgers WL. *The quality of American life: perceptions, evaluations, and satisfactions.* New York: Russell Sage Foundation, 1976.

18. Patrick DL, Erikson P. What constitutes quality of life? Concepts and dimensions. *Clin Nutr* 1988; **7**[2]: 53–63. Pleasantville, NJ, Nutrition Publications.

19. Chatterjee A, Anderson K, Moskowitz C, Hauser W, Marder K. A comparison of self-report and caregiver assessment of depression, apathy, and irritability in Huntington's disease. *J Neuropsychiatr Clin Neurosci* 2005; **17**[3]: 378–383.

20. Deckel A, Morrison D. Evidence of a neurologically based "denial of illness" in patients with Huntington's disease. *Arch Clin Neuropsychol* 1996; **11**[4]: 295–302.

21. Duff K, Paulsen JS, Beglinger LJ, Langbehn DR, Wang C, Stout JC et al. "Frontal" behaviors before the diagnosis of Huntington's disease and their relationship to markers of disease progression evidence of early lack of awareness. *J Neuropsych Clin N.* 2010; **22**(2): 196–207.

22. Hoth K, Paulsen J, Moser D, Tranel D, Clark L, Bechara A. Patients with Huntington's disease have impaired awareness of cognitive, emotional, and functional abilities. *J Clin Exp Neuropsychol* 2007; **29**[4]: 365–376.

23. Snowden J, Craufurd D, Griffiths H, Neary D. Awareness of involuntary movements in Huntington disease. *Arch Neurol* 1998; **55**[6]: 801–805.

24. Clancy C, Eisenberg J. Outcomes research: measuring the end results of health care. *Science* 1998; **282**[5387]: 245–246.

25. Guyatt G, Feeney D, Patrick D. Measuring health-related quality of life. *Ann Int Med* 1993; **118**: 622–629.

26. Shoulson I, Fahn S. Huntington disease: clinical care and evaluation. *Neurology* 1979; **29**[1]: 1–3.

27. Huntington Study Group. Unified Huntington's Disease Rating Scale: Reliability and Consistency. *Movement Disord* 1996; **11**[2]: 136–142.

28. de Tommaso M, Di Fruscolo O, Sciruicchio V et al. Efficacy of levetiracetam in Huntington disease. *Clin Neuropharmacol* 2005; **28**[6]: 280–284.

29. Mayeux R, Stern Y, Herman A, Greenbaum L, Fahn S. Correlates of early disability in Huntington's disease. *Ann Neurol* 1986; **20**[6]: 727–731.

30. Nehl C, Paulsen JS, The Huntington Study Group. Cognitive and psychiatric aspects of Huntington disease contribute to functional capacity. *J Nerv Ment Dis* 2004; **192**[1]: 72–74.

31. van Vugt JPP, Siesling S, Piet KKE et al. Quantitative assessment of daytime motor activity provides a responsive measure of functional decline in patients with Huntington's disease. *Movement Disord* 2001; **16**[3]: 481–488.

32. Nance MA. Comprehensive care in Huntington's disease: a physician's perspective. *Brain Res Bull* 2007; **72**: 175–178.

33. Frank SA, Marshall F, Plumb S et al. Functional decline due to chorea in Huntington's disease. *Neurology* 2004; **62**[5].

34. Hamilton JM, Salmon DP, Corey-Bloom J et al. Behavioural abnormalities contribute to functional decline in Huntington's disease. *J Neurol Neurosurg Psychiatry* 2003; **74**: 120–122.

35. Benton AL, des Hamsher KD. *Multilingual Aphasia Examination Manual.* Iowa City, IA: University of Iowa, 1978.

36. Smith A. *Symbol Digit Modalities Test Manual.* Los Angeles: Western Psychological Services, 1973.

37. Stroop JR. Studies of interference in serial verbal reactions. *J Exp Psychol* 1935; **18**: 643–662.

38. Hogarth P, Kayson E, Kieburtz K, et al. Interrater agreement in the assessment of motor manifestations of Huntington's disease. *Movement Disord* 2005; **20**: 293–297.

39. Klempir J, Klempirova O, Spackova N, Zidovska J, Roth J. Unified Huntington's disease rating scale: clinical practice and critical approach. *Funct Neurol* 2006; **21**[4]L 217–221.

40. Ware JE, Kosinski M, Keller SD. *SF-36 Physical and Mental Health Summary Scales: A User 's Manual.* Boston, MA: The Health Institute, New England Medical Center, 1994.

41. Bergner M, Bobbitt RA, Carter WB, Gilson BS. The Sickness Impact Profile: development and final revision of a health status measure. *Med Care* 1982; **19**[8]: 787–805.

42. Ho AK, Robbins AOG, Walters SJ, Kapotoge S, Sahakian B, Barker RA. Health-related quality of life in Huntington's disease: a comparison of two generic instruments, SF-36 and SIP. *Movement Disord* 2004; **19**[11]: 1341–1348.

43. Ho AK, Gilbert AS, Mason SL, Goodman AG, Barker RA. Health-related quality of life in Huntington's disease: which factors matter most? *Movement Disord* 2008; **24**[4]: 574–578.

44. Kaptein AA, Scharloo M, Helder DI et al. Quality of life in couples living with Huntington's disease: the role of patients' and partners' illness perceptions. *Qual Life Res* 2007; **16**: 793–801.

45. Cubo E, Shannon KM, Tracy D et al. Effect of donepezil on motor and cognitive function in Huntington disease. *Neurology* 2006; **67**[1 of 2]: 1268–1271.

46. Helder DI, Kaptein AA, van Kempen GMJ, van Houwelingen JC, Roos RAC. Impact of Huntington's disease on quality of life. *Movement Disord* 2001; **16**[2]: 325–330.

47. Kaptein AA, Helder DI, Scharloo M et al. Illness perceptions and coping explain well-being in patients with Huntington's disease. *Psychol Health* 2006; **21**[4]: 431–446.

48. Folstein MF, Folstein SE, McHugh PR. Mini-Mental State: a practical method for grading the cognitive state of patients for the clinician. *J Psychiatr Res* 1975; **12**: 189–198.

49. Soloman AC, Stout JC, Johnson SA et al. Verbal episodic memory declines prior to diagnosis in Huntington's disease. *Neuropsychologia* 2007; **45**[8]: 1767–1776.

50. Schmitz N, Hartkamp N, Franke G. Assessing clinically significant change: application to the SCL-90-R. *Psychol Rep* 2000; **86**[1]: 263–274.

51. Logsdon RG, Gibbons LE, McCurry SM, Teri L. Assessing quality of life in older adults with cognitive impairment. *Psychosom Med* 2002; **64**[3]: 510–519.

52. The ALS CNTF Treatment Study (ACTS) Phase 1–2 Study Group. The Amyotrophic Lateral Sclerosis Functional Rating Scale. *Arch Neurol* 1996; **53**: 141–147.

53. Tibben A, Frets PG, van de Kamp JJP et al. Presymptomatic DNA-testing for Huntington disease: pretest attitudes and expectations of applicants and their partners in the Dutch program. *Am J Med Genet (Neuropsychiatr Genet)* 1993; **48**: 10–16.

54. Tibben A, Frets PG, van de Kamp JJP et al. On attitudes and appreciation 6 months after predictive DNA testing for Huntington disease in the Dutch program. *Am J Med Genet (Neuropsychiatr Genet)* 1993; **48**: 103–111.

55. Van Der Linden WJ, Hambleton RK. *Handbook of Modern Item Response Theory*. New York, NY: Springer, 1997.

56. Cella D, Yount S, Rothrock N et al. The Patient-Reported Outcomes Measurement Information System (PROMIS): Progress of an NIH roadmap cooperative group during its first two years. *Med Care* 2007; **45**[5, Supplement 1].

57. Ho AK, Hocaoglu MB. Impact of Huntington's disease on health-related quality of life. Paper presented at the European Huntington's Disease Network Conference. Lisbon, Portugal, 2008.

8

Measuring quality of life in dementia

Rebecca E. Ready

Quality of life (QoL) is an elusive concept. It differs on the basis of culture, values, attitudes, and circumstances. There are as many definitions of QoL as there are individuals. Tensions and dualities in assessment of QoL are plentiful. QoL is agreed to be highly subjective, evaluative, and emotionally laden (1); yet, there are strong pressures and sound reasons to develop standardized measures of QoL, for example, as outcome measures in therapeutic trials. QoL will be an increasingly important outcome measure to justify health care expenditures in the treatment of dementia (1, 2, 3). Consideration of QoL also is critical in calling attention to humanistic perspectives on disease and treatment (3, 4).

The complexities of the QoL construct are omnipresent in the context of dementia, where, by definition, individuals suffer impairments in cognition, insight, and self-awareness that can interfere with self-report QoL data from patients. It is almost universally agreed that self-report is the gold standard for QoL assessment (3); thus, the challenges involved in measuring QoL in dementia can seem, at times, insurmountable.

Despite the difficulties, investigators have forged ahead, recognizing that assessment of QoL in dementia is too critical to be avoided, just for fear that it is an ill-defined, difficult to measure entity. It has been agreed that, whatever it is, QoL is a necessary construct because it is distinct from *symptoms* of dementia (5); rather, QoL relates more closely to the evaluative and subjective *impact* that symptoms have on one's life. The goals of this chapter are to critically evaluate the current state of the literature on the assessment of QoL in dementia, and to review dementia-specific QoL instruments with a particular focus on two new instruments.

Conceptions of QoL in dementia

No consensus definition of QoL in dementia has been identified.[1] As a result, QoL research in dementia is criticized as being atheoretical (6). This is not an entirely a valid criticism because research teams for some QoL measures have based their ideas on particular theoretical models or conceptual frameworks (7, 8). However, it is true that the field is lacking overarching theoretical guidance. Different perspectives on QoL abound and are manifest in the many different available instruments to assess QoL (Table 8.1). In the absence of *a priori* definitions and theoretical guidance, investigators have increasingly turned to patients with mild to moderate dementia to help identify constructs that are important for their QoL (9, 10, 11, 12, 13).

[1] The term Health-Related Quality of Life (HRoL) often is favored when discussing QoL that is specific to a particular disease or condition. The terms QoL and HRoL are interchangeable in the current piece.

Quality of Life Measurement in Neurodegenerative and Related Conditions, eds., Crispin Jenkinson, Michele Peters, and Mark B. Bromberg. Published by Cambridge University Press. © Cambridge University Press 2011.

The result of patient-centered measurement development is less arm-chair hypothesizing as to what constitutes QoL in dementia from "experts" or outside observers. If nothing else, the tendency to turn to patients for guidance in understanding life quality is validating of their unique experiences and perspectives.

As noted earlier, it is widely agreed that, in ideal circumstances, it is best to gather QoL data directly from the patient. The basis for this argument is that QoL is a subjective construct. However, Carr and Higginson (6) aptly point out that, even though data may be gathered from patients with some QoL instruments, this approach does not exactly capture subjectivity because the instruments are standardized, that is, although many instruments were developed based in part on patient review and input, eventually, a predefined and rigid set of items was created for the instrument, which functions to constrain the subjectivity that can be introduced into an assessment (3). A problem with the standardized approach is that it does not allow patients to indicate which aspects of QoL are most important for their lives at any particular time. Whitehouse and colleagues (14) found an interesting way around this problem by using a standardized instrument to assess for QoL but then adapting the instrument to allow individuals to indicate how important each item is to their QoL (14). Most dementia QoL instruments, however, are standardized, and the degree of subjectivity that is introduced into the measurement is limited to respondents' interpretation and rating of the predetermined items.

QoL measures in dementia

At least 11 dementia-specific measures of QoL are available (Table 8.1). They vary widely in breadth and depth in conceptualization of QoL. Broad consensus indicates that quality of life is emotionally salient, subjective, and evaluative (15). QoL is about how a person *feels* about particular life circumstances and not about the circumstances (e.g., symptoms, limitations) themselves. Common features of dementia QoL instruments are assessment of positive and negative emotions, self-esteem, enjoyment of activities, aesthetic sense, physical and mental health, feeling useful, social attachments and contact, and engagement in enjoyable activities. Ettema et al. (16) concluded that the greatest overlap in dementia QoL scales was noted for social relations or interaction, self-esteem, and mood or affect.

Consensus indicates that QoL in dementia is multi-dimensional (3). It is interesting to observe, however, that despite agreement about multidimensionality, only 6 of 11 measures have subscales that allow for assessment of multiple components of QoL (i.e., DQoL, BASQUID, ADRQL, DCM, Patient Activity Scale-AD, and the Modified Apparent Emotion Scale, QUALIDEM). Total scores often are preferred for research and program evaluation, but more fine-grained information gathered from subscales may be preferable in other situations (e.g., to determine differential change in components of QoL over time) (17). Instruments that have the versatility to allow for a total QoL score *and* subscale scores may be most useful, but to date, only two measures have both features (i.e., BASQUID, Patient Activity Scale-AD & the Modified Apparent Emotion Scale).

Instruments listed in Table 8.1 are organized by source of information (i.e., patient self-report only, patient-and proxy-report, proxy-report only); for other detailed reviews of dementia QoL measures, see (3, 18, 19). It can be assumed that all proxy-report instruments can theoretically be used in severe dementia (although not all of these instruments have been *evaluated* in severe dementia, see "Other Information" column Table 8.1), whereas exclusively self-report measures are appropriate for mild to moderate dementia.

Source of data for QoL measurement

The source of QoL data in dementia is a controversial topic. Tension exists between recognition that the best source of QoL data is self-report and knowledge that symptoms of dementia may interfere with

Table 8.1. Review of dementia-specific quality of life (QoL) measures

Measure	No. of items	Time frame	Total versus subscales	Reliability	Validity	Other information
Patient-Report Only						
D-QoL (9)	30	Recently	Five subscales: 1. Positive Affect 2. Negative Affect 3. Feelings of Belonging 4. Self-esteem 5. Sense of Aesthetics	Internal consistency reliability Mdn = .80 (range, .67 to .89); 2-week test-retest reliability Mdn = .72 (range, .64 to .90)	All subscales exhibit modest correlation (rs = .42 to .64) with depressive symptoms except Aesthetics	Evaluated in sample of mild to moderate dementia; takes 10 minutes to administer
BASQUID (12)	14	Not specified	Total score plus two subscales: 1. Life Satisfaction 2. Feelings of Positive QoL	Total internal consistency reliability alpha = .89 (.84–.83 for subscales); total 2-week test-retest reliability = .85	Moderate correlations with depressive symptoms and proxy-report generic QoL, no significant correlations with age or cognition	Self-report measure for mild to moderate AD
Patient & Proxy Report						
QoL-AD (10, 43, 58)	13	Past few weeks	Total score	Internal consistency reliability alpha = .84 to .88; 1-week test-retest reliability .76 (patients) and .92 (caregivers)	Low to moderate correlation with cognition, functioning, depressive symptoms, and engagement in pleasant events; patient-caregiver agreement ranges from .19 to .40	Responsive to change over time; takes 10 minutes or less to complete; used with mild to severe dementia
CBS (59)	19	Past month	Total score	Interrater reliability = .90; internal consistency reliability = .63	Total score negatively correlated with dementia severity –.35	Ratings are made by a clinician after a joint interview with patient and a caregiver; evaluated only with mild-moderate dementia patients
QOLAS (60)	10	Now	Total score	Internal consistency reliability alpha = .78	QoL higher for patients with less disability; convergent correlation with generic QoL measure Mdn r = .45 (range, .09 to .67)	Respondent picks and rates 10 issues (2 each from domains of physical, psychological, social/family, usual activities, cognitive functioning that are most important for his/her QoL); evaluated only in very small sample of mild-moderate dementia

Instrument	Items	Time frame	Subscales/Domains	Reliability	Validity	Comments
DEMQoL (7, 32, 52, 61)	28–31 items; plus one global QoL rating	Past week	Total score	Self-report internal consistency-reliability alpha = .87, 2-week test-retest reliability = .76; proxy-report internal consistency alpha=.87, test-retest reliability = .76	Self-report convergence with QoL-AD (r = .54) and DQoL (rs = .29–45); proxy-report convergence with QoL-AD (r = .52) and with depressive symptoms (r = −.61)	Self-report version has 28 items and can be used in mild-moderate dementia; proxy-report has 31 items and can be used in mild-severe dementia; both versions are interviewer administered

Proxy/Observer Report Only

Instrument	Items	Time frame	Subscales/Domains	Reliability	Validity	Comments
ADRQL (62, 63)	47 items	Past 2–4 weeks	Five domains: 1. Social Interaction 2. Awareness of Self 3. Feelings and Mood 4. Enjoyment of Activities 5. Response to Surroundings	Internal consistency alpha > .80 for 54/61 participants	Correlates with cognition (r = .51), functional impairment (r = .43), depressive symptoms (r = .43), and behavior disorder (r = .38)	Items weighted differently (but in a standardized manner) based on family caregiver data; developed to be used with all dementia severity levels
DCM (64, 65, 66)	26 items	Codes made every 5 minutes for 1 to 6 hours	Subscales: 1. Well-being 2. Activity	Activity and well-being correlated (Mdn = .53), supporting internal consistency; 1- to 4-week test-rest reliability for well-being = .55 and for activities = .40	Correlations between DCM and quality assurance audit measures of nursing homes; well-being item shows better convergence with generic QoL measure than activities	Observational scale that is appropriate for moderate-severe patients in residential settings; high face validity and staff acceptability
Patient Activity Scale-AD & the Modified Apparent Emotion Scale (67, 68, 69)	15 items	Past 2 weeks	Two subscales: 1. Activity 2. Affect; Plus, overall composite can be calculated	One-week test-retest reliability for affect Mdn = .77; above .60 for 12 of 15 activities	Activity decreases with dementia severity	Responsive to change over time

(cont.)

Table 8.1. (cont.)

Measure	No. of items	Time frame	Total versus subscales	Reliability	Validity	Other information
QUALID (70)	11 items	Past 7 days	Total score	Internal consistency reliability alpha = .77; 2- to 3-day test-retest reliability was .81; interrater reliability was .83	No significant correlations with cognition or ADLs but with depressive symptoms (r = .36) and neuropsychiatric symptoms (r = .40)	Subset of observable items from Albert et al.'s affect and activity measure (described above) for severe dementia; 5 minutes to administer
QUALIDEM (16, 53)	37 items	Past 2 weeks	Nine subscales: 1. Care Relationships 2. Positive Affect 3. Negative Affect 4. Restless Tense Behavior 5. Positive Self-image 6. Social Relations 7. Social Isolation 8. Feeling at Home 9. Having Something to Do	Subscale internal consistency reliabilities alphas=.62 to .89	Some association with dementia severity	Observational assessment of QoL in residential settings; 15 minutes to administer

Note. D-QoL = Dementia Quality of Life; BASQUID = Bath Assessment of Subjective Quality of Life in Dementia; AD = Alzheimer's disease; QoL-AD = Quality of Life in Alzheimer's Disease; CBS = Cornell Brown Scale for Quality of Life in Dementia; QoLAS = Quality of Life Assessment Schedule; DEMQoL = instrument to assess QoL in dementia; ADRQL = Alzheimer's Disease Health-Related Quality of Life Scale; DCM = Dementia Care Mapping.

the reliability, validity, or both of self-report data. In fact, the potential risks to patient-report data are plentiful. First, patients change over time. Whereas they might be able to provide self-report data at the beginning of a longitudinal study, they may not be able to continue to provide data for the duration of the project, risking significant loss of data. Second, patients may lack insight into their symptoms and current situation (20). Third, persons with dementia suffer from impairments in memory, language, and comprehension that might adversely affect QoL assessment.

However, despite these risks, Ready (15) reviewed the literature and concluded that compelling data are available to support the assertion that patients with mild to moderate dementia can provide reliable and valid data about their needs, preferences, and life quality (10, 21, 22). Even some patients with advanced dementia can complete self-report scales (10, 23) or use single-item QoL rating scales (24). As noted earlier, several QoL instruments were developed based in part on patient input (e.g., DQoL, QoL-AD, DEMQoL, BASQUID) (9, 10, 11, 13). Many patients also can understand that there is a difference in how they perceive their QoL and how another person might judge their QoL (24), which is a rather complex judgment. Further, with regard to longitudinal studies and risk for loss of data, most clinical trials last less than 6 months (25), a time frame that is too short for many patients to deteriorate so significantly as to lose the ability to provide QoL data over time.

Evidence of convergent validity of patient-report data has been found (26). The validity of patient-report QoL data also is supported by significant associations with behavioral and neuropsychiatric symptoms, particularly depression (10, 23, 26, 27, 28, 29). The QoL reports of patients with moderate to severe dementia also have been associated with functional impairment (10). Few to no associations between self-report QoL and cognition are shown (30).

As a general rule, persons with dementia who are unable to provide QoL data have Mini-Mental State Exam (MMSE) scores below 10 (10, 24, 26). Although

MMSE scores lower than 10 should not represent an *automatic* exclusion from reporting QoL outcomes, persons with scores as low as 4 completed the QoL-AD in research studies (10, 23) – it can be a useful benchmark.

Proxy-reports about QoL in persons with dementia often are favored, not because they are a more valid or reliable source of QoL data, but because they are easier to obtain, and proxies are more likely to be able to provide data throughout the duration of a longitudinal study. It is an unfortunate truth that when patients are in institutional settings or are experiencing severe dementia, many cannot participate in assessment of their QoL (17, 31, 32).

Whereas some might believe that proxy data are more reliable or valid than self-reports from persons with mild to moderate dementia, no empirical support for this assumption is available. Internal consistencies and test-retest reliabilities tend to be comparable for patient and caregiver report data (see Table 8.1). As for validity of proxy-reports, associations have been noted between QoL and neuropsychiatric symptoms and functional impairment similar to results for data provided by patients (10, 23). However, caregiver report QoL data are significantly influenced by caregiver burden and depression (10, 28, 33). Caregivers also routinely rate patient QoL lower than patients (5, 10, 22, 23, 26, 28, 34). (Of note, proxies tend to rate QoL lower than patients with many different types of disorders and diseases, not just for dementia (35, 36, 37, 38).) Further, patient-proxy agreement for quality of life tends be moderate at best, suggesting that the two sources of data are unique and non-overlapping to a significant degree. Agreement tends to be greater for more observable relative to less observable dimensions (39), which is a general finding in the self-other agreement literature and again is not specific to dementia (40, 41). A recent study elegantly demonstrated that, whereas patients and caregivers can mostly agree as to the important components of QoL, their *thinking* about these components is different (42). Thus, caregiver-reported QoL should never be considered a "substituted" judgment for a patient. The most reasonable perspective is to view self-report and proxy-report data as distinct with unique risks for error and as providing QoL from two different yet valid perspectives. In fact, data are beginning to emerge that multiple perspectives are needed for a comprehensive assessment of QoL in dementia (34).

Featured measures

A good variety of measures are available to assess QoL in dementia (Table 8.1). Two studies performed head-to-head comparisons of select dementia QoL measures (17, 18). Schölzel-Dorenbos et al. (18) compared several scales, many of which were dementia-specific, and concluded that no scale was appropriate for all patients in all care settings. The particular focus of these researchers was on instruments that would be useful for professional caregivers providing daytime activities or 24-hour care. If self-report data are not feasible to collect, they recommended the QUALIDEM observational scale, which can be used for mild to severe dementia. For self-report, the QoL-AD was recommended.

Sloane et al. (17) evaluated different dementia-specific QoL measures in long-term care settings. Completion rates for self-reported QoL from residents who carried diagnoses of dementia were poor (25% to 30%), whereas few data from caregivers were missing (17). Again, investigators concluded that no instrument could claim superiority but that observational measures offered greater disadvantages (e.g., floor effects, poor reliability, lack of variation, lack of multi-dimensionality) than self- or proxy-report scales.

The most popular instrument is Logsdon and colleagues' QoL-AD (10). It has been used to evaluate cognitive interventions (43) and as an outcome in controlled, randomized trials (e.g. (44)), and it has been translated for use in the United Kingdom (26), Taiwan (45), Japan (27), France (46), and China (47). It is brief and allows for self- and proxy-report about the patient's QoL. The QoL-AD has been modified by one team of investigators to allow for standard-ized rating of the items as well as an importance "weighting" of each item so respondents can indicate the extent to which different QoL factors affect their lives (14). The QoL-AD is a sound and versatile measure. One potential drawback to the QoL-AD is that the item content is broad and includes symptoms of dementia (e.g., memory, functioning); compelling data show that QoL is not (and probably should not be) equated with symptoms of disease (48).

Brod and colleagues' DQoL also is a popular instrument (9) and the first that was developed to assess QoL in dementia expressly and exclusively from the patient's perspective (see BASQUID from Trigg and colleagues (Table 8.1) for the second measure of this kind). The DQoL has been translated for use in the United Kingdom (49), the Netherlands (50), and Japan (51). Ready et al. (15) modified the DQoL for caregiver report and found evidence that patient and caregiver report conformed to very similar factor structures, supporting, in part, the construct validity of data from patients.

Thus, the QoL-AD and the DQoL have been influential instruments. They are the standard against which newer measures often compare themselves (12, 32). Rather than highlight the QoL-AD, which has a large and sound research base that is easily accessible, or the DQoL, which is a favored but limited instrument because of its exclusive reliance on patient report, an in-depth focus will instead be devoted to two new dementia QoL instruments. These are the DEMQoL (7, 11, 32, 52), which constitutes a pair of self- and proxy-report measures for mild to severe dementia, and the QUALIDEM (16, 53), an observational measure to be used in residential settings.

The DEMQoL

The conceptual framework for the DEMQoL is that QoL is a multidimensional construct that includes involvement in activities, autonomy and choice, social and family relationships, health and well-being, and life satisfaction (7). QoL reflects individual, subjective perceptions of the impact of a health condition on life quality (54). The authors developed the DEMQoL instruments because of a perceived need for broad, scientifically rigorous, self- and proxy-report measures of the overall impact of dementia that could be used at all stages of dementia and in a range of care settings (32). The intent was to create QoL measures for randomized clinical trials and observational research studies.

Scale development began by conducting in-depth interviews with persons suffering from dementia (n = 19) and caregivers (n = 20), review of the relevant literature, expert opinion, and development team discussion (11, 32). Caregivers were observed to have difficulty distinguishing between their feelings and problems and those of the person with dementia. Differences in perception of QoL were noted between caregivers and patients (7, 11). Persons with dementia focused on the "here and now" and were more concrete in their thinking than caregivers. They were positive, accepting of symptoms and associated limitations, and evaluated themselves favorably relative to other persons. Caregivers were more negative than patients, more reflective, and focused on changes over time. They also focused upon their own limitations. These different perspectives prompted investigators to develop two DEMQoL instruments – one for patients and one for caregivers – and to allow these instruments to have different item content.

Items were developed on the basis of results of interviews with patients and caregivers and were piloted in 12 patient-caregiver dyads. A potential 73 items had four-point response scales (a lot, quite a bit, a little, not at all) (32). Next, a preliminary field test (n = 130 persons with dementia, n = 126 caregivers) was conducted. The DEMQoL is an interviewer-administered scale. Items were eliminated based on pilot testing using missing data rates, endorsement frequencies, redundancy, and analysis of item-total correlations, factor analyses, and convergent and discriminant correlations. These efforts resulted in a 28-item self-report version and a 31-item caregiver or proxy-report version of the scale.

The final self-report DEMQoL version includes different groups of item types with different stems (7). Thirteen items pertain to positive and negative emotions, and persons rate the extent to which they have felt these emotions over the past week; the five positive emotion items are reverse scored. Six items pertain to memory and cognition, and participants rate how worried they have been about these issues. Nine items inquire about a variety of everyday life issues (e.g., social interaction, communication, toileting, overall health), and again persons rate their degree of worry about each item. A single, global QoL rating has four response options (very good, good, fair, poor). In the final proxy-report DEMQoL, 11 items pertain to emotion (including 5 positive emotion items), 9 items pertain to memory and cognition, 11 items pertain to everyday life issues, and the stems are similar to the self-report version; a global QoL item is also included.

The completed inventories were evaluated in 101 persons with dementia and 99 caregivers (32). Patients with severe dementia were largely unable to complete the self-report version, and so analyses on self-report data were restricted to persons with mild to moderate dementia. In patient data, factor analyses revealed a four-factor solution: daily activities, memory, negative emotion, and positive emotion. Thus, the measure did not conform to the hypothesized five-factor conceptual model. Internal consistency reliability for self-report data was .87, and 2-week test-retest reliability was .76.

The QoL-AD and DQoL were included in validity analyses because they were regarded as "best available" measures. Missing self-report data on the DEMQoL was 13.9%, which is somewhat better than for the QoL-AD (16.6%) and the DQoL (50%). Self-report on the DEMQoL correlated significantly with self-report on the QoL-AD (r = .54) and DQoL subscales (rs = .29 to .45). A positive correlation of the DEMQoL with age was noted (r = .39).

For proxy-report data, factor analyses revealed a two-factor solution of functioning and emotion. Internal consistency reliability was .87, and test-retest reliability was .67. Convergence with the QoL-AD was r = .52, and a strong negative correlation with depressive symptoms was found ($r = -.61$). Again, there was a positive correlation with age ($r = .34$). Proxy QoL scores did not significantly correlate with cognition or functional status, but associations with several neuropsychiatric symptoms, including agitation, anxiety, disinhibition, and irritability, were seen (52). Poorer caregiver mental health was associated with decreased ratings of QoL for the person with dementia.

Good dispersion or distribution of scores occurred at all levels of dementia severity, leading the authors to speculate that good QoL is possible at all stages of dementia (52). They also noted that, even though QoL does not exhibit significant correlations with cognition, it is not accurate to conclude that improving cognitive abilities will not have an impact on QoL.

The DEMQoL is a new and untested instrument, but preliminary data are intriguing. It has not yet been evaluated or used by investigators besides the test developers, and it has been developed, tested, and evaluated only in community-dwelling samples (32). Responsiveness to change is unknown, but preliminary pilot data are encouraging (52). More attention to the factor structure of the instrument(s), particularly in light of the original conceptual model of QoL, appears needed. Given the rapid pace of QoL research in dementia, more data about the DEMQoL are likely to be available in the near future.

The DEMQoL questionnaires have some distinguishing features. The self- and proxy-report versions have different item content. For example, only 9 of 13 emotion items, 4 of 6 cognitive items, and 2 of 9 everyday items from the self-report DEMQoL are found on the proxy-version. This feature was motivated, as noted previously, by the fact that persons with dementia have different perspectives on QoL than their caregivers (7), but it is unclear if differing item content will prove to be a strength or weakness of the instrument. At minimum, patient-caregiver comparisons of QoL are not possible, and lack of comparablility could be a limitation for some studies. Another unique feature is that the DEMQoL is very emotionally laden. Many items pertain to positive and negative emotions, and items that have non-emotional item content have a stem that pertains to "worry" about the item; thus, every single item is about an emotional experience. Whether the emotional content of the DEMQoL is an asset or a liability likely will pertain to the context in which the instrument will be used. As reviewed earlier, there is broad consensus that QoL is an emotionally laden construct, and in this sense, the DEMQoL may strongly measure a core aspect of QoL. Along these lines, a benefit of the DEMQoL is that measurement of QoL is clearly distinguished from *symptoms* of dementia.

The QUALIDEM

The QUALIDEM is a dementia-specific QoL measure that is intended to be rated by professional caregivers about patients with dementia in residential settings (16). It was developed because QoL is an essential outcome for treatment effectiveness (53). Item formulation began by focusing on the seven adaptive tasks of dealing with disability, developing adequate care relationships with staff, preserving emotional balance, preserving a positive self-image, preparing for an uncertain future, developing and maintaining social relationships, and dealing with the nursing home environment. The authors strove to incorporate a focus on *adaptation* in their assessment of QoL, which they judged to be missing from other existing instruments (3). The authors noted that it was hard to develop item content for "coping with disability" and "preparing for the future." Experts reviewed potential items, and 49 items were used in a pilot study (n = 238). Mokken scale analysis was used to reduce items. The final version of the scale is multi-dimensional and includes 37 items (21 of which are reverse scored) of observable behavior with 9 homogeneous subscales (care relationship, positive affect, negative affect, restless tense behavior, positive self-image, social relations, social isolation, feeling at home, having something to do). Each item has four response options: never, seldom, sometimes, often. Internal consistency reliabilities for the scales are moderate to strong (rho = .60 to

.90, alpha = .62 to .89). Interrater reliability is moderate to weak (rs = .47 to .79, Mdn = .72). Subscales are correlated significantly but to a modest degree (rs = −.33 to .59, Mdn = .27). Six of nine subscales are appropriate for very severe dementia; positive self-image, feeling at home, and having something to do were not observed because of loss of function in severe dementia.

The QUALIDEM is unique and represents a step forward for the field in some respects. It fills the need for an observational measure of QoL, especially for severe dementia, and calls more attention to QoL issues in long-term care settings. Research using the QUALIDEM was recently published demonstrating that aspects of QoL can be measured in the final stages of dementia (55), and, as mentioned above, it was recommended for adoption in a comparative study of dementia QoL measures (18). It includes item content that is missing from many other dementia-specific QoL measures such as a focus on care relationships and coping with residential treatment environments; further, an eye toward adaptive aspects of QoL in dementia was forefront in the conceptual development of the instrument. A limitation of the QUALIDEM is that some items measure behaviors that are less evident as dementia progresses; thus, there is some confounding of QoL assessment with disease severity. This may be corrected by using only select subscales with certain populations. Another limitation is that interrater reliability is modest at best, and further development along these lines appears warranted.

Evolution of the field and a view to the future

Measurement development and research into QoL in dementia have been conducted for approximately 15 years. In this relatively short time span, there has been an explosion of literature, and instrument development has advanced rapidly. Conceptualizations of QoL are more nuanced, sophisticated, and patient-focused than ever before. There is a trend for QoL research to be focused more on severe dementia, which is heartening, because it is recognized that QoL can be detected and enhanced even in advanced stages of disease.

Thus, the future for QoL research in dementia looks bright. Three issues would be particularly fruitful to address to advance research. First, it would be useful to know how to best gather reliable and valid self-report data from patients because it is widely agreed that self-report is the best source of QoL data. The impact of patient insight and awareness on self-report QoL data is a largely unanswered question and it will be tricky to address given the multi-dimensional nature of insight (56, 57). That is, one should not ask if awareness is impaired for any particular patient but rather to what *extent* is awareness altered for cognition, change over time, performance of activities of daily living, emotion, etc., and then one should examine impact on self-report data (15). Second, it will be important to determine the extent to which strong, existing measures of QoL in dementia are sensitive to change because QoL is increasingly valued as an outcome measure in intervention studies (30). Third, predictors of QoL in dementia are poorly understood beyond depressive symptoms and perhaps some other neuropsychiatric symptoms (15). Cognitive and functional measures are weak explanatory variables (30). Hoe et al. (5) suggest that living environment and acetylcholinesterase inhibitors (AChEIs) might be associated with higher QoL, but more information is needed. These data will be invaluable for determining how to maximize QoL for patients at every stage of disease severity and will help clinicians and investigators focus on salient patient-centered issues in dementia care and research.

REFERENCES

1. Mack JL, Whitehouse PJ. Quality of life in dementia: State of the Art – Report of the International Group for Harmonization of Dementia Drug Guidelines and the Alzheimer's Society Satellite Meeting. *Alzheimer Dis Assoc Disord* 2001; 15: 69–71.
2. Frank LB. Commentary on 'Health economics and the value of therapy in Alzheimer's disease.' Report from

the Alzheimer's Association Research Roundtable on patient-reported outcomes and dementia research. *Alzheim Dement* 2007; **3**: 162–165.

3. Ettema TP, Droes R-M, de Lange J, et al. A review of quality of life instruments used in dementia. *Qual Life Res* 2005; **14**: 675–686.

4. Gerritsen DL, Ettema TP, Boelens E, et al. Quality of life in dementia: do professional caregivers focus on the significant domains? *Am J Alzheimer's Dis* 2007; **22**: 176–183.

5. Hoe J, Katona C, Orrell M, et al. Quality of life in dementia: care recipient and caregiver perceptions of quality of life in dementia. The LASER-AD study. *Int J Geriatr Psychiatry* 2007; **22**: 1031–1036.

6. Carr AJ, Higginson IJ. Measuring quality of life: are quality of life measures patient centered? *BMJ* 2001; **322**: 1357–1360.

7. Smith SC, Lamping DL, Banerjee S, et al. Measurement of health-related quality of life for people with dementia: development of a new instrument (DEMQoL) and an evaluation of current methodology. *Health Technol Assess* 2005; **9**: 1–107.

8. Brod M, Stewart AL, Sands L. Conceptualization of quality of life in dementia, In: Albert SM, Logsdon RG, eds. *Assessing Quality of Life in Alzheimer's Disease.* New York: Springer, 2000; 3–16.

9. Brod M, Stewart AL, Sands L, et al. Conceptualization and measurement of quality of life in dementia: the dementia quality of life instrument (DQoL). *Gerontologist* 1999; **39**: 25–35.

10. Logsdon RG, Gibbons LE, McCurry SM, et al. Assessing quality of life in older adults with cognitive impairment. *Psychosom Med* 2002; **64**: 510–519.

11. Smith SC, Murray J, Banerjee S, et al. What constitutes health-related quality of life in dementia? Development of a conceptual framework for people with dementia and their carers. *Int J Geriatr Psychiatry* 2005; **20**: 889–895.

12. Trigg R, Skevington SM, Jones RW. How can we best assess the quality of life of people with dementia? The Bath Assessment of Subjective Quality of Life in Dementia (BASQID). *Gerontologist* 2007; **47**: 789–797.

13. Trigg R, Jones RW, Skevington SM. Can people with mild to moderate dementia provide reliable answers about their quality of life? *Age Ageing* 2007; **36**: 663–669.

14. Whitehouse P, Patterson MB, Sami SA. Quality of life in dementia: ten years later. *Alzheimer Dis Assoc Disord* 2003; **17**: 1999–200.

15. Ready RE. Patient-reported outcomes in clinical trials for Alzheimer's disease. *Alzheimer Dement* 2007; **3**: 172–176.

16. Ettema TP, Droes R-M, de Lange J, et al. QUALIDEM: development and evaluation of a dementia specific quality of life instrument – validation. *Int J Geriatr Psychiatry* 2007; **22**: 424–430.

17. Sloane PD, Zimmerman S, Williams CS, et al. Evaluating the quality of life of long-term care residents with dementia. *Gerontologist* 2005; **45**: 37–49.

18. Schölzel-Dorenbos CJM, Ettema TP, Bos J, et al. Evaluating the outcome of interventions on quality of life in dementia: selection of the appropriate scale. *Int J Geriatr Psychiatry* 2007; **22**: 511–519.

19. Ready RE, Ott BR. Quality of life measures for dementia. *Health Qual Life Outcomes* 2003; **1**: 11.

20. Ready RE, Ott BR, Grace J. Insight and self-reported QOL from memory disorder patients. *Am J Alzheimer Dis* 2006; **21**: 242–248.

21. Feinberg LF, Whitlatch CJ. Are persons with cognitive impairment able to state consistent choices? *Gerontologist* 2001; **47**: 374–382.

22. Ready RE, Ott BR, Grace J. Patient versus informant perspectives of quality of life in mild cognitive impairment and Alzheimer's disease. *Int J Geriatr Psychiatry* 2004; **19**: 256–265.

23. Shin IS, Carter M, Masterman D, et al. Neuropsychiatric symptoms and quality of life in Alzheimer's disease. *Am J Geriatr Psychiatry* 2005; **13**: 469–474.

24. James BD, Xie SX, Karlawish JHT. How do patients with Alzheimer's disease rate their overall quality of life? *Am J Geriatr Psychiatry* 2005; **13**: 484–490.

25. Behl P, Lanctot KL, Streiner DL, et al. Cholinesterase inhibitors slow decline in executive functions, rather than memory, in Alzheimer's disease: a 1-year observational study in Sunnybrook Dementia Court. *Curr Alzheimer Res* 2006; **3**: 147–156.

26. Thorgrimsen L, Selwood A, Spector A, et al. Whose quality of life is it anyway? The validity and reliability of the Quality of Life-Alzheimer's Disease (QoL-AD) Scale. *Alzheimer Dis Assoc Disord* 2003; **17**: 201–108.

27. Matsui T, Nakaaki S, Murata Y, et al. Determinants of the quality of life in Alzheimer's disease patients as assessed by the Japanese Version of the Quality of Life – Alzheimer's Disease scale. *Dement Geriatr Cogn Disord* 2006; **21**: 182–191.

28. Sands LP, Ferreira P, Stewart AL, et al. What explains differences between dementia patients' and their

caregivers' ratings of patient's quality of life? *Am J Geriatr Psychiatry* 2004; **12**: 272–280.

29. Snow AL, Dani R, Souchek J, et al. Comorbid psychosocial symptoms and quality of life in patients with dementia. *Am J Geriatr Psychiatry* 2005; **13**: 393–401.

30. Banerjee S, Samsi K, Petrie CD, et al. What do we know about quality of life in dementia? A review of the emerging evidence on the predictive and explanatory value of disease specific measures of health related quality of life in people with dementia. *Int J Geriatr Psychiatry* 2009; **24**: 15–24.

31. Hoe J, Hancock G, Livingston G, et al. Quality of life of people with dementia in residential care homes. *Br J Psychiatry* 2006; **188**: 468–464.

32. Smith SC, Lamping DL, Banerjee S, et al. Development of a new measure of health-related quality of life for people with dementia: DEMQOL. *Psychol Med* 2007; **37**: 737–746.

33. Rosenberg PB, Mielke MM, Lyketsos CG. Caregiver assessment of patients' depression in Alzheimer's disease: Longitudinal analysis in a drug treatment study. *Am J Geriatr Psychiatry* 2005; **13**: 822–826.

34. Arlt S, Hornung J, Eichenlaub M, et al. The patient with dementia, the caregiver and the doctor: Cognition, depression and quality of life from three perspectives. *Int J Geriatr Psychiatry* 2008; **23**: 604–610.

35. Sneeuw KCA, Aaronson NK, Osoba D, et al. The use of significant others as proxy raters of the quality of life of patients with brain cancer. *Med Care* 1997; **35**: 490–506.

36. Phillips WT, Alexander JL, Pepin V, et al. Cardiac rehabilitation patient versus proxy quality-of-life perceptions. *Clin Nurs Res* 2003; **12**: 282–293.

37. Kubler A, Winter S, Ludolph AC, et al. Severity of depressive symptoms and quality of life in patients with Amyotrophic Lateral Sclerosis. *Neurorehabil Neural Repair* 2005; **19**: 182–193.

38. Sandgren AK, Mullens AB, Erickson SC, et al. Confidant and breast cancer patient reports of quality of life. *Qual Life Res* 2004; **13**: 155–160.

39. Jones CA, Feeny DH. Agreement between patient and proxy responses of health-related quality of life after hip fracture. *J Am Geriatr Soc* 2005; **53**: 1227–1233.

40. Funder DC. Accuracy in personality judgment: Research and theory concerning an obvious question. In: Roberts BW, Hogan R, eds. *Personality Psychology in the Workplace*. Washington, DC: American Psychological Association, 2001.

41. Ready RE, Clark LA, Watson D, et al. Self- and peer-reported personality: agreement, trait ratability, and the "self-based heuristic." *J Res Personality* 2000; **34**: 208–224.

42. Droes R-M, Boelens-Van der Knoop ECC, Bos J, et al. Quality of life in dementia in perspective: an exploratory study of variations in opinions among people with dementia and their professional caregivers, and in literature. *Dementia* 2006; **5**: 533–558.

43. Spector A, Thorgrimsen L, Woods B, et al. Efficacy of an evidence-based cognitive stimulation therapy programme for people with dementia. *Br J Psychiatry* 2003; **183**: 248–254.

44. McCarney R, Fisher P, Iliffe S, et al. Ginkgo biloba for mild to moderate dementia in a community setting: a pragmatic, randomised, parallel-group, double-blind, placebo-controlled trial. *Int J Geriatr Psychiatry* 2008; **23**: 1222–1230.

45. Fuh JL, Wang SJ. Assessing quality of life in Taiwanese patients with Alzheimer's disease. *Int J Geriatr Psychiatry* 2006; **21**: 103–107.

46. Wolak A, Novella J-L, Drame M, et al. Transcultural adaptation and psychometric validation of a French-language version of the QoL-AD. *Citation only available. Aging Ment Health* 2009; **13**(4): 593–600.

47. Hao-ying H, Guo-dong M, Mou-ni T. Reliabilities and validities of the Quality of Life-Alzheimer's Disease (QOL-AD) scale. *Chin J Clin Psychol* 2005; **13**: 402–404.

48. Banerjee S, Smith SC, Lamping DL, et al. Quality of life in dementia: more than just cognition. An analysis of associations with quality of life in dementia. *J Neurol Neurosurg Psychiatry* 2006; **77**: 146–148.

49. Karim S, Ramanna G, Petit T, et al. Development of the Dementia Quality of Life questionnaire (D-QOL): UK version. *Aging Ment Health* 2008; **12**: 144–148.

50. Van Der Steen JT, van Campen C, Bosboom PR, et al. Quality of life and dementia. II. Selection of a measurement instrument for well-being appropriate for the reference model. *Tijdschrift voor Gerontologie an Geratrie* 2001; **32**: 259–264.

51. Suzuki M, Uchida A, Kanamori M, et al. Development of the Dementia Quality of Life Instrument-Japanese version. *Nippon Ronen Igakkai Zasshi* 2005; **42**.

52. Banerjee S. Commentary on "Health economics and the value of therapy in Alzheimer's disease." Quality of life in dementia: Development and use of a

disease-specific measure of health-related quality of life in dementia. *Alzheimer Dement* 2007; **3**: 166–171.

53. Ettema TP, Droes R-M, de Lange J, et al. QUALIDEM: development and evaluation of a dementia specific quality of life instrument. Scalability, reliability and internal structure. *Int J Geriatr Psychiatry* 2007; **22**: 549–556.

54. Bullinger M, Anderson R, Cella D, et al. Developing and evaluating cross-cultural instruments from minimum requirements to optimal models. *Qual Life Res* 1993; **2**: 451–459.

55. Koopmans RTCM, Van Der Molen M, Raats M, et al. Neuropsychiatric symptoms and quality of life in patients in the final phase of dementia. *Int J Geriatr Psychiatry* 2009; **24**: 25–32.

56. Kotler-Cope S, Camp CJ. Anosognosia in Alzheimer disease. *Alzheimer Dis Assoc Disord* 1995; **9**: 52–56.

57. Vasterling JJ, Seltzer B, Watrous WE. Longitudinal assessment of deficit unawareness in Alzheimer's disease. *Neuropsychiatry Neuropsychol Behav Neurol* 1997; **10**: 197–202.

58. Logsdon RG, Gibbons LE, McCurry SM, et al. Quality of life in Alzheimer's disease: patient and caregiver reports. *J Ment Health Aging* 1999; **5**: 21–32.

59. Ready RE, Ott BR, Grace J, et al. The Cornell-Brown Scale for Quality of Life in Dementia. *Alzheimer Dis Assoc Disord* 2002; **16**: 109–115.

60. Selai CE, Trimble MR, Rossor M, et al. Assessing quality of life in dementia: preliminary psychometric testing of the Quality of Life Assessment Schedule (QOLAS). *Neuropsychol Rehabil* 2001; **11**: 219–243.

61. Smith TL, Toseland RW, Rizzo VM, et al. Telephone caregiver support groups. *J Gerontol Social Work* 2004; **44**: 151–172.

62. Rabins PV. Measuring quality of life in persons with dementia. *Int Psychogeriatr* 2000; **12**: 47–49.

63. Rabins PV, Kasper JD, Kleinman L, et al. Concepts and methods in the development of the ADRQL: an instrument for assessing health-related quality of life in persons with Alzheimer's disease. *J Ment Health Aging* 1999; **5**: 33–48.

64. Fossey J, Lee L, Ballard C. Dementia care mapping as a research tool for measuring quality of life in care setting: psychometric properties. *Int J Geriatr Psychiatry* 2002; **17**: 1064–1070.

65. Brooker D, Foster N, Banner A, et al. The efficacy of dementia care mapping as an audit tool: report of a 3-year British NHS evaluation. *Aging Ment Health* 1998; **2**: 60–70.

66. Beavis D, Simpson S, Graham I. A literature review of dementia care mapping: methodological considerations and efficacy. *J Psychiatr Ment Health Nurs* 2002; **9**: 725–736.

67. Albert SM, Castillo-Castanada C, Jacobs DM, et al. Proxy-reported quality of life in Alzheimer's patients: comparison of clinical and population-based samples. *J Ment Health Aging* 1999; **5**: 49–58.

68. Albert SM, Castillo-Castaneda CD, Sano M, et al. Quality of life in patients with Alzheimer's disease as reported by patient proxies. *J Am Geriatr Soc* 1996; **44**: 1342–1347.

69. Albert SM, Jacobs DM, Sano M, et al. Longitudinal study of quality of life in people with advanced Alzheimer's disease. *Am J Geriatr Psychiatry* 2001; **9**: 160–168.

70. Weiner MF, Martin-Cook K, Svetlik DA, et al. The Quality of Life in Late-Stage Dementia (QUALID) Scale. *J Am Med Dir Assoc* 2000; **1**: 114–116.

9

Condition-specific instruments to measure the quality of life (QoL) of children and adolescents with cerebral palsy (CP)

Elizabeth Waters, Amy Shelly, and Elise Davis

Introduction

Cerebral palsy (CP) is the leading cause of physical disability in children. Defined as "a group of permanent disorders of the development of movement and posture" (1), CP occurs in approximately 2 to 2.5 per 1,000 live births (2). In recent years, the concept of good health has moved from the "absence of disease" to a more positive concept, which embraces quality of life (QoL). QoL is a multi-dimensional construct including both health (i.e., physical health, emotional health, social health) and nonhealth domains (i.e., finances, school, autonomy) (3). In pediatrics and child health, there is growing awareness that mortality and morbidity are not the only important outcome variables to be considered. Within the area of childhood CP, clinicians and researchers are more aware than ever that CP-related interventions need to go beyond treating physical functioning and must take a holistic approach to increase a child's QoL.

What is CP?

Cerebral palsy is the most common physical disability in childhood. Caused by "nonprogressive disturbances that occurred in the developing fetal or infant brain" (1), CP is characterized by limited functional ability and is often accompanied by "disturbances of sensation, perception, cognition, communication, and behavior, by epilepsy, and by secondary musculoskeletal problems" (1). During the past three decades, cases of CP have been on the increase, likely because of advances in neonatal care and improved documentation of confirmed cases (4). The costs of medical care for disabled children have been estimated to be 2.5 to 20 times the average costs of caring for nondisabled children (5).

The severity of CP ranges from mild to severe motor impairment (6). CP is generally categorized using the Gross Motor Function Classification System (GMFCS) (7). Although placing emphasis on sitting and walking, this classification system also distinguishes between functional limitations, the need for assistive technology, and, to a lesser extent, the quality of self-initiated movement (7). The GMFCS is classified into five age-specific categories (i.e., 0 to 2 years, 2 to 4 years, 4 to 6 years, 6 to 12 years), with I being mild impairment (i.e., can walk unaided) and V being severe impairment (i.e., has difficulty controlling head and body posture in most positions) (7). Treatment of the motor disorder alone may involve a range of therapies and interventions such as physiotherapy, the use of orthoses, orthopedic surgery, and medications for spasticity such as Botulinum toxin A (BTX-A) and oral and intrathecal baclofen (8).

Quality of Life Measurement in Neurodegenerative and Related Conditions, eds., Crispin Jenkinson, Michele Peters, and Mark B. Bromberg. Published by Cambridge University Press. © Cambridge University Press 2011.

QoL versus health-related QoL

To date, there is no universally accepted definition of QoL, and as such, QoL is variously defined. One commonly cited definition of QoL is the World Health Organization's definition, which states that QoL is "the individual's perception of their position in life, in the context of culture and value systems in which they live and in relation to their goals, expectations, standards and concerns" (9). Although many researchers adopt this definition, others often develop their own definitions for child QoL, such as "QoL includes, but is not limited to the social, physical and emotional functioning of the child, and when indicated, his or her family, and it must be sensitive to the changes that occur throughout development" (10). Although there are many different definitions, one core theme is that QoL refers to satisfaction with a variety of domains, including both health and nonhealth domains (3).

Within child QOL literature, there is often confusion between QoL and health-related QoL (HRQoL). Like QoL, there is currently no universally accepted definition of HRQoL; however, HRQoL has been defined as "a multidimensional functional effect of an illness or a medical condition and its consequent therapy upon the child" (11). It is useful to look at the definitions in adult QoL literature to distinguish between QoL and HRQoL. QoL generally refers to satisfaction with a range of domains such as physical well-being, emotional well-being, intimacy, material well-being, productivity, community, and safety (12), whereas HRQoL refers to individual perceptions of health (13). Therefore, it is reasonable to conceptualize HRQoL as a subset of the more global construct of QoL (14).

Why are researchers and clinicians interested in QoL?

More recently, QoL and HRQoL have become core outcome variables in clinical (15) and public health research for children with CP (15, 16, 17, 18, 19, 20, 21, 22). Within the area of childhood CP, as in other areas of pediatrics and child health, awareness is growing that traditional outcome measures such as survival or reduction of symptoms do not capture the range of ways in which a child may be affected by illness or treatment. Inclusion of outcomes such as measures of QoL and HRQoL is gaining increasing importance.

A range of medical and public health population-based interventions are now available for children and adolescents with CP. Over the past decade, the need to demonstrate empirically that interventions are effective in improving the QoL of children and adolescents with CP has gained increasing recognition. As such, a range of outcome measures are now available; however, they are often focused on outcomes at the level of body structure and physical function. These outcomes on their own are inadequate for evaluating medical interventions that have an impact not only on symptoms but on a child's whole life. For example, some interventions may result in discomfort, pain, inconvenience, or embarrassment for the child, as well as increased well-being, self-esteem, and happiness or improved sleeping. Furthermore, research suggests that, although physical function has been shown to be correlated with the physical domains of QoL, there is only a weak or nonsignificant relationship between physical function and the psychosocial domains of QoL (16, 23, 24). Therefore, there is increasing awareness that, in addition to measures of physical function, QoL instruments must measure other facets of a child's life such as emotional and social well-being.

Measuring QoL for children with CP

The area of QoL measurement for children in general as well as for children with CP remains underdeveloped. Unique challenges in measuring the QoL of children and adolescents may be further complicated if the child or adolescent has a disability such as CP (i.e., communication difficulties). Researchers have been hesitant to apply the principles and definitions of adult QoL to child QoL given consensus that the language and content of children's QoL measures need to be appropriate to children's development and experiences (25).

Generic versus condition-specific instruments

Two major types of instruments are commonly recommended and available to measure QoL: generic and condition-specific. Generic instruments are designed to be applicable to all population subgroups and are useful for comparing outcomes of subgroups (15) such as the QoL of children with CP compared with the QoL of children with diabetes. They are not as useful when evaluating the effectiveness of interventions for children with a specific illness or disability such as CP because they do not include domains that are specific to the illness or disability (i.e., symptoms, pain and discomfort, communication). Hence, if a child with CP completed a generic QoL instrument, the scores might not completely capture QoL because some important domains that have an impact on his or her life (i.e., medication) would not be assessed. Condition-specific instruments are designed to be applicable to one illness/disease (i.e., children with CP) and are useful for detecting small changes in a condition following an intervention (15). Because condition-specific instruments include domains that are specific to an illness, it is more likely that, if a change occurs as the result of an intervention, it will be detected. Increasingly, instrument developers are producing QoL instruments that have both a generic core and additional condition-specific modules. This allows comparisons between condition-specific groups and the general population.

Child self-report versus parent-proxy report

Although in the adult QoL literature, self-report questionnaires are regarded as the primary method of assessing QoL, in the child QoL literature, it is proposed that parents may be more capable of rating some aspects of their child's QoL than the children themselves because of children's cognitive immaturity, limited social experience, and continued dependency. Instrument developers are now producing child/adolescent self-report and parent-proxy report versions of instruments to allow for both proxy and self-report (i.e., Cerebral Palsy Quality of Life Questionnaire for Children; proxy-report for children aged 4 to 12 years; and self-report for children aged 9 to 12 years). A majority of child self-report instruments start around the age of 8 to 9 years. The explanation for starting around this age stems from Piaget's theory that at 7 years of age, children are in their preoperational stage of development, which means that their understanding is limited by their inability to carry out a variety of logical operations (26), limiting their ability to self-report.

Although it is generally accepted that parents are able to estimate their child's well-being (daily monitoring of a child's well-being can alert parents to small behavioral changes or physical symptoms), parents may easily overestimate or underestimate the importance their child's attributes to certain aspects of his or her well-being at a specific point in time. For example, peer-related issues may be far more important to an adolescent than parents might think they are. Furthermore, parental views of their child's current health state and QoL may be influenced by their expectations and previous experiences with their child.

Research has begun to examine the level of concordance between proxy and child self-report scores. A recent systematic review found that 14 studies assessing the relationship between parent-proxy and child self-reported QoL demonstrated that the level of agreement between parents and children is dependent on the domain (27). Overall there was good agreement (correlations >0.5) between parents and children for domains reflecting physical activity, physical function, and symptoms; however, poor agreement (correlations <0.30) was found for domains that reflected more social or emotional domains.

Within the area of CP, difficulties may arise when only parent-proxy data can be collected for a variety of reasons such as the child's age, severity of illness, type of disease, cognitive ability, or communication ability. It is important to understand how and why scores differ between proxy and self-reported QoL, especially when parent/proxy-reported QoL is used to guide clinical decisions.

Parents and children may report QoL differently for numerous reasons. Parents and children may reflect about different events that have happened or may interpret events differently. Additionally, parents and children may use different response styles (i.e., approach questions, items, response scales). Finally, parents and children may also differ in their understanding and interpretation of the items. A recent qualitative study conducted with parents and children to examine possible reasons for discordance found that the major reasons for discordance were that parents and children were providing different reasons for the answers and had different response styles (28).

Condition-specific measures of QoL for children and adolescents with CP DISABKIDS CP disease module

DISABKIDS is designed to measure HRQoL and includes a generic module, a chronic generic module, and condition-specific modules (29). The generic module is the KIDSCREEN, a HRQoL instrument that has both self-report and proxy report versions. It is designed to measure the HRQoL of healthy and chronically ill children and adolescents aged 8 to 18 years. The chronic generic module is suitable for use with children and adolescents who suffer from any chronic medical condition. The condition-specific modules are called the DISABKIDS Disease Modules and include instruments for arthritis, asthma, atopic dermatitis, cerebral palsy, cystic fibrosis, diabetes, and epilepsy (29). The DISABKIDS CP Disease Module includes 14 disease-specific questions focused on the domain impact of the condition, as well as two additional items on communication about the condition (29). Early analysis suggests that the DISABKIDS CP Disease Module has good internal consistency, ranging from 0.72 to 0.82; however this must be further explored given the small sample size used (n = 43) (29).

Caregiver priorities and Child Health Index of Life with Disabilities (CPCHILD)

The CPCHILD is a condition-specific instrument for children and adolescents aged 5 to 18 years with severe CP (30). It focuses on measuring caregivers' perspective of the activity limitations, health status, well-being, and ease of care of their children. It consists of 37 items in six sections: personal care; positioning, transfers, and mobility; communication and social interaction; comfort, emotions, and behavior; health; and overall QoL. Items are rated on degree of difficulty ("no problem" to "impossible") and level of assistance ("independent" to "total assistance"). Early analysis of the CPCHILD suggests that it has sound psychometric properties, where 2-week test-retest reliability ranged from $r = 0.88$ to $r = 0.96$ (30).

Although the CPCHILD purports to measure QoL, many of its domains are measures of functioning. The CPCHILD includes items such as how difficult is it for the adolescent to eat or be fed, have a bath, and move about in the house (30). Additionally, this instrument actually measures perspectives of the caregiver rather than those of the child, limiting its usefulness as an instrument intended to measure the QoL of children and adolescents with CP.

Pediatric QoL Inventory (PedsQL) – CP Module

The Pediatric QoL Inventory – CP Module (PedsQL – CP Module) (31) is a condition-specific HRQoL instrument for children and adolescents with CP. Available in both proxy and self-report versions (5+ years), the PedsQL – CP Module is available for children aged 2 to 4 years, 5 to 7 years, and 8 to 12 years, and for adolescents aged 13 to 18 years. The instrument provides seven domain scores, including daily activities, school activities, movement and balance, pain and hurt, fatigue, eating activities, and speech and communication (31). The PedsQL – CP Module has good internal consistency ranging from 0.79 to 0.91 (31).

When using the PedsQL – CP Module to measure QoL, researchers and clinicians must be aware that it measures physical function rather than feelings about life. For example, the PedsQL – CP Module assesses daily activities according to whether adolescents can put on their own shoes, button their own shirt, and brush their own hair, whereas social activities are measured by whether an adolescent has difficulty using scissors and difficulty writing or drawing with a pen (31).

Cerebral Palsy Quality of Life Questionnaire for Children (CP QoL-Child)

The CP QoL-Child is designed to measure the QoL of children with CP aged 4 to 12 years (22). This questionnaire, consistent with Bjornson and McLaughlin's definition of QoL (15), is designed to assess well-being rather than ill-being. Three features are notable about the design of the questionnaire: (1) it is based on the International Classification of Function (ICF); (2) it has been developed with international expertise; and (3) it recognizes the importance of obtaining the views of the child and primary caregivers in developing and completing the questionnaire. Two versions of CP QoL – Child are available: a child self-report version (9+ years) and a parent-proxy version. The parent-proxy version assesses seven domains of QoL, including social well-being and acceptance, feelings about functioning, participation and physical health, emotional well-being, access to services, pain, and feeling about disability and family health. The child self-report version assesses all of the above domains except access to services and family health. Almost all of the items have the following

item stem: "How do you think your child feels about..." with a 9-point rating scale, where 1 = very unhappy, 3 = unhappy, 5 = neither happy nor unhappy, 7 = happy, and 9 = very happy. The few items where this stem or rating scale is not appropriate, such as pain, have the stem and rating scale (e.g., "How does your child feel about the amount of pain that they have?"), where 1 = not upset at all to 9 = very upset. The parent-proxy version of this questionnaire is psychometrically sound, and early results of the child self-report version suggest that it has good psychometric properties (22).

Development of the CP QoL – Child

The CP QoL-Child was developed in two stages. First, qualitative thematic analysis was undertaken to determine the themes of QoL relevant for children with CP aged 4 to 12 years, followed by the piloting of the draft CP QoL – Child with children with CP, their parents, and health professionals. And second, the psychometric properties of the CP QoL – Child were tested.

Thematic analysis and piloting of the CP QoL – Child

The first stage of development of the CP QoL – Child involved qualitative interviews with primary caregivers and children (3), reviewing and developing items and response scales used in other QoL questionnaires (32), and piloting the CP QoL – Child using interviews with both primary caregivers and children as well as with health professionals (3). A sample of 28 families was purposely selected from the Victorian Cerebral Palsy Register maintained by the Department of Developmental Medicine at the Royal Children's Hospital, Melbourne, Australia (33). The sample was representative of age, functional severity, socioeconomic status, and geographic location. Functional severity was classified by the GMFCS (7). Of the 28 families who participated in the study, 16 were parents of children aged 4 to 8 years and 12 were parents of children aged 9 to 12 years. Of 12 children who could possibly be involved in self-report, five children with mild impairment were able to be involved (3). Interview questions were derived from a review of the QoL literature. The questions were designed to prompt discussion and elicit new information relevant to QoL.

Interviews with children and parents provided significant information about the daily lives of children with cerebral palsy and their families. Thirteen themes of QoL were extracted from discussions with parents and children about their child's life (3). According to families, to have a high QoL, children need to have the following:

- *Physical health* – refers to adequate gross motor skills and fine motor skills, the ability to use aides (if required), and good overall physical health.
- *Absence of body pain and discomfort* – refers to absence of stiffness and soreness in joints and pain associated with therapy.
- *Daily living tasks* – refers to the ability to carry out normal daily living tasks, including dressing, feeding, and toileting, and being independent.
- *Participation in regular physical and social activities* – refers to participating in school activities, sporting activities, and community activities.
- *Emotional well-being and self-esteem* – refers to being happy, being able to achieve goals, and being satisfied with one's body and emotions.
- *Interaction with the community* – refers to being socially accepted, being a valued member of the community, and being treated "normally."
- *Communication* – refers to having good communication skills with family, peers, and people in the general community.
- *Family health* – refers to good parental emotional health, good family relations, and few restrictions on the family to go out socially.
- *Supportive physical environment* – refers to a supportive school environment, family environment, and community environment. These environments need to have the required equipment and devices.
- *Future QoL* – refers to having the opportunities to do everything that they desire, being able to do

things as well as their peers, and being able to make choices in their life.
- *Provision of, and access to, services* – refers to having access to therapy, respite, and having the support required.
- *Financial stability* – refers to the earning capacity of parents and the ability to cover the expenses of equipment and treatment.
- *Social well-being* – refers to the ability to interact with family members, peers, and people in the general community.

Consultations with children with cerebral palsy and their parents about their QoL provided some insight into the daily lives of such families and confirmed and enhanced the previous evidence-based impression of the key themes of QoL. Although all domains of health identified by the WHO, including physical well-being, mental well-being, and social well-being emerged as themes, these were complemented by themes that were specific to children, such as family health, and themes that were specific to cerebral palsy, including body pain and discomfort, daily living tasks, and communication (3). The remaining themes differed somewhat from the traditional QoL literature and included satisfaction with access to services, supportive physical environments, financial stability of the family, and acceptance in the broader community, appearing to address the practicalities of having a child with cerebral palsy (36). Items included in the CP QoL – Child were based on these themes.

Psychometric analysis of the CP QoL – Child

The aim of this study was to explore the dimensional structure of the CP QoL – Child and then to examine construct validity (using other measures of QoL, health, and functioning), internal consistency, and test-retest reliability (22). It was anticipated that scores on the CP QoL – Child would be moderately positively correlated with other measures of QoL, health, and functioning, contributing evidence to its validity. Given that only a proportion of children in the study were able to complete the questionnaire because of their age or severity of impairment, the factor structure was explored using primary caregiver-proxy data. This factor structure was used to construct scales for the child self-report data. The relationship between primary caregiver-proxy and child self-report scores was examined, and it was hypothesized that their scores would be moderately correlated.

Of 695 families of children with CP aged 4 to 12 years on the Victorian Cerebral Palsy Register, 205 families agreed to participate. Questionnaire I was completed by 205 primary caregivers. Because only a proportion of children were able to complete the questionnaire given their age and severity of impairment, 53 children aged 9 to 12 years completed questionnaire I. One hundred and twenty families were allocated to the 2-week retest group, and 105 families to the 2-month retest group. Of the first group (the 2-week retest group), 110 out of 120 families returned questionnaire I (91%) and 86 returned questionnaire II (78%). Of the second group (the 2-month retest group), 95 of 105 families returned questionnaire I (86%) and 85 returned questionnaire II (89%). Two questionnaires were given to parents. The first questionnaire included demographic questions, child QoL (CP QoL – Child and KIDSCREEN (34)), child health (Child Health Questionnaire, CHQ (35)), and functioning (Gross Motor Function Classification System, GMFCS). The second questionnaire included the CP QoL – Child and questions on life events (22).

The CP QoL – Child is designed to provide several domain scores, and items, therefore, are aggregated and averaged. Domain scores range from 0 to 100. The parent-proxy version of this questionnaire is psychometrically sound, whereas early results of the child self-report version suggest that it has good psychometric properties (22). For parent-proxy, the 2-week test-retest reliability ranged from r=0.76 to 0.89, and internal consistency ranged from 0.74 to 0.92 (22). The questionnaire was also moderately correlated with the CHQ (35) and KIDSCREEN (34), supporting the validity of the CP QoL – Child parent-proxy version.

A review of condition-specific (n = 25) and generic (n = 14) QoL questionnaires for children demonstrated that the most common domains of QoL are those that refer to emotions, social interactions, physical health/functioning, symptoms, medical/treatment, cognition, activities, school, family, independence/autonomy, pain, behavior, future, leisure, and body image (32). The seven domains that were identified in the CP QoL – Child are comparable to the domains used in other QoL questionnaires, as demonstrated by this review. It is encouraging that the domains identified for the CP QoL – Child are similar to other instruments, which are often based on the opinions of clinicians, given that this instrument was primarily based on interviews with primary caregivers and children.

A separate principal components analysis is currently under way to examine the structure of the child self-report questionnaire; however, early results suggest that the structure of the primary caregiver questionnaire and the child questionnaire may be similar. Consistent with past QoL studies (27), good concordance was found between primary caregiver proxy and child self-report data (r = 0.52–Q.77). Past studies have suggested that there is better agreement (>0.5) between primary caregivers and children for domains on physical health, functioning, and symptoms, and poorer agreement (<0.30) for domains on social or emotional issues (27). Although this expected variation across domains was not observed in this study, further analyses with a larger sample are required.

The CP QoL – Child is the first condition-specific QoL measure for children with CP that is designed to assess well-being. It can be used to gain further understanding about the determinants of QoL and, once sensitivity to change is established, it can be used to evaluate the effectiveness of interventions for children with CP.

Conclusion

The use of QoL as an outcome measure for children and adolescents with CP is essential within

Table 9.1. Comparison of condition-specific instruments for children and adolescents with CP

Instrument	DISABKIDS-CP Module	The Caregiver Priorities and Child Health Index of Life with Disabilities (CPCHILD)	Pediatric QoL Inventory (PedsQL)-CP Module	Cerebral Palsy Quality of Life Questionnaire for Children (CP QoL-Child)
Purpose of instrument	Health-related QoL	Caregiver perspectives of activity limitation, health status, well-being, and ease of care	Health-related QoL	QoL
Country of origin	Europe (7 countries)	Canada	USA	Australia
Age range (years)	8–18	5–18	2–18	4–12
Proxy report	Yes	Yes	Yes	Yes
Self-report (age)	Yes (8+)	No	Yes (5+)	Yes (9+)
GMFCS level	I-V	IV and V	I-V	I-V
Number of items	16	36	35	52 (self-report), 66 (proxy report)
Domains	Generic module, a chronic generic module, and a condition-specific module	Personal care; positioning, transfers, and mobility; communication and comfort, emotions and behavior; health; and overall QoL	Daily activities, school activities, movement and balance, pain and hurt, fatigue, eating activities, and speech and communication	Social well-being and acceptance, functioning, participation and physical health, emotional well-being, access to services, pain and feelings about disability and family health
Reliability/validity tested for CP	Yes (29)	Yes (30)	Yes (31)	Yes (22)
Sensitivity to change	No	No	No	No

pediatric and child health. The measurement of QoL within child health and, more specifically, within the area of childhood CP has gained significant advancement within the last decade. Although several condition-specific instruments are now in use for children and adolescents with CP, researchers and clinicians must understand the challenges associated with measuring the QoL of children and adolescents while understanding the limitations of some QoL instruments. Continued exploration of the QoL of children and adolescents with CP is essential, not only to inform intervention devel-

opment aimed at improving QoL, but also to assist program and service planning and delivery (Table 9.1).

REFERENCES

1. Rosenbaum P, Paneth N, Leviton A, Goldstein M, Bax M, Damiano D, Dan B, Jacobsson B. A report: the definition and classification of cerebral palsy April 2006. *Dev Med Child Neurol* 2007; **109**: 8–14.

2. Blair E, Watson L, Badawi N, Stanley FJ. Life expectancy among people with cerebral palsy in Western Australia. *Dev Med Child Neurol* 2001; **43**: 508–515.

3. Waters E, Maher E, Salmon L, Reddihough D, Boyd R. Development of a condition-specific measure of quality of life for children with cerebral palsy: empirical thematic data reported by parents and children. *Child Care Hlth Dev* 2005; **31**(2): 127–135.

4. Rumeau-Rouquette C, Grandjean H, Cans C, du Mazaubrum C, Verrier A. Prevalence and time trends of disabilities in school-age children. *Int J Epidemiol* 1997; **26**: 137–145.

5. Brehaut JC, Kohen DE, Raina P, Walter SD, Russell DJ, Swinton M, O'Donnell M, Rosenbaum P. The health of primary caregivers of children with cerebral palsy: how does it compare with that of other Canadian caregivers? *Pediatrics* 2004; **114**(2): e182–e191.

6. Koman LA, Smith BP, Shilt JS. Cerebral palsy. *Lancet* 2004; **363**(9421): 1619–1631.

7. Palisano R, Rosenbaum P, Walter S, Russell D, Wood E, Galuppi B. Development and reliability of a system to classify gross motor function in children with cerebral palsy. *Dev Med Child Neurol* 1997; **39**: 214–223.

8. Boyd RN, Hays RM. Current evidence for the use of botulinum toxin type A in the management of children with cerebral palsy: a systematic review. *Eur J Neurol* 2001; **8**: 1–20.

9. Division of Mental Health, World Health Organization. *Measuring Quality of Life: The Development of the World Health Organization Quality of Life Instrument (WHOQOL)*. Geneva, Switzerland: World Health Organization; 1993.

10. Bradlyn AS, Ritchey AC, Harris CV, Moore IM, O'Brien RT, Parsons SK, Patterson K, Pollock BH. Quality of life research in pediatric oncology: research methods and barriers. *Cancer* 1996; **78**: 1333–1339.

11. Ronen GM, Rosenbaum P, Law M. Health-related quality of life in childhood disorders: a modified focus group technique to involve children. *Qual Life Res* 2001; **10**: 71–79.

12. Cummins RA, Eckersley R, Pallant J, Misajon R. Developing a national index of subjective wellbeing: the Australian Unity Wellbeing Index. *Soc Indic Res* 2004; **64**(2): 159–190.

13. Irrgang JJ, Anderson AF. Development and validation of health-related quality of life measures of the knee. *Clin Orthop* 2002; **1**: 95–109.

14. Spilker B, Revicki DA. Taxonomy of quality of life, In: Spilker B, ed. *Quality of Life and Pharmacoeconomics*. Philadelphia: Lippincott-Raven, 1996; 25–31.

15. Bjornson KF, McLaughlin JF. The measurement of health-related quality of life (HRQL) in children with cerebral palsy. *Eur J Neurol* 2001; **8**: 183–193.

16. Vargus-Adams J. Health-related quality of life in childhood cerebral palsy. *Arch Phys Med Rehabil* 2005; **86**(5): 940–945.

17. Varni JW, Burwinkle TM, Sherman SA, Hanna K, Berrin SJ, Malcarne VL, Chambers HG. Health-related quality of life of children and adolescents with cerebral palsy: hearing the voices of the children. *Dev Med Child Neurol* 2005; **47**(9): 592–597.

18. Hodgkinson I, d'Anjou MC, Dazord A, Berard C. Quality of life of a population of 54 ambulatory children with cerebral palsy: a cross-sectional study. *Ann Readaptation Med Physique* 2002; **45**(4): 154.

19. Tüzün E, Eker L, Daskapan A. An assessment of the impact of cerebral palsy on children's quality of life. *Fizyoterapi Rehabilitasyon* 2004; **15**(1): 3–8.

20. Dickinson HO, Parkinson KN, Ravens-Sieberer U, Schirripa G, Thyen U, Arnaud C, Beckung E, Fauconnier J, McManus V, Michelsen SI, Parkes J, Colver AF. Self-reported quality of life of 8–12-year-old children with cerebral palsy: a cross-sectional European study. *Lancet* 2007; **369**(9580): 2171–2178.

21. Shelly A, Davis E, Waters E. Measuring the quality of life (QOL) of children with cerebral palsy (CP): comparing the conceptual underpinnings and psychometric properties of three instruments. *Dev Med Child Neurol* (Submitted Oct 2007).

22. Waters E, Davis E, Boyd R, Reddihough D, Graham HK, Mackinnon A, Lo SK, Wolfe R, Stevenson R, Bjornson K, Blair E, Hoare P, Ravens-Sieberer U. Cerebral Palsy Quality of Life Questionnaire for Children (CP QOL – Child): psychometric properties of parent proxy questionnaire. *Dev Med Child Neurol* 2007; **49**(1): 49–55.

23. Shelly A, Davis E, Waters E, Mackinnon A, Reddihough D, Boyd R, et al. The relationship between quality of life (QOL) and functioning for children with cerebral palsy: does poor functioning equate with poor QOL? *Dev Med Child Neurol* 2007; **50**(3): 199–203.

24. Pirpiris M. Function and well-being in ambulatory children with cerebral palsy. *J Pediatr Orthop* 2006; **26**(1): 119–124.

25. Gerharz EW, Eiser C, Woodhouse CRJ. Current approaches to assessing the quality of life in children and adolescents. *BJU International* 2003; **91**: 150–154.

26. Piaget J. *The Child's Conception of the World*. New York: Harcourt, Brace Jovanovich, 1929.

27. Eiser C, Morse R. Can parents rate their child's health-related quality of life? Results of a systematic review. *Qual Life Res* 2001; **10**: 347–357.

28. Davis E, Nicolas C, Waters E, Cook K, Gibbs L, Gosch A, Ravens-Sieberer U. Parent-proxy and child self-reported health-related quality of life: using qualitative methods to explain the discordance. *Qual Life Res* 2007; **16**(5): 863–871.

29. Baars RM, Atherton CI, Koopman HM, Bullinger M, Power M. The European DISABKIDS project: development of seven condition-specific modules to measure health related quality of life in children and adolescents. *Health Qual Life Outcomes* 2005; **3**: 70.

30. Narayanan UG, Fehlings D, Weir S, Knights S, Kiran S, Campbell K. Initial development and validation of the Caregiver Priorities and Child Health Index of Life with Disabilities (CPCHILD). *Dev Med Child Neurol* 2006; **48**(10): 804–812.

31. Varni JW, Burwinkle TM, Berrin SJ, Sherman SA, Artavia K, Malcarne VL, Chambers HG. The PedsQL in pediatric cerebral palsy: reliability, validity, and sensitivity of the Generic Core Scales and Cerebral Palsy Module. *Dev Med Child Neurol* 2006; **48**(6): 442–449.

32. Davis E, Waters E, Mackinnon A, Reddihough D, Graham HK, Mehmet-Radji O, Boyd R. Paediatric quality of life instruments: a review of the impact of the conceptual framework on outcomes. *Dev Med Child Neurol* 2006; **48**: 311–318.

33. Reid S, Lanigan A, Alstab J, Reddihough D. *Third Report of the Victorian Cerebral Palsy Register*. Melbourne: Department of Child Development and Rehabilitation, Murdoch Childrens Research Institute, Royal Children's Hospital; 2005.

34. Ravens-Sieberer U, Gosch A, Rajmil L, Erhart M, Bruil J, Duer W, Auquier P, Power M, Abel T, Czemy L, Mazur J, Czimbalmos A, Tountas Y, Hagquist C, Kilroe J. KIDSCREEN-52 quality-of-life measure for children and adolescents. *Expert Rev Pharmacoeconomics Outcomes Res* 2005; **5**(3): 353–356.

35. Landgraf JM, Abetz L, Ware JA. *The CHQ User's Manual*. First edition. Boston: The Health Institute, New England Medical Centre, 1996.

Appendix 1: CP QOL-Child (Proxy)

Cerebral Palsy
Quality of Life Questionnaire for Children (CP QOL-Child)

Primary Caregiver Questionnaire (4-12 years)

We want to ask you some questions about how you think your child FEELS about aspects of their life such as family, friends, health and school. Each question begins with "How do you think your child FEELS about.....?"

It is important for you to report how you believe your child feels. Sometimes it is difficult to know how your child is feeling. Please just try and answer as best as you can.

For each question we want you to (circle) the best number that shows how you think your child FEELS. You can circle any number from 1 (Very unhappy) to 9 (Very happy).

This questionnaire is measuring how your child feels, not what they can do.

How do you think your child feels about ...

	Very Unhappy	Unhappy	Neither happy nor unhappy	Happy	Very Happy
their ability to play games with other children	1 2	3 4	5 6	(7) 8	9

How do you think your child feels about ...

Friends and family

	Very Unhappy	Unhappy	Neither happy nor unhappy	Happy	Very Happy
the way they get along with people, generally?	1 2	3 4	5 6	7 8	9
the way they get along with you?	1 2	3 4	5 6	7 8	9
the way they get along with their brothers and sisters? OR ☐ My child does not have any brothers or sisters	1 2	3 4	5 6	7 8	9
the way they get along with other children at preschool or school? (If your child attends more than one school, please think about the school where your child spends the most time). OR ☐ My child does not attend preschool or school	1 2	3 4	5 6	7 8	9
the way they get along with other children outside of preschool or school?	1 2	3 4	5 6	7 8	9
the way they get along with adults?	1 2	3 4	5 6	7 8	9
the way they get along with their teachers and/or carers?	1 2	3 4	5 6	7 8	9
their ability to play on their own?	1 2	3 4	5 6	7 8	9
their ability to play with friends?	1 2	3 4	5 6	7 8	9
going out on trips with the family?	1 2	3 4	5 6	7 8	9
how they are accepted by their family?	1 2	3 4	5 6	7 8	9
how they are accepted by other children at preschool or school? (If your child attends more than one school, please think about the school where your child spends the most time). OR ☐ My child does not attend preschool or school	1 2	3 4	5 6	7 8	9

Cerebral Palsy **Quality of Life Questionnaire for Children** (CP QOL-Child)

Primary Caregiver Questionnaire (4-12 years)

How do you think your child feels about ...

	Very Unhappy		Unhappy		Neither happy nor unhappy		Happy		Very Happy
how they are accepted by other children outside of preschool or school?	1	2	3	4	5	6	7	8	9
how they are accepted by adults?	1	2	3	4	5	6	7	8	9
how they are accepted by people in general?	1	2	3	4	5	6	7	8	9
being able to do the things they want to do?	1	2	3	4	5	6	7	8	9

Participation

	Very Unhappy		Unhappy		Neither happy nor unhappy		Happy		Very Happy
their ability to participate at preschool or school? (If your child attends more than one school, please think about the school where your child spends the most time) OR ☐ My child does not attend preschool or school	1	2	3	4	5	6	7	8	9
their ability to participate in recreational activities?	1	2	3	4	5	6	7	8	9
their ability to participate in sporting activities? (this question is asking how your child feels about their ability to participate in sport, not whether they can participate).	1	2	3	4	5	6	7	8	9
their ability to participate in social events outside of preschool or school?	1	2	3	4	5	6	7	8	9
their ability to participate in their community?	1	2	3	4	5	6	7	8	9

Communication

	Very Unhappy		Unhappy		Neither happy nor unhappy		Happy		Very Happy
the way they communicate with people they know well? (using any means of communication)	1	2	3	4	5	6	7	8	9
the way they communicate with people they don't know well? (using any means of communication)	1	2	3	4	5	6	7	8	9
the way other people communicate with them?	1	2	3	4	5	6	7	8	9

Health

	Very Unhappy		Unhappy		Neither happy nor unhappy		Happy		Very Happy
their physical health?	1	2	3	4	5	6	7	8	9
the way they get around?	1	2	3	4	5	6	7	8	9
how they sleep?	1	2	3	4	5	6	7	8	9
the way they look?	1	2	3	4	5	6	7	8	9
their ability to keep up academically with their peers?	1	2	3	4	5	6	7	8	9
their ability to keep up physically with their peers?	1	2	3	4	5	6	7	8	9
their life in general?	1	2	3	4	5	6	7	8	9
themselves?	1	2	3	4	5	6	7	8	9
their future?	1	2	3	4	5	6	7	8	9
their opportunities in life?	1	2	3	4	5	6	7	8	9

Cerebral Palsy **Quality of Life Questionnaire for Children** (CP QOL-Child)

Primary Caregiver Questionnaire (4-12 years)

The next 3 questions are asking how your child feels about using parts of their body, not whether your child can use part of their body.

How do you think your child feels about ...

	Very Unhappy		Unhappy		Neither happy nor unhappy		Happy		Very Happy
the way they use their arms?	1	2	3	4	5	6	7	8	9
the way they use their legs?	1	2	3	4	5	6	7	8	9
the way they use their hands?	1	2	3	4	5	6	7	8	9

The next 3 questions are asking how your child feels about their ability to complete daily activities, not whether your child can complete the activities.

How do you think your child feels about ...

	Very Unhappy		Unhappy		Neither happy nor unhappy		Happy		Very Happy
their ability to dress themselves?	1	2	3	4	5	6	7	8	9
their ability to eat or drink independently?	1	2	3	4	5	6	7	8	9
their ability to use the toilet by themselves?	1	2	3	4	5	6	7	8	9

Special Equipment

	Very Unhappy		Unhappy		Neither happy nor unhappy		Happy		Very Happy
the special equipment they have at home? (eg. special seating, standing frames, wheelchairs, walkers) OR ☐ My child does not need any special equipment at home	1	2	3	4	5	6	7	8	9
the special equipment they have at their school? (eg. special seating, standing frames, wheelchairs, walkers) OR ☐ My child does not need any special equipment at school	1	2	3	4	5	6	7	8	9
the special equipment that is available in the community? (ramps, escalators, wheelchair access) OR ☐ My child does not need any special equipment in the community	1	2	3	4	5	6	7	8	9

Pain and bother

The next few questions ask about things that may bother your child.

	Not at all bothered								Very bothered
Is your child bothered by hospital visits?	1	2	3	4	5	6	7	8	9
Is your child bothered when they miss school for health reasons?	1	2	3	4	5	6	7	8	9
Is your child bothered by being handled by other people?	1	2	3	4	5	6	7	8	9

	Never	Rarely	Sometimes	Often	Always
Does your child worry about who will take care of them in the future?	1	2	3	4	5

Cerebral Palsy **Quality of Life Questionnaire for Children** (CP QOL-Child)

Primary Caregiver Questionnaire (4-12 years)

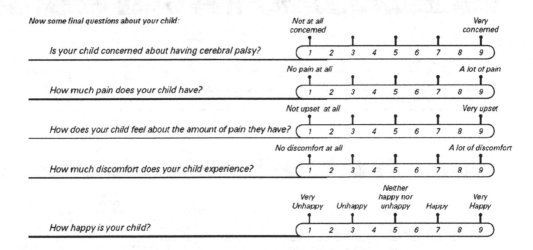

Now some final questions about your child:

	Not at all concerned								Very concerned
Is your child concerned about having cerebral palsy?	1	2	3	4	5	6	7	8	9

	No pain at all								A lot of pain
How much pain does your child have?	1	2	3	4	5	6	7	8	9

	Not upset at all								Very upset
How does your child feel about the amount of pain they have?	1	2	3	4	5	6	7	8	9

	No discomfort at all								A lot of discomfort
How much discomfort does your child experience?	1	2	3	4	5	6	7	8	9

	Very Unhappy		Unhappy		Neither happy nor unhappy		Happy		Very Happy
How happy is your child?	1	2	3	4	5	6	7	8	9

The next set of questions are about YOU and how you feel about your access to services

How do you feel about ...

<u>Access to services</u>	Very Unhappy		Unhappy		Neither happy nor unhappy		Happy		Very Happy
your child's access to treatment?	1	2	3	4	5	6	7	8	9
your child's access to therapy? (for example, physiotherapy, speech therapy, occupational therapy)	1	2	3	4	5	6	7	8	9
your child's access to specialised medical or surgical care?	1	2	3	4	5	6	7	8	9
your ability to get advice from a paediatrician?	1	2	3	4	5	6	7	8	9
your access to respite care? OR ☐ *I have never tried to access respite care (please skip the next two questions on respite)*	1	2	3	4	5	6	7	8	9
the amount of respite care you receive?	1	2	3	4	5	6	7	8	9
how easy it is to get respite?	1	2	3	4	5	6	7	8	9
your child's access to community services and facilities? (eg. kindergarten, childcare, after-school programs, holiday programs, community-based groups such as cubs and brownies).	1	2	3	4	5	6	7	8	9
your child's access to extra help with learning at preschool or school?	1	2	3	4	5	6	7	8	9

Cerebral Palsy **Quality of Life Questionnaire for Children** (CP QOL-Child)

Primary Caregiver Questionnaire (4-12 years)

Now some questions about you.

How do you feel about ...

<u>*Parents' health*</u>

	Very Unhappy		Unhappy		Neither happy nor unhappy		Happy		Very Happy
your physical health?	1	2	3	4	5	6	7	8	9
your work situation?	1	2	3	4	5	6	7	8	9
your family's financial situation?	1	2	3	4	5	6	7	8	9
How happy are you?	1	2	3	4	5	6	7	8	9

	Not at all confident								Very confident
How confident are you that you can report how your child feels?	1	2	3	4	5	6	7	8	9

Appendix 2: CP QOL (Self-report version)

Cerebral Palsy
Quality of Life Questionnaire for Children (CP QOL-Child)

Child Report Questionnaire (9-12 years)

We want to ask you some questions about your life such as your family, your friends, your health and your school.

Each question begins with 'How do you FEEL about...?'.

For each question we want you to (circle) the best number that shows how you FEEL.

You can circle any number from 1 (Very unhappy) to 9 (Very happy).

This questionnaire is measuring how you feel, not what you can do.

Here is an example:

How do you feel about ...

	Very Unhappy	Unhappy	Neither happy nor unhappy	Happy	Very Happy
your ability to play games with other children	1 2 3	4	5 6	(7)	8 9

How do you feel about ...

Friends and family

	Very Unhappy	Unhappy	Neither happy nor unhappy	Happy	Very Happy
the way you get along with people, generally?	1 2	3	4 5 6	7	8 9
the way you get along with the person who looks after you	1 2	3	4 5 6	7	8 9
the way you get along with your brothers and sisters? OR ☐ *I do not have any brothers or sisters*	1 2	3	4 5 6	7	8 9
the way you get along with other children at school? (If you attend more than one school, please think about the school where you spend the most time).	1 2	3	4 5 6	7	8 9
the way you get along with other children outside of school?	1 2	3	4 5 6	7	8 9
the way you get along with adults?	1 2	3	4 5 6	7	8 9
the way you get along with your teachers and/or carers?	1 2	3	4 5 6	7	8 9
your ability to play on your own?	1 2	3	4 5 6	7	8 9
your ability to play with friends?	1 2	3	4 5 6	7	8 9
going out on trips with your family?	1 2	3	4 5 6	7	8 9
how you are accepted by your family?	1 2	3	4 5 6	7	8 9
how you are accepted by other children at school? (If you attend more than one school, please think about the school where you spend the most time).	1 2	3	4 5 6	7	8 9
how you are accepted by other children outside of school?	1 2	3	4 5 6	7	8 9

Cerebral Palsy **Quality of Life Questionnaire for Children** (CP QOL-Child)

Child Report Questionnaire (9-12 years)

How do you feel about ...

	Very Unhappy	Unhappy	Neither happy nor unhappy	Happy	Very Happy
how you are accepted by adults?	1 2	3 4	5 6	7 8	9
how you are accepted by people in general?	1 2	3 4	5 6	7 8	9
being able to do the things you want to do?	1 2	3 4	5 6	7 8	9

Participation

	Very Unhappy	Unhappy	Neither happy nor unhappy	Happy	Very Happy
your ability to participate at school? (If you attend more than one school, please think about the school where you spend the most time)	1 2	3 4	5 6	7 8	9
your ability to participate in recreational activities?	1 2	3 4	5 6	7 8	9
your ability to participate in sporting activities? (this question is asking how you feel about your ability to participate in sport, not whether you can participate).	1 2	3 4	5 6	7 8	9
your ability to participate in social events outside of school?	1 2	3 4	5 6	7 8	9
your ability to participate in your community?	1 2	3 4	5 6	7 8	9

Communication

	Very Unhappy	Unhappy	Neither happy nor unhappy	Happy	Very Happy
the way you communicate with people you know well? (using any means of communication)	1 2	3 4	5 6	7 8	9
the way you communicate with people you don't know well? (using any means of communication)	1 2	3 4	5 6	7 8	9
the way other people communicate with you?	1 2	3 4	5 6	7 8	9

Health

	Very Unhappy	Unhappy	Neither happy nor unhappy	Happy	Very Happy
your physical health?	1 2	3 4	5 6	7 8	9
the way you get around?	1 2	3 4	5 6	7 8	9
how you sleep?	1 2	3 4	5 6	7 8	9
the way you look?	1 2	3 4	5 6	7 8	9
your ability to keep up academically with your peers?	1 2	3 4	5 6	7 8	9
your ability to keep up physically with your peers?	1 2	3 4	5 6	7 8	9
your life in general?	1 2	3 4	5 6	7 8	9
yourself?	1 2	3 4	5 6	7 8	9
your future?	1 2	3 4	5 6	7 8	9
your opportunities in life?	1 2	3 4	5 6	7 8	9

Cerebral Palsy **Quality of Life Questionnaire for Children** (CP QOL-Child)

Child Report Questionnaire (9-12 years)

The next 3 questions are asking how you feel about using parts of your body, not whether you can use parts of your body.

How do you feel about ...

	Very Unhappy	Unhappy	Neither happy nor unhappy	Happy	Very Happy
the way you use your arms?	1 2 3	4	5 6	7	8 9
the way you use your legs?	1 2 3	4	5 6	7	8 9
the way you use your hands?	1 2 3	4	5 6	7	8 9

The next 3 questions are asking how you feel about your ability to complete daily activities, not whether you can complete the activities.

How do you feel about ...

	Very Unhappy	Unhappy	Neither happy nor unhappy	Happy	Very Happy
your ability to dress yourself?	1 2 3	4	5 6	7	8 9
your ability to eat or drink independently?	1 2 3	4	5 6	7	8 9
your ability to use the toilet by yourself?	1 2 3	4	5 6	7	8 9

Special Equipment

	Very Unhappy	Unhappy	Neither happy nor unhappy	Happy	Very Happy
the special equipment you have at home? (eg. special seating, standing frames, wheelchairs, walkers) OR ☐ *I do not need any special equipment at home*	1 2 3	4	5 6	7	8 9
the special equipment you have at your school? (eg. special seating, standing frames, wheelchairs, walkers) OR ☐ *I do not need any special equipment at my school*	1 2 3	4	5 6	7	8 9
the special equipment that is available in the community? (ramps, escalators, wheelchair access) OR ☐ *I do not need any special equipment in the community*	1 2 3	4	5 6	7	8 9

Pain and bother

The next few questions ask about things that may bother you.

	Not at all bothered				Very bothered
Are you bothered by hospital visits?	1 2 3	4	5 6	7	8 9
Are you bothered when you miss school for health reasons?	1 2 3	4	5 6	7	8 9
Are you bothered by being handled by other people?	1 2 3	4	5 6	7	8 9

	Never	Rarely	Sometimes	Often	Always
Do you worry about who will take care of you in the future?	1	2	3	4	5

Cerebral Palsy **Quality of Life Questionnaire for Children** (CP QOL-Child)

Child Report Questionnaire (9-12 years)

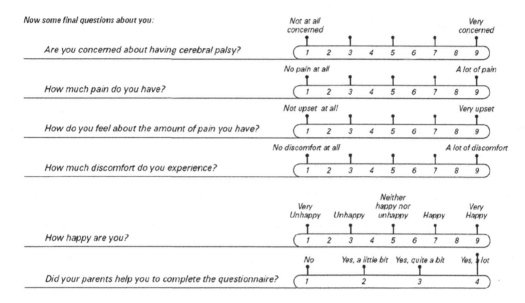

Now some final questions about you:

Are you concerned about having cerebral palsy?
Not at all concerned — 1 2 3 4 5 6 7 8 9 — *Very concerned*

How much pain do you have?
No pain at all — 1 2 3 4 5 6 7 8 9 — *A lot of pain*

How do you feel about the amount of pain you have?
Not upset at all — 1 2 3 4 5 6 7 8 9 — *Very upset*

How much discomfort do you experience?
No discomfort at all — 1 2 3 4 5 6 7 8 9 — *A lot of discomfort*

How happy are you?
Very Unhappy (1) — *Unhappy* (3) — *Neither happy nor unhappy* (5) — *Happy* (7) — *Very Happy* (9)

Did your parents help you to complete the questionnaire?
No (1) — *Yes, a little bit* (2) — *Yes, quite a bit* (3) — *Yes, a lot* (4)

Thanks for helping us with our questions. Well Done!

10

Outcome measures for informal carers of individuals with neurodegenerative conditions

Michele Peters

The impact of a disease on a patient has become an important outcome measure in medicine and health care. More recently, increasing attention has also been paid to the impact on informal caregivers of someone with a long-term disease. Carers or caregivers play an important role in the care of chronically ill patients, particularly because there is an increase in the number of people with a long-term condition. Vitaliano et al. (1) define informal carers as "caregivers who are not financially compensated for their services." Informal carers tend to be family members, often the patient's spouse, or friends, and provide significant amounts of support to the patient who may have difficulties because of physical, cognitive, or emotional impairments (1). Caring for someone with ill health poses challenges, including psychological, physical, financial, and social factors (2). It is increasingly recognized that caring for someone can be stressful and difficult and that it can lead to adverse physical and psychological outcomes for the carer.

Two types of outcome measures have been used to assess carer burden: generic and carer-specific outcome measures. Using generic instruments is an indirect approach to assessing carer outcomes, whereas using a carer-specific instrument is a direct approach to the assessment of carer outcomes (3). Generic instruments provide broad insight into health, but they do not provide information on the burden resulting from being a carer. Generic outcome measures tend to have been tested extensively, but mostly not in a carer population. On the other hand, carer-specific instruments provide a more direct measure of carer burden by focusing specifically on carers' experiences.

Carer-specific instruments can be generic in that they have been developed for carers generally, or they can be disease-specific in that they have been developed for the carers of patients with a specific condition. Generic carer instruments (e.g., the Carer Strain Index (4)) provide a more specific measure of carer burden than generic instruments, but these may not capture disease-specific burden. Thus some instruments have been developed to assess disease-specific carer burden, such as the Coping with Multiple Sclerosis Caregiving Inventory (5). Disease-specific measures are sometimes used for conditions other than the condition the instrument was developed for because the items on disease-specific carer instruments mostly do not refer to the specific condition. For example, the Carer Strain Index (CSI) was developed for carers of patients who have recently been discharged from hospital after surgery, but the CSI has been used in dementia (6). However, frequently these instruments will not have been tested for that particular population of carers, and the usefulness of using instruments in this way has been questioned by Vitaliano and colleagues (6).

Quality of Life Measurement in Neurodegenerative and Related Conditions, eds., Crispin Jenkinson, Michele Peters, and Mark B. Bromberg. Published by Cambridge University Press. © Cambridge University Press 2011.

Outcome measures can also vary in the number of dimensions that they measure. Dimension-specific instruments may measure fatigue or depression (often these are generic rather than carer-specific), whereas other instruments measure several dimensions, including, for example, physical health, psychological health, and social functioning. Many studies use a combination of several outcome measures to assess carer burden. This can be a combination of one or several generic, carer-specific, dimension-specific instruments, or all three. For example, a Japanese study used a generic quality of life questionnaire (WHOQoL), a carer-specific questionnaire (Zarit Burden Interview [ZBI]), and a dimension-specific questionnaire (Beck Depression Inventory) (7).

It is challenging to provide an overview of psychometric properties of outcome measures used in carers for several reasons. First, different types of instruments (generic, disease-specific, and dimension-specific) have been used in carers of a person with a neurodegenerative condition; however, few generic instruments have been formally tested in this population. The psychometric information presented in this chapter on generic instruments is largely extrapolated from surveys rather than being information from formal psychometric evaluations of the instrument. Second, many different instruments have been used, of which the majority have not undergone thorough psychometric testing. Third, different versions of the same instrument have been used, making it difficult to draw overall conclusions on the psychometric properties of any instrument. Fourth, some disease-specific instruments have been used, but have not necessarily been tested, in neurodegenerative conditions other than the condition the instrument was developed for. Finally, some instruments that have been developed and tested in a condition other than a neurodegenerative condition have been used in studies on carers of someone with a neurodegenerative condition. Given all these challenges, this chapter reviews psychometric information on multidimensional generic and carer-specific instruments that have been developed or tested for informal carers of an individual with a neurodegenerative con-

dition. It is beyond the scope of this chapter to discuss dimension-specific carer outcome measures; however, they are widely used, as will be evident from the information given on the validity of some of the generic or carer-specific instruments. This chapter differs from other chapters in this book in that, because of these challenges, the psychometric information had to be largely extrapolated from surveys rather than presented as a review of psychometric evaluation studies. This applies to both the generic instruments and the carer-specific instruments, including the Zarit Burden Interview, which is reviewed more extensively. The various studies used in this chapter are outlined in several tables in the various sections to give information on the study population and on the version of the instrument that was used.

Generic instruments

A wide range of generic outcome measures are available, some of which have been used to assess carer burden. However, few studies have evaluated the psychometric properties for carers of someone with a neurodegenerative condition. The four instruments for which psychometric information is available are the SF-36 (or SF-12), the General Health Questionnaire (GHQ), the World Health Organization Quality of Life (WHOQoL and WHOQoL-bref), the EQ-5D, and the schedule for evaluation of individual quality of life (SEIQoL). The WHOQoL (7, 8) and the EQ-5D (9, 10) were evaluated in only two studies, and the SEIQoL in one study (8). Because of limited information on these three instruments, their psychometric properties will not be discussed in greater detail in this chapter. The SF-36 (including the SF-12) and the GHQ have been evaluated more frequently, and their respective psychometric properties will be outlined in this section.

SF-36 and SF-12

The SF-36 is a generic self-administered health measure that can be used within different

Table 10.1 Evaluative studies related to the SF-36 or the SF-12 when completed by carers of someone with a neurodegenerative condition

Author, date	Disease	Sample	Country	Version
Bell et al. (2001) (12)	Alzheimer's disease	679 carers	Canada	SF-36
Berg-Weger et al. (2003) (13)	Alzheimer's disease	102 former carers whose family member died at least 1 year prior to the study	USA	SF-36
Lyons et al. (2004) (14)	Parkinson's	311 spouse carers	USA	Physical Subscale of SF-36
Argimon et al. (2005) (15)	Dementia	181 carers	Spain	SF-36
McConaghy and Caltabiano (2005) (16)	Dementia	42 carers	Australia	SF-12
Van Den Berg et al. (2005) (17)	Amyotrophic lateral sclerosis (ALS)	208 patients and carers	The Netherlands	SF-36
Patti et al. (2007) (18)	Multiple sclerosis	445 patients and their carers	Italy	SF-36
Martinez-Martin et al. (2007) (19)	Parkinson's	80 patients and 79 carers	Spain	SF-36
Argimon et al. (2004) (20)	Dementia	181 carers	Spain	SF-36
Jenkinson et al. (2000) (21)	Amyotrophic lateral sclerosis (ALS)	451 patients and 415 carers	15 European countries	SF-36

populations (11). It mostly uses Likert-style response scales, but some questions are dichotomous (yes/no). The SF-36 has eight dimensions, including physical function, social function, role physical, role mental, pain, mental health, energy, and health perception. It has been suggested that two summary scales can be derived, namely, a physical component summary score (PCS) and a mental component summary score (MCS). The SF-12 is a shorter, 12-item version of the SF-36, from which the two summary scales (PCS and MCS) can also be derived.

Table 10.1 provides a summary of different evaluative studies on the SF-36 and the SF-12. Half of these studies were carried out in a sample of carers of someone with dementia. Psychometric information mainly relates to issues of validity, and few studies give information on reliability, responsiveness, or precision. No information on feasibility, interpretability, or acceptability is available.

Reliability

Only four studies have evaluated the internal consistency of the SF-36 or SF-12. Good internal consistency for the SF-36 was found in carers of patients with amyotrophic lateral sclerosis (ALS) (21) and for Alzheimer's disease (13). Good internal consistency was also found for the physical subscale of the SF-36, with Chronbach's alpha being 0.89 for the baseline and after 2 years, and 0.91 after 10 years (14).

However, weak internal consistency was found for both the physical and mental component scales of the SF-12 (version 2) in a sample of dementia carers (16).

Validity

Convergent and discriminant validity

The PCS and MCS scores of the SF-36 have been found to be lower in ALS carers than in the general population in a Europe-wide study (21). A total of 49.7% of carers scored below the mean on PCS and 71.6% below the mean for MCS in comparison with the general population (21). Significant differences in the SF-36 scores of carers and the scores of the Italian normative sample were found on all dimensions of the SF-36, expect for physical functioning (18). In this study, all dimension scores, apart from physical functioning and bodily pain, were significantly lower in carers than in normal subjects. Mental health was the dimension that was most affected in carers, especially among men, followed by vitality and general health. Bodily pain was slightly higher in carers than in normal subjects, especially among women.

Carers with higher pessimism had significantly lower scores on physical health than carers with lower levels of pessimism (14).

Carer instruments

Significant correlations of the dimensions of the SF-36 have been found with the Zarit Burden Interview (ZBI) (19). The correlations were strong for the mental health, mental component, and social functioning dimensions of the SF-36, whereas for the other SF-36 dimensions, the correlations were weak to moderate.

Predictive validity

The MCS scale of the SF-36 has been found to predict the results of the Health Utilities Index Mark 2 (HUI2) in carers of a person with Alzheimer's disease (12).

Sociodemographic variables

Older PD caregivers had significantly poorer physical health at baseline and faster rates of decline (14). Age and sex, in a regression model, were found to be the strongest predictors of a carer's quality of life (18).

Female carers scored lower than male carers on seven of the eight dimensions of the SF-36 in two

studies (18, 20). The dimension for which the men scored higher than the women differed between the two studies, with men scoring higher on physical functioning (20) or male spousal carers scoring higher on mental health in comparison with female spousal carers (18). Male spousal carers have also been found to have higher scores than parent carers on physical functioning, role physical, social functioning, bodily pain, mental health, vitality, and general health (18).

Patient variables

Carers of patients who had been placed in a nursing home had significantly lower scores on the two subscales (physical functioning and physical role) and five dimensions (bodily pain, general health, vitality, emotional role, and mental health) of the SF-36, after controlling for confounding variables (15). The type of care received has not been found to lead to a significant difference in quality of life in carers of ALS patients who had received multi-disciplinary care versus patients receiving general care (17).

Precision

Floor and ceiling effects were investigated in only one study for ALS carers, and floor effects were found in 19.3% of carers for role physical and in 23.4% for role mental (21). Ceiling effects were found in 32.7% for physical function, 50.6% for role physical, 49.0% for role mental, and 38.2% for pain.

Responsiveness

Only one study gives information about responsiveness, finding that SF-36 scores for the physical health subscale declined by approximately 13 points over a period of 10 years (14).

General Health Questionnaire

The General Health Questionnaire, or GHQ, is a self-administered questionnaire that focuses on two

Table 10.2 Evaluative studies related to the GHQ when completed by carers of someone with a neurodegenerative condition

Author, date	Disease	Sample	Country	Version
Jackson et al. (1991) (24)	Dementia	24 carers	Ireland	GHQ-30
Draper et al. (1992) (25)	Stroke and dementia	99 co-resident carers (stroke 48 and dementia 51)	Australia	GHQ-30
O'Reilly et al. (1996) (26)	Parkinson's	154 carer spouses and 124 noncarer spouses	Ireland	GHQ-12
Donaldson et al. (1998) (27)	Alzheimer's	100 community dwelling patients and their carers	UK	GHQ-28
Rosenvinge et al. (1998) (28)	Dementia and chronic depression	57 carers (32 dementia and 25 depression)	UK	GHQ-30
Matsuda (1999) (29)	Dementia	Carers of elderly relatives	Japan	GHQ-60
Nagatomo et al. (1999) (30)	Dementia	62 relative carers	Japan	GHQ-30
Groom et al. (2003) (31)	Multiple sclerosis	49 carers (27 of community-dwelling patients and 22 of patients at rehabilitation unit)	UK	GHQ-12
Woods et al. (2003) (32)	Dementia	104 carers	UK	GHQ-28
Prince (2004) (33)	Dementia	706 carers	India, China, South East Asia, Latin America and the Caribbean, and Africa	GHQ-22
Secker and Brown (2005) (34)	Parkinson's	30 carers, 15 treatment and 15 control	UK	GHQ-28
Love et al. (2005) (35)	Motor neuron disease	75 carers	Australia	GHQ-12
Roud et al. (2006) (36)	Dementia	45 carers	New Zealand	GHQ-30

major areas – the inability to carry out normal functions and the appearance of new and distressing psychological phenomena (22, 23). The GHQ is available in several different versions: GHQ-60 (the fully detailed 60-item questionnaire), GHQ-30 (a short form without items related to physical illness), GHQ-28 (a scaled version that assesses somatic symptoms, anxiety and insomnia, social dysfunction, and severe depression), and GHQ-12 (a quick, reliable, and sensitive short form).

No formal evaluation studies of the GHQ in carers of someone with a neurodegenerative condition have been conducted, thus psychometric information is limited and needs to be extrapolated from research studies. Mainly, it is only information on

validity that is available, although one study also gives information on responsiveness. Table 10.2 outlines studies that give psychometric information on the GHQ in carers, highlighting that most of the studies have been conducted with carers of dementia patients.

Validity

Convergent and discriminant validity

Parkinson's carer spouses did not show significant increase in the risk of psychiatric morbidity, as measured by the GHQ-12, in comparison with controls, but those providing extensive care had an almost five-fold increased risk (26). In a sample of carers of a hospitalized MS patient and carers of a community-dwelling person with MS, the GHQ-12 score was significantly correlated the SODS (Signs of Depression Scale), which was developed to assess mood in stroke patients with communication difficulties (31).

The GHQ-30 was positively correlated with carer burden (30). The GHQ-30 score has also been found to be significantly higher in a group of carers of someone with dementia than in controls (24), and in carers of someone with dementia in comparison with carers of someone with depression (28). However, no significant differences in the score of the GHQ-28 were found between carers of someone with dementia versus someone who had a stroke (25). The GHQ-30 was found to be significantly and positively correlated with carer burden assessed by the Relatives Stress Scale for both dementia and stroke (25). Strong negative correlations were found between the GHQ-30 and the Life Satisfaction Questionnaire (25). The depression and anxiety subscales of the GHQ-30 were found to be moderately related to the negative impact subscale of the COPE (Carers of Older People in Europe) Index, but the positive value subscale of COPE was not significantly related to either of the GHQ-30 subscales (36). The COPE index assesses the role perceptions of older carers.

In a study comparing conventional nurse services versus Admiral Nurse (AN) services (treatment group), a nonsignificant trend for higher GHQ total scores and depression subscales was found for carers who had used AN teams at baseline (32). On follow-up after 8 months, carers who had used AN services had a significantly higher score on the anxiety and insomnia subscale in comparison with carers who had used conventional services.

Carer instruments

The Japanese version of the GHQ-60 was used to validate the subjective burden scale for family carers of elderly with dementia (29). A significant, medium, and positive correlation was found between the two instruments.

Sociodemographic variables

Differences in the GHQ-12 score have been found between different developing countries and regions, including India, China and South East Asia, Latin America and the Caribbean, and Africa (33). However, it is not clear if these differences were statistically significant.

GHQ-12 scores were found to be related to time as a carer, with those who reported having been a carer for less than 2 years having lower average scores than those who reported caring for longer than 2 years (35).

Household income has been found to be significantly (26) or not significantly (35) related to GHQ-12. The significant difference found by O'Reilly et al. (26) was no longer significant after adjusting for variables such as age, gender, and social class.

Living arrangements have been found to not influence the GHQ score (27, 35); however, another study reported better outcomes for carers who were not co-residents of the patient (32). No significant correlations were found between the GHQ score and the length of time the carer and the patient had lived together (30) or whether dependent or adult children were living at home (35).

Two studies found that the relationship of the carer to the person he or she cared for did not influence the GHQ score (27, 35). However, another study found that the GHQ score was significantly worse for spouses than for offspring carers (30).

One study found no significant correlation between the GHQ and the carer's gender (28), whereas another found that distress as measured by the GHQ-28 was significantly higher in women than in men (27). No significant correlation was found for the carer's age.

Patient variables

A number of patient variables have been found to be significantly related to the carer's GHQ score, including patient depression, some aspects of behavior disturbance, and psychotic symptoms (27). The GHQ is negatively correlated with the age of the patient with dementia and was positively correlated with the Dementia Behaviour Disturbance Scale (30).

However, a number of patient variables have been found not to be significantly related to the carer's GHQ score, including the dependent's behavioral and mood disturbance (24), patient severity ratings (measured by the MMSE [Mini-Mental State Examination] and the Brief Psychiatric Rating Scale), the behavior rating schedule of the COPE or the Montgomery–Asberg Depression Rating Scale (28), cognitive impairment, and any category of the Activities of Daily Living (ADL) scale, expect for self-expression (30).

Responsiveness

Both conventional and Admiral Nurse services led to lower scores on one of the GHQ subscales (the anxiety and insomnia) over an 8-months period (32). In a randomized controlled trial, it was found that the GHQ-28 score was reduced in both the cognitive behavioral therapy (CBT) group and the control group after 3 months, but the improvement in the CBT group was significantly greater (34).

Carer-specific instruments

Carer-specific instruments could potentially be of two different types: those developed for carers but not for a specific disease, and those developed for carers of someone with a specific disease. In reality, many carer-specific instruments have been developed in one disease, but they are used across conditions. They are suitable for use in that they do not contain any reference in the items to the disease they were developed for. However, they often have not been extensively validated in other diseases, and it could therefore be argued that they may not be suitable for use.

This section will give an overview of carer outcome measures developed in neurodegenerative

conditions, including instruments evaluated in single studies and instruments evaluated in multiple studies. The most commonly evaluated carer outcome measure is the ZBI, and its psychometric properties will be described in greater detail.

The overall picture for carer outcome measures (from both single and multiple studies) is that most have been developed for dementia (including Alzheimer's disease). The second most common condition for single-study instruments is Parkinson's disease. Some carer-specific instruments that have been developed in multiple diseases, such as the Caregiver Burden Scale in stroke and dementia (37) and the Burden of Caregiver Index in Japan, included carers of people with a variety of neurological conditions (38). Most instruments were developed in English-speaking countries, predominantly the United States. A handful of instruments were developed in Asia, but there do not seem to be any from Africa or South America. The sample sizes are mostly small, with approximately two-thirds of the single-study instruments having sample sizes below 100 (range 10–946). For the ZBI, it is "only" about half of the studies that had a sample size below 100 (range 29–770).

As far as the content of carer outcome measures is concerned, some concepts are similar to those of generic outcome measures, such as physical function, mental health, and social health. Symptoms and social support, which are concepts of interest in generic outcome measures, are rarely, if at all, assessed. Additional questions, making the instrument more carer-specific, are questions about existential issues (including personal issues, financial security, or personal costs), time-dependence burden, and demands on the carer. Most instruments assess several of these aspects, and some studies have conducted factor analysis to identify the underlying structure of the instrument (e.g., the Burden Index of Caregivers (38)). The number of items or questions is predominantly between 20 and 30, although a large number of studies do not report how many items their instrument contains. Furthermore, there also is a lack of clarity in a minority of studies on the content of the questionnaire, beyond the authors' describing that the instrument measures carer burden.

A majority of carer outcome measures have been used in one study only, and usually little information is available on the development and psychometric evaluation. Instruments that have been evaluated and used in multiple studies are the ZBI (developed in the United States), the PIXEL instrument (France) (39, 40), the Elmstahl questionnaire (Sweden) (37, 41, 42, 43, 44), and the Glozman (Russia and Spain) (10, 45). The ZBI will be described in greater detail below because this is the instrument that has been more widely evaluated than any other carer-specific outcome measure. It is important to note that, even with the more extensively evaluated outcome measures, psychometric information is limited, usually to reliability (mostly internal consistency) and validity. Frequently, the validity of carer instruments is not formally assessed, but information on an instrument's validity can be extrapolated from studies where the instrument is used in conjunction with other instruments.

Zarit Burden Interview

The Zarit Burden Interview was first developed in the United States with carers of a person with senile dementia living in the community (46). The Zarit Burden Interview is mostly referred to as the ZBI but also sometimes as the BI (burden interview) (47), CBI (Carer Burden Inventory) (48), BIS (Burden Interview Scale) (49), ZS (Zarit Scale) (50), or ZBS (Zarit Burden Scale) (51). For the purposes of this chapter, it will be referred to as the ZBI.

The ZBI is reported to be the most widely used instrument in carers of a person with dementia (2, 52), including senile dementia, cognitive impairment, and Alzheimer's disease. However, the ZBI has also been used in conditions other than dementia, such as Parkinson's disease (53) and multiple sclerosis (54); elderly in need of care (55); muscular dystrophy (56); and stroke, chronic obstructive pulmonary disease, and general disability (57).

The ZBI, as originally described, consists of 29 questions that measure the degree of burden experienced by a carer (46). Items were developed on the basis of the authors' clinical experience and prior studies. The items refer to the spouse, despite the original study sample also including daughters who were carers. None of the items refer to dementia. From the item scores, a total score was calculated, with four items scored negatively (and hence subtracted from the total score). The items were scored on a scale from "not at all" to "extremely," but it is not clear how many points were on the scale, nor what score was given to "not at all" or "extremely." No formal testing of the ZBI was reported at this point in time.

The original ZBI included 29 questions (46), but was later modified to a 22-item version (93). The ZBI was developed to evaluate subjective impact of caregiving and contains questions on the carer's health, psychological well-being, finances, and social life, and on the carer's relationship with the patient (46, 93). The authors report that the instrument has primarily been used in research but may also be useful for health care practitioners as a way of estimating how much stress the carer is experiencing. The ZBI is scored on a 5-point Likert-type scale (0 = never and 4 = nearly always), with a higher score meaning a higher burden (58). If the extent of the burden on the carer has been assessed before an intervention, then administering the interview again after the intervention will indicate the degree of burden of success or improvement in the caregiver's situation.

The original ZBI was interviewer-administered, and mostly, this has been the method of administration of the questionnaire. Despite this, it has been reported that the ZBI is a self-administered questionnaire (56), and a number of studies (as shown in Table 10.3) have used the ZBI as a self-administered questionnaire.

Versions

As already indicated above, there are a number of different versions of the ZBI, in terms of the number

Table 10.3 Evaluative studies related to the Zarit Burden Interview (ZBI) when completed by carers of someone with a neurodegenerative condition

Author, date	Disease	Sample	Country	Version	Administration
Zarit et al. (1980) (46)	Senile dementia	29 patients in the community and their carers (18 spouses and 11 daughters)	USA	29-item	Interview
Zarit et al. (1986) (58)	Dementia	64 spouse carers (community)	USA	20-item	Interview
Zarit et al. (1987) (59)	Dementia	119 family carers (community)	USA	22-item	Interview
Anthony-Bergstone et al. (1988) (60)	Dementia	184 caregivers (community)	USA	22-item	Not specified
Whitlatch et al. (1991) (47)	Dementia	113 primary carers of a non-institutionalized patient	USA	22-item	Interview
Hébert et al. (1993) (61)	Dementia	40 carers of patients living in the community	France	22-item	Not specified
Magone et al. (1993) (62)	Dementia	25 patient-carer dyads	Argentina	21-item	Self-administered
Hadjistavropoulos et al. (1994) (63)	Dementia	136 patients and their carer (community)	Canada	22-item	Interview
Rankin et al. (1994) (64)	Cognitive impairment	140 patients and their carers (community)	USA	22-item	Not specified
Majerovitz (1995) (65)	Dementia	54 spouse carers currently residing with patient and who are primary carer	USA	22-item	Interview
Molloy et al. (1996) (66)	Cognitive impairment	108 adult- carer dyads	Canada	22-item	Not specified
Arai et al. (1997) (55)	Elderly in need of care	66 carers	Japan	22-item	Self-administered
Coen et al. (1997) (67)	Alzheimer's	50 patients and their primary carers	Ireland	22-item	Not specified
Coen et al. (1999) (68)	Alzheimer's	50 patients and their primary carers	Ireland	25-item	Not specified
Schneider et al. (1999) (48)	Alzheimer's	20 carers for preliminary study, 280 carers for main study	14 European countries	29-item	Semistructured interview for preliminary study Not specified for main study
Hébert et al. (2000) (69)	Dementia	312 carers of an elderly person with dementia	Canada	22-item	Interview
Knight et al. (2000) (70)	Dementia	Sample 1: 220 carers of demented elderly; sample 2: 108 carers	USA	22-item	Interviews
Bedard et al. (2001) (71)	Cognitive impairment	413 carers	Canada	22-item and 4-item	Not specified

Table 10.3 (*cont.*)

Author, date	Disease	Sample	Country	Version	Administration
Colvez et al. (2002) (72)	Alzheimer's disease	322 informal carers	European (Denmark, Germany, Belgium, Spain, Sweden, and France)	29-item	Interview
Edwards and Ruettiger (2002) (73); Edwards and Scheetz (2002) (74)	Parkinson's disease	41 couples in which one spouse or partner had Parkinson's disease	USA	22-item	Self-report
Gallicchio et al. (2002) (75)	Dementia	327 carers of patients living in the community	USA	22-item	Interview
Miyamoto et al. (2002) (76)	Dementia	379 primary caregivers of people with dementia living at home	Japan	21-item	Not specified
O'Rourke and Tuokko (2003) (77)	Dementia	770 carers of community-dwelling patients	Canada	12-item	Interview
Rivera-Navarro et al. (2003) (54)	Multiple sclerosis	91 patients and their carers	Spain	22-item	Interview
Dooley and Hinojosa (2004) (78)	Alzheimer's	40 patients and their carers	USA	29-item	
Taub et al. (2004) (79)	Dementia	50 carers	Brazil	22-item	Interview
Ankri et al. (2005) (80)	Dementia	152 community-dwelling patients and their caregivers	France	22-item	Not specified
Mc Conaghy and Caltabiano (2005) (16)	Dementia	42 carers	Australia	22 -item	Mixture of mailed questionnaire and face-to-face interviews
Spurlock (2005) (49)	Alzheimer's	150 African American or Caucasian caregivers related to the community-dwelling patient	USA	29-item	Self-administered
Boyer et al. (2006) (56)	Muscular dystrophy	56 patients and their family carers	France	22-item	Self-administered
Cifu et al. (2006) (53)	Parkinsonism	49 patients and their carers	USA	22-item	Not specified
Serrano-Aguilar et al. (2006) (81)	Alzheimer's disease	237 carers	Spain	25-item	Self-administered
Arai et al. (2007) (82)	Early-onset dementia (EOD) and late-onset dementia (LOD)	68 patient-carer dyads (14 EOD and 54 LOD)	Japan	22-item	Self-administered

(cont.)

Table 10.3 (*cont.*)

Author, date	Disease	Sample	Country	Version	Administration
Bridges-Webb et al. (2007) (83)	Dementia	107 carers of patients living in the community	Australia	Modified ZBI	Not specified
Boutoleau-Bretonniere et al. (2008) (84)	Alzheimer's (AD) and frontotemporal dementia (FTD)	26 FTD and 28 AD patients and their carers	France	22-item	Interview
Bruce et al. (2008) (85)	Mild cognitive impairment	51 patients and their carers	USA	22-item	Interview
Dias et al. (2008) (51)	Dementia	81 patients and their principal carers (41 for intervention and 40 as control)	India	29-item	Interview
Gaugler et al. (2008) (86)	Alzheimer's	406 spouse carers of community-dwelling patients	USA	15-item	Interview
Ko et al. (2008) (87)	Dementia	181 patient-carer dyads	China	22-item	Self-report
Choo et al. (2003) (88)	Dementia	70 carers of a family member with dementia	Malaysia	22-item	Interview
Prince (2004) (33)	Dementia	706 people with dementia living in their own home with their principal caregivers; 179 from India, 91 China and South East Asia, 416 Latin America and the Caribbean, and 20 Nigeria	Multi-country	22-item	Interview
Takahashi et al. (2005) (7)	Dementia	23 informal home-based carers, 24 professional carers, and 31 controls	Japan	22-item	Self-report
Onishi et al. (2005) (89)	Elderly people some with dementia	116 carers of elderly patients, some with dementia, but not clear how many had dementia	Japan	21-item	Self-report
Goldstein et al. (2006) (90)	Amyotrophic lateral sclerosis	50 spouse carers	UK	22-item	Interview
Kim et al. (2006) (91)	Elderly in need of care including some with cognitive impairment	484 carers of the elderly, of which 61 (13%) had dementia	Korea	22-item	Interview
Roud et al. (2006) (36)	Dementia	45 primary carers	New Zealand	18-item, 12-item personal strain subscale and 6-item role strain subscale	Interview
Gort et al. (2007) (50)	Dementia	66 carers of dementia patients who were not in residential care	Spain	22-item	Self-report
Martinez-Martin et al. (2007) (19)	Parkinson's	88 carers of hospital outpatients	Spain	22-item	Self-report

of items or the language used. The original version of the ZBI had 29 items, but a subsequent 22-item version, a short 12-item version, and a 4-item screening version have followed. However, other versions (i.e., with different numbers of items) have also been used (see Table 10.3), and these modifications to the ZBI have been carried out by the authors of specific studies to suit the needs of that particular study, for example, Roud et al. (36).

Reviewing and comparing psychometric properties of the ZBI are challenging because of the number of different versions and because not all studies make it clear which version was used (e.g., (49)), and some such as Cifu et al. (53) report using the 22-item version but reference the 29-item version. In their meta-analysis on the ZBI, Bachner and O'Rourke (52) found that the range of ZBI total items was 7 to 33 (only studies with ZBI items over 6 were included) with almost half of studies (49.3% or 68 out of 138 studies) using the "standard" 22-item scale; 10% used the 29-item version. In four articles, authors had added items to either the 22- or the 29-item scale, and the remaining studies (n = 138) used various abridged versions of the ZBI (52). In Australia, a "modified ZBI" was used (83), but it was not clear what these modifications were, or how many questions this version had.

The ZBI has been used in a number of different countries (Table 10.3); therefore, different language versions exist. Often studies that describe the translation and validation of the translated version are not published in English. Not all translations and evaluations have been carried out in carers of someone with a neurodegenerative condition; the 22-item Japanese version was developed in a sample of carers of the elderly (55), or an 8-item Japanese version of the ZBI was developed in carers of the elderly (93). The 22-item Japanese ZBI was later used in a study with carers of someone with dementia (82).

Psychometrics

The ZBI was originally developed by Zarit et al. (46), but formal evaluation studies were not carried out until later. Mostly, psychometric informa-

tion remains limited to internal consistency reliability, and validity information can be extrapolated from studies that have used other instruments (carer, patient, or proxy reported). Some more formal evaluation studies were carried out at a later date. The reliability and validity of the ZBI were studied by Hébert and colleagues nearly 20 years after initial development of the instrument (69). The various versions of the ZBI make it challenging to establish, summarize, and compare the psychometric properties of the ZBI from different studies.

Reliability

Mostly, reliability information remains limited to internal consistency (Cronbach's alpha). Overall, internal consistency is the most frequently given psychometric information on the ZBI. For their meta-analysis on the reliability of the ZBI, Bachner and O'Rourke (52) included articles that had used a range of different versions of the ZBI (studies using 6 or fewer ZBI items were excluded). Of the 258 studies found, 149 (57.8%) did not report reliability information in relation to their respective samples, and the remaining 138 articles were included in the study. For internal consistency, the average was Chronbach's alpha = 0.86 (SD = 0.006, median 0.88, range 0.62 to 0.95). Five studies (each using an abridged ZBI version) reported an alpha below the acceptable level of 0.69. Using regression analysis, a large number of variables (such as sample size, mean age of carers) failed to significantly predict the ZBI's internal consistency. Only three variables contributed significantly and uniquely to the regression equation, including the number of ZBI items (with fewer item versions being found to be less reliable), residence of the care recipient (ZBI completed by community-dwelling carers had higher reliability), and language format (Hebrew version statistically lower reliability estimates relative to the English language version). The Hebrew version was the 29-item version, which generally has lower reliability.

Even though it is not clear whether the ZBI is a multi-dimensional outcome measure (see below), internal consistency has been assessed on the dimensions of the ZBI that have been identified in a study by Whitlatch et al. (47), with personal strain having an alpha coefficient of 0.80 and role strain an alpha of 0.81 (47).

Although the meta-analysis by Bachner and O'Rourke (52) shows good internal consistency for the ZBI, it is not clear from the article which studies were included and what information relates to which article. Presumably, studies using the ZBI that were not carried out in dementia were also included in the sample. From the studies included in this chapter (Table 10.3), internal consistency (Cronbach's alpha) ranged from 0.79 to 0.93. Differences in internal consistency have been found between men (alpha 0.82) and women (0.85) for the 12-item version (77), but both these alphas are within the acceptable range.

The meta-analysis also provided information on test-retest reliability. Of the 102 studies included (52), only 11 studies reported test-retest reliability, with the mean correlation coefficient being $r = 0.59$ (SD = 0.22) (range $r = 0.24$–0.89) over an interval of 31.56 (SD 27.72) months on average (ranging from a few days to 5 years). Bachner and O'Rourke (52) believed that the variability in the correlation coefficient may have been due to the large range of time and may therefore reflect sensitivity to change as opposed to suspect reliability. The test-retest coefficient was 0.89 in a French study (69) and 0.88 in a Chinese study (87). The time span between testing was 2 weeks in the Chinese study in a small sample of 36 carers (87).

Construct validity

The factor structure of the ZBI was analyzed in eight studies (47, 63, 64, 69, 70, 71, 77, 80). The first of these studies was carried out more than 10 years after the development of the original 29-item ZBI. The samples in these studies were carers of non-institutionalized dementia patients (47, 80), carers of dementia patients (63, 69, 77), and carers of cog-

nitively impaired elderly (71). The ZBI's structure was examined by factor analysis in four studies and by principal component analysis in three studies. The ZBI structure was mostly studied for the 22-item questionnaire apart from the two studies on the 12-item version (69, 77). When the structure of the 22-item ZBI was analyzed, item 22, an overall general burden factor, was generally omitted.

An initial study found two factors: personal strain (12 items) and role strain (6 items) (47). Thus, four items were not contained in either of the two factors. A second study analyzed the ZBI's structure by creating subscales based on the findings by Whitlatch et al. (47) and then calculating Pearson's correlation coefficient between the scores of the subscales. It was found that the two factors were significantly correlated, which led the authors to suggest a unifactorial solution (63). The unifactorial solution found accounted for 40% of the variance (63).

A small study found a two-factor solution, based on factor analysis, with the first factor being "uncertainty and inability for caring," and the second "a familial and social life impact" factor (62). The authors list seven items included for each factor, but it is not clear if these are examples or all the items in that particular factor.

A further study found a five-factor solution accounting for 64% of the variance of the ZBI (64). No further information on this is given, but this finding, together with findings from the factor analysis of the Impact of Caregiving Scale, was used to reduce the total number of items for a burden screen (containing items and factors of both the ZBI and the Impact of Caregiving Scale).

The factor model by Whitlatch (47), as well as two other models (a one-factor and a three-factor solution), was tested by Knight and colleagues (70). Item 22, a global measure of burden, was omitted from the three confirmatory factor analyses. With two different samples, neither the first nor the second model fitted the data. Exploratory analysis revealed a five-factor solution, but two factors had only one item loading on them. Therefore the authors proposed a three-factor solution on 14 of the 22 items, with the factors being embarrassment/anger (nine items), patient's dependency (two items), and self-criticism (three items). The three-factor solution was confirmed in a second sample, and shifting one item from factor 1 to factor 2 resulted in an improved fit of the model (70). These findings led the authors to conclude that the ZBI does not have a clear factor structure.

A further study used principal component analysis on 21 items (again, item 22 was omitted) of the ZBI and found support for a two-factor solution (personal strain and role strain) (71). From this, the 12-item version was determined by selecting the six items for each factor with the highest factor loading and the highest item-total correlation. Four items were selected according to the highest ranking item-total correlations while respecting factor weighting of the 12-item version (3:1 ratio) to create a screening version of the ZBI. When the short version was used with a two-way ANOVA, the results obtained were identical to those produced with the full version (71).

The viability of the two-factor solution of the 12-item version was further tested by O'Rourke and Tuokko (77) with an initial factor analysis with 200 carers and a second confirmatory factor analysis with 895 carers. Initial factor analysis revealed three factors, but one factor explained less than 10% of the variance and thus was omitted from further analysis. Further analysis of the two remaining factors produced results similar to those of Bedard et al. (71), with each of the 12 items loading on its respective factors. However, four items loaded significantly across factors, and one factor loading in this sample was greater on "personal strain" than on "role strain," which was not in agreement with the findings of Bedard et al. (71). The second confirmatory factor analysis showed good fit of the data for the two-factor solution, and the authors concluded that their findings show that the two-factor solution was viable (77).

Ankri et al. (80) found a five-factor solution for the 22-item ZBI through principal component analysis. Three of the factors were retained because they were clinically relevant, and two factors were discarded (one because it contained only one item, and

the second because there was overlap with another factor). The factors for the 22 items represented "consequences on the carer's daily social and personal life" (factor 1 accounted for 41.5% of variance), "psychological burden and emotional reactions" (factor 2, 8.6% of variance), and "guilt" (factor 3, 6.2% of variance).

Another five-factor solution was found for the Chinese version of the ZBI, including the factors of "caregiver's feelings of oversacrifice" (eight items), "patient's dependence on the caregiver" (four items), "negative emotions due to caring" (four items), "caregiver's feelings of inadequacy" (two items), and "uncertainty about the patient's future" (three items) (87). Item 22, a general item often not included in the factor analysis, was included in this factor analysis and loaded on the first factor.

The factor structure of the ZBI was not part of the development process of the ZBI. To date, there is no agreement as to the dimensionality of the ZBI, with some studies having shown that it is multifactorial and other studies having found that it is unidimensional. Studies that have found multiple factors do not necessarily agree on the number of factors, and to date, the factor structure of the ZBI remains unclear.

Validity

Few studies have directly investigated the validity of the ZBI, but some information can be extrapolated from the findings of studies that have used multiple instruments. Predictive validity can be extrapolated from data on the patient or the carer. These data were gained from generic, disease-specific, or dimension-specific outcome measures, and in some cases, carer-specific outcome measures. Associations between the ZBI and personal characteristics of the patient or carer, or with the patient's disease characteristics, have also been studied. Associations between the ZBI and other instruments have mostly been studied through correlations, although some studies have carried out regression analysis or multi-factorial analysis.

Carer variables

Carer characteristics

The type of carer (e.g., formal vs. informal, male vs. female) has in some, but not all, studies been found to have an effect on burden. The ZBI score is statistically significant higher for informal versus professional carers, and this difference remains for the two factors by Whitlatch: "personal strain" and "role strain" (47). No statistically significant relationship was found between ZBI score and the gender of the carer (50, 91), but another study found that female spouses reported almost twice the mean burden of male spouses (74). When the cutoff score was 33 or above as high burden, and below 33 as low to normal burden, it was found that a significantly higher percentage of women reported a high burden score in comparison with male carers (75). Other studies found no significant difference in ZBI score, depending on the carer's gender (47, 88, 89).

With respect to the carer's age, it has been found that there is no significant difference in the burden measured by the ZBI according to the carer's age (50, 88, 89, 94) and that there is a higher burden with increasing age of the carer (81, 91). Using logistic regression, with the ZBI score above 21 as a cutoff score, significant relationships were found between the ZBI and the age of the carer (younger than 48 years of age, or 48 years of age or older) (56). However, another study found that when dichotomizing carers into low or high burden (as determined by the median), no difference in ZBI according to carer's age was noted (94).

Higher burden was significantly associated with lower levels of education (81).

Significant associations of the ZBI score were found with financial dissatisfaction (48), but not with household income (88). Spouse carers in the lowest financial category (<$25,000/year) reported more than twice the burden of spouse carers in other financial categories (74).

No significant difference in ZBI was found for work outside the house (dichotomized yes or no) (50) or location of residence (rural vs. urban) (74). However, in a later study, the ZBI score was found

to be related to location of residence, with carers living in rural areas having a higher burden than carers living in urban areas (91).

After 2 years, patients whose carers had reported higher burden at baseline were more likely to have been placed in a nursing home (58). A variation of ZBI scores was found, depending on whether patients lived in an institution or in the community (86). However, it is questionable whether this information is useful to assess the ZBI, as this study used a modified 15-item version of the ZBI, and it was not clear whether these are all ZBI items, or whether some items are from the original ZBI; some items are newly generated for this study. Another study found that living in an institution was significantly associated with lower ZBI (72).

Four studies report on the effect of ethnicity or country in relation to the ZBI. Differences in burden were found between Korean and American carers of elderly parents with dementia, with Koreans reporting significantly more developmental, social, and emotional burden (95). The authors reported an overall higher burden for Americans, but this difference was small and not significant. Differences in ZBI scores have been found between the countries of India and South Asia; China and South East Asia; Taiwan and Hong Kong; Latin America and the Caribbean; and Nigeria (range, 25.9–50.3) (33), but the authors do not report whether these differences are statistically significant. A significant difference in burden was found between Malays, Chinese, and Indians in Malaysia, with the Malays having a lower score than the Chinese or Indian respondents (88), and between African Americans and Caucasians, with African Americans reporting lower burden (49).

Family relationship

The findings on associations between the ZBI score and the relationships of carers to the persons they care for are conflicting. Some studies found no significant differences in total burden score for child versus spouse carers (46, 91), between a variety of family carers (89), or between different (unspecified) carers (7, 50, 76, 88). However, other studies have found a significant relationship between ZBI score and the relationship between the caregiver and the care recipient. A European study found that spouses (both husbands and wives) expressed significantly more burden than the other types of informal carers (72), and another study found that higher burden was significantly associated with family relationships (81).

The association between ZBI score and family relationships has been found to change over time, with husbands who were carers reporting less burden than wives who were carers at baseline, but after 2 years, average scores for husbands and wives were about the same (58). In a study that has found that the ZBI is multi-factorial, the scores of two of the three ZBI factors were related to the carer's family status (80). For factor 1 ("consequences on the carer's daily social and personal life"), spouses had higher scores than children. For factor 3 ("guilt"), children had higher scores than spouses. Scores on factor 2 ("psychological burden and emotional reactions") were independent of the carer's family status.

However, associations have been examined not only for the type of relationship between the carer and the person being cared for but for the quality of the relationship or the carer's perception of social support. Carers' subjective social support and quality of relationship before the onset of dementia were both significantly and negatively correlated with carer burden (58). The significant correlation between the ZBI and the quality of the premorbid relationship between the carer and the person who is cared for was not found in another study (89). Marital satisfaction significantly predicted ZBI scores (74).

Social support

Full-time carers have been found to have higher ZBI scores than carers who share the caring responsibility with a sibling (88), but no correlation was found between the ZBI scores and paying for caring services by a nurse or a maid (88). A significant relationship between the ZBI and having no alternative carer has also been found (91). However, there is

also evidence that having an alternative carer does not make a significant difference to the carer's burden (7, 89). Furthermore, no significant difference in ZBI was found according to the help provided to the carer (50).

Social support assessed with the Social Support Appraisals Scale significantly predicted carer burden (68), as did perceived social support (measured by the Perceived Social Support-Family Scale) (74).

Caring variables

Significant correlations were found between the ZBI score and a number of caring variables, including years of caring (80, 89, 96); hours spent caring (19, 80, 88), including number of hours helping the patient with ADLs; number of hours helping with instrumental tasks; the carer's hours of sleep (19); the carer's ability to cope (36, 53, 65); and the number of hours invested in care. The ZBI subscales of "personal strain" and "role strain" have also been found to be weakly to moderately and significantly correlated with the "negative impact" and "positive value" subscales of the COPE Index (36).

Health status and quality of life

It has mostly been found that there is a significant association between carer burden and quality of life. The carer's quality of life has been assessed by a number of different outcome measures. Burden was found to be significantly and inversely correlated with the carer's well-being, as measured by the Satisfaction with Life Scale (65). Individual quality of life (measured by the SEIQoL) was significantly and negatively correlated with burden measured by the ZBI (68). When health status was assessed by the EQ-5D, it was found that carers who reported higher burden had significantly lower quality of life (81).

The ZBI showed low to moderate correlations with the different dimensions of the SF-36 (10). The Chinese ZBI has been found to be significantly related to the Chinese Health Questionnaire and the Caregiver Activity Survey (87).

When the cutoff score was 33 or above as high burden, and below 33 as low to normal burden, carers with worse perceived health had higher odds of reporting a high burden score than carers with good perceived health, although the levels were not statistically significant ($p = 0.07$) (75). For this study, a single question was used to assess health status with 5- point Likert-style response options. Another study which also found no significant correlation with the ZBI had used a single question rated on a 6-point Likert-style scale on which carers reported their health status (53).

Dimension-specific

A significant correlation has been found between the ZBI score and the carer's distress (53), the carer's anxiety (10, 82), depression (10), spiritual well-being (49), and insomnia (82). Furthermore, for a late onset of dementia group (but not an early onset of dementia group), the ZBI was significantly correlated with the carer's somatic symptoms and perceived difficulties due to the patient's behavioral disturbances (82). The role strain factor of the ZBI has been found to be significantly correlated with the Beck Depression Inventory (7).

Patient variables

Patient characteristics

When carers were dichotomized into low or high burden, it was found that the high-burden group tended to be caring for older patients and for a longer duration (94). Using logistic regression (cutoff score above 21), significant relationships were found between the ZBI and the age of the patient ($<$or$> = 26$ years of age) (56). One study found significant but weak correlations between the ZBI and the Parkinson's disease patient's age and age of onset of PD (19). No significant correlation was found between the ZBI and the patient's education, age, gender, or estimated premorbid intelligence, or living situation (living independently vs. living with the carer) (85). One study did not find any sig-

nificant relationships between patient demographic variables and the ZBI (76).

Type of condition

Only information on dementia and Parkinson's in relation to the ZBI score is available. ZBI scores have been found to be significantly higher in carers of elderly with dementia in comparison with carers of elderly without dementia (91). For both the early-onset dementia group and the late-onset group (i.e., age of onset of 65 years and older), the ZBI score was significantly correlated with the Neuropsychiatric Inventory (NPI), but no significant difference in total burden score was found between the early-onset and late-onset groups (82). However, when frontotemporal dementia was compared with Alzheimer's, the ZBI score was found to be significantly higher when the person cared for had frontotemporal dementia (84). Also, the ZBI score significantly increases with the severity of dementia (80). Parallel to an increase in burden with dementia severity, the progression of Parkinson's disease has been found to be significantly related to carer burden (19).

Illness severity

The relationship with the ZBI has been assessed in a number of studies that have used a range of different instruments to assess the patient's illness severity. For some instruments (the Barthel Index and the Hoehn and Yahr Scale), both significant and nonsignificant correlations have been found.

Significant correlations of total burden have been found between various measures of the patient's impairments (46), including decreasing patient function (66). Significant correlations have been found between all the subscales of the Brief Symptoms Inventory and the ZBI, with the anxiety and hostility subscale being the most strongly correlated with the ZBI (60). Significant correlations were also found between the Direct Assessment of Functional Status Scale (to measure abilities in different functional domains) (62) and some domains of the

Functional Assessment of Multiple Sclerosis questionnaire (including mobility, general contentment, thinking and fatigue, family/social well-being, and the total score) (54), and with the severity of dementia (89), the degree of dependency of the patient (KATZ questionnaire) (56), the "motor examination" of the Unified Parkinson's Disease Scale (53), the Barthel Index (19), the Hoehn and Yahr Scale (19), and the clinical global impression-severity scale (19), as well as the Mattis Dementia Rating Scale for Alzheimer's disease but not for frontotemporal dementia (84).

However, the ZBI score did not differ according to the Barthel Index in another study (55). Other variables that were not significantly related to the ZBI were duration of illness (46), pain measured by a visual analogue scale (53), the Hoehn and Yahr Staging Scale (53), the dementia rating scale (53), disability (measured by the Functional Disability Scale) (84), and the patients' neuropsychological test performance (85).

Patient behavior

Patient behavior or activity has been found to be mostly significantly related to carer burden as measured by the ZBI. Significant associations have been found between the ZBI and behavioral disturbance of the person cared for (48, 50, 55, 58, 69). Carers of patients with behavioral disturbances had significantly higher ZBI scores than those who cared for patients without behavioral disturbances (as measured by the Behavioral Disturbances Scale) (55). Furthermore, patient behavior disturbance, as measured by the Baumgarten Behavior Disturbance questionnaire, significantly predicted carer burden (68).

A significant positive linear relationship has been found between the total score of the Dysfunctional Behaviour Rating Instrument (DBRI) and the ZBI score (66), and three of the seven domains ("acting out," "disruptive behavior," and "frustration") of the DBRI and the ZBI were strongly significantly associated. Other domains of the DBRI were significantly, but weakly, related to the ZBI, including "hallucinations" and "other behaviors," but no significant association was found with the domains of "delusions" and "repeating."

The ZBI has been found to be significantly related to ADL (Activities of Daily Living) (62, 66, 80), IADL (Instrumental Activities of Daily Living) performance (66, 80), IADL involvement (80), and SMS-ADL (Activities of Daily Living Subscale of the SCOPA-Motor scale) (19). The ZBI is also significantly correlated with some other (specific) items of ADL, including incontinence, grooming, toileting, and feeding (62). The relationship between IADL (instrumental ADL) and burden has been found to be stronger than that between basic ADL and burden (66). The amount of assistance needed with ADLs was found to be the single strongest predictor of burden, with the burden increasing with the greater need for assistance of the person with Parkinson's (74). When patient behavior was assessed by proxy, it was also found to be significantly related to carer burden (85). Only one study did not find a significant difference in ZBI score between carers of patients with no IADL impairment and those with any IADL impairment (91).

One study examined how ZBI factors are related to patient behavior (80) and found that the ZBI has five factors; investigators examined how the scores of the factors are related to patient behavior. The scores of factor 1 were found to be related to degree of difficulty on ADL and IADL performance or involvement. The scores of factor 1 were also related to the patient's aggressiveness, verbal aggressiveness, wandering, and communication problems (80). Scores on factor 2 were related to the patient's verbal aggressiveness, sadness, and depression, with lack of IADL involvement and with progression of dementia (80).

Correlations between carer burden and patient behavior have been found to be related to the severity of illness. For mobile patients, there was a significant correlation for the degree of care needed in dressing and the ZBI but not for any other ADLs (76). There was no significant correlation for any ADLs and the ZBI for nonmobile patients (76). For the two groups together (mobile and nonmobile), two ADL items (feeding and ambulating) were significantly related to the ZBI score (76). In the mobile group, there was a significant relationship between the ZBI and frequency of 13 out of 14 individual behaviors, and in the nonmobile group, there was a significant relationship only for six individual behaviors (such as "interfering with family conversations" or "physical and/or verbal aggression") (76). In the mobile group, "wandering" was the strongest predictor of carer burden, accounting for 16% of the variance. Other predictors of carer burden for the mobile group were "interfering with family conversation," "physical and/or verbal aggression," and "repetition and/or clinging." In the nonmobile group, "repetition and/or clinging" was the only predictor of carer burden (76).

Patient mental state

The relationship between carer burden and the patient's mental state has been frequently investigated. It has been found that the patient's mental state after 2 years was significantly related to carer burden (58). Various aspects of mental state have been assessed, including cognition, depression, and memory of the patient. Frequently, the Mini-Mental State Examination (MMSE) has been used to assess the patient's mental state. The ZBI has been found to be significantly correlated with cognitive decline (as assessed by the Blessed Dementia Scale) (48, 62), the patient's cognitive impairment (48), the patient's mental state as assessed by the MMSE (80) and the Folstein MMSE (53), and cognitive difficulties (as measured by the Cognitive Difficulties Scale) (85). Furthermore, ZBI scores were significantly higher in carers of patients with moderate to severe cognitive impairment (according to MMSE) than in carers of individuals with mild cognitive impairment (91). A significant negative correlation was found between the MMSE and the ZBI for mobile patients, but not for the nonmobile group (76).

However, some studies failed to find significant correlations with the patient's mental state; for example, no significant correlations were found for the ZBI with the Global Deterioration Scale, which measures cognitive decline (62), the MMSE (62), and the standardized MMSE (66). One study has examined how ZBI factors are related to the patient's mental status (80), and the scores of factor 1 were found not to be related to severity of dementia as measured by MMSE or the Clinical Dementia Rating scale.

The patient's mental state in terms of depression has been assessed in a number of studies, all of which have found significant associations between the patient's depression and the carer's burden, despite the fact that a variety of different outcome measures were used to assess the patient's depression. Significant relationships between burden and depression were found with the Geriatric Depression Scale (66), the Hospital Anxiety and Depression Scale (19), and the Beck Depression Inventory (85). Scores on factor 2 of the ZBI were related to the patient's sadness and depression, irrespective of MMSE score or CDR (clinical dementia rating) measurement (80). Significant relationships between burden and patient depression were also found when the carer reported that the patient was depressed or unhappy (89), or when the carer completed the Beck Depression Inventory by proxy (85).

As far as the patient's memory was concerned, it has been found to be significantly related to carer burden (both at baseline and at 2-year follow-up) (58). Furthermore, the ZBI was significantly correlated with the subscales of the revised memory and behavior problems checklist, as well as the total score (69).

Longitudinal

Variation in ZBI scores was found, depending on whether patients were in the treatment versus the nontreatment group and whether they lived in an institution or in the community (86). Again, this information is based on a modified 15-item version of the ZBI, and it was not clear whether these are all ZBI items or whether some items were from the original ZBI or were newly generated for this study.

Responsiveness to change

The association between ZBI score and family relationship has also been found to change over time, with husbands who were carers reporting less burden than wives who were carers at baseline, but after 2 years, the average scores for husbands and wives were about the same (58).

At baseline, there was a difference in burden between husband and wife carers, but this difference did not exist after 2 years (59).

No changes in ZBI score were found as a result of an intervention, which was a community-based program focusing on supporting the carer by providing information on dementia, guidance on behavior management, a psychiatric assessment and psychotropic medication if needed (51).

Cut-off scores

The first study that aimed to establish clinical cutoffs for carer burden was conducted by Rankin et al. (64). The authors concluded that they did not find a definite cutoff, but even if they had, it probably would not have been useful in terms of providing information on a cut-off score for the ZBI because the instrument used to establish the cut-off score was based on items from two carer burden outcome measures: the ZBI and the Impact of Caregiving inventory.

Bedard et al. (71) suggest a cutoff score of 17 for the 12-item ZBI, and of 8 on the 4-item ZBI. This cutoff represents the top quartile of the burden score; however, the authors point out that their data cannot be assumed as normative. In their study, O'Rourke and Tuokko (77) further tested the cutoff score first suggested by Bedard et al. They found that a score of above 16 on the ZBI identified less than half of the carers presenting with clinically significant depression, as measured by the Center for Epidemiologic Studies Depression Scale (CED-S). A cut-off score of above 10 increased sensitivity to 75% relative to the CED-S but reduced specificity to 68%.

This led the authors to conclude that it is premature to propose a definite clinical cutoff.

Two further studies use cut-off scores for their analysis. The first study used a cut-off score of 33 or higher to signify "high burden" and a score below 33 as "low to normal burden" (75). Boyer et al. (56), for the purposes of their study, classed a ZBI score of below 21 as absent to slight burden, and a ZBI of 21 and above as moderate to severe burden. For both studies, no information is available on how this cut-off score was derived.

Feasibility

One study (12-item version) found a significantly higher response rate from female carers in comparison with male carers (77).

Floor and ceiling effects

One study described having 90% of computable scores with 1.3% of ceiling and floor effects (19).

Conclusion

To summarize, carer burden in long-term conditions is being increasingly assessed, including in neurodegenerative conditions. A wide range of instruments have been used, but little formal psychometric testing has been undertaken, and psychometric information mostly needs to be extrapolated from studies using the instruments. This means that little, if any, psychometric information is available for generic instruments, and for most generic instruments, the information is derived from a single study. The largest number of studies for generic instruments giving some psychometric information are related to the SF-36 (and SF-12) and the GHQ. Mostly, only information on validity is available, although information on responsiveness is available from one study for each measure. Additionally, some reliability and precision information is available for the SF-36. Because generic outcome measures have been assessed and validated widely, it is likely that these instruments are useful in the assessment of carer health-related quality of life. However, more formal and extensive psychometric testing would need to be carried out to confirm this.

As far as carer-specific instruments are concerned, many different instruments have been used, but few have been formally developed and tested. The instruments have mostly been developed for dementia, including the ZBI, which has been reviewed more extensively in this chapter. The ZBI is thought to be the most commonly used carer burden instrument for dementia (2). Available psychometric information is predominantly validity information, which is similar to the evaluation information available for generic instruments. Some evaluation studies, such as those evaluating the dimensionality of the ZBI, were carried out many years after the first development of the ZBI. Additionally, some evidence is conflicting, such as the evidence on whether the ZBI is unidimensional or multi-dimensional. However, evidence from a wide range of studies indicates that the ZBI is a valid instrument. The ZBI also fared favorably in a review by Moniz-Cook et al. (97), who rated the ZBI well, despite the paucity of intervention outcome data, and concluded that the ZBI will probably stand the test of time. Similarly, because generic instruments are increasingly used in carer populations for which they have not been validated, the ZBI is commonly used for populations for whom it has neither been intended nor validated (52). The conclusion regarding the value of using ZBI in carers of someone with a neurodegenerative condition other than dementia has to be the same as for generic instruments. Given evidence of the psychometric properties of the ZBI, it is likely that it is useful for assessing carer burden in neurodegenerative conditions generally, and not only in dementia, for which it was originally developed. As for generic instruments, more formal and extensive testing of the ZBI is required to confirm this.

REFERENCES

1. Vitaliano PP, Zhang J, Scanlan JM. Is caregiving hazardous to one's physical health? A meta-analysis. *Psychol Bull* 2003 Nov; **129**(6): 946–972.
2. Dillehay RC, Sandys MR. Caregivers for Alzheimer's patients: what we are learning from research. *Int J Aging Hum Dev* 1990; **30**(4): 263–285.
3. Fitzpatrick R, Bowling A, Gibbons E, Jenkinson CP, Mackintosh A, Peters M. A structured review of patient-reported measures in relation to selected chronic conditions, percpetions of quality of carer and carer impact. Oxford: Report to the Department of Health; November 2006.
4. Robinson BC. Validation of a caregiver strain index. *J Gerontol* 1983; **38**(3): 344–348.
5. Pakenham KI. Development of a measure of coping with multiple sclerosis caregiving. *Psychol Health* 2002; **17**(1): 97–118.
6. Vitaliano PP, Young HM, Russo J. Burden: a review of measures used among caregivers of individuals with dementia. *Gerontologist* 1991 Feb; **31**(1): 67–75.
7. Takahashi M, Tanaka K, Miyaoka H. Depression and associated factors of informal caregivers versus professional caregivers of demented patients. *Psychiatry Clin Neurosci* 2005 Aug; **59**(4): 473–480.
8. Lo Coco G, Lo Coco D, Cicero V, Oliveri A, Lo VG, Piccoli F, et al. Individual and health-related quality of life assessment in amyotrophic lateral sclerosis patients and their caregivers. *J Neurol Sci* 2005 Nov 15; **238**(1–2): 11–7.
9. Wade DT, Gage H, Owen C, Trend P, Grossmith C, Kaye J. Multidisciplinary rehabilitation for people with Parkinson's disease: a randomised controlled study. *J Neurol Neurosurg Psychiatry* 2003 Feb; **74**(2): 158–162.
10. Martinez-Martin P, ito-Leon J, Alonso F, Catalan MJ, Pondal M, Zamarbide I, et al. Quality of life of caregivers in Parkinson's disease. *Qual Life Res* 2005 Mar; **14**(2): 463–472.
11. Ware JE, Jr., Sherbourne CD. The MOS 36-item short-form health survey (SF-36). I. Conceptual framework and item selection. *Med Care* 1992 Jun; **30**(6): 473–483.
12. Bell CM, Araki SS, Neumann PJ. The association between caregiver burden and caregiver health-related quality of life in Alzheimer disease. *Alzheimer Dis Assoc Disord* 2001 Jul; **15**(3): 129–136.
13. Berg-Weger M, Rauch SM, Rubio DM, Tebb SS. Assessing the health of adult daughter former caregivers for

elders with Alzheimer's disease. *Am J Alzheimer Dis Other Dementias* 2003; **18**(4): 231–239.

14. Lyons KS, Stewart BJ, Archbold PG, Carter JH, Perrin NA. Pessimism and optimism as early warning signs for compromised health for caregivers of patients with Parkinson's disease. *Nurs Res* 2004 Nov; **53**(6): 354–362.

15. Argimon JM, Limon E, Vila J, Cabezas C. Health-related quality-of-life of care-givers as a predictor of nursing-home placement of patients with dementia. *Alzheimer Dis Assoc Disord* 2005 Jan; **19**(1): 41–44.

16. McConaghy R, Caltabiano ML. Caring for a person with dementia: exploring relationships between perceived burden, depression, coping and well-being. *Nurs Health Sci* 2005 Jun; **7**(2): 81–91.

17. Van Den Berg JP, Kalmijn S, Lindeman E, Veldink JH, de VM, Van Der Graaff MM, et al. Multidisciplinary ALS care improves quality of life in patients with ALS. *Neurology* 2005 Oct 25; **65**(8): 1264–1267.

18. Patti F, Amato MP, Battaglia MA, Pitaro M, Russo P, Solaro C, et al. Caregiver quality of life in multiple sclerosis: a multicentre Italian study. *Mult Scler* 2007 Apr; **13**(3): 412–419.

19. Martinez-Martin P, Forjaz MJ, Frades-Payo B, Rusinol AB, Fernandez-Garcia JM, Ito-Leon J, et al. Caregiver burden in Parkinson's disease. *Mov Disord* 2007 May 15; **22**(7): 924–931.

20. Argimon JM, Limon E, Vila J, Cabezas C. Health-related quality of life in carers of patients with dementia. *Fam Pract* 2004 Aug; **21**(4): 454–457.

21. Jenkinson CP, Fitzpatrick R, Swash M, Peto V. The ALS Health Profile Study: quality of life of amyotrophic lateral sclerosis patients and carers in Europe. *J Neurol* 2000 Nov; **247**(11): 835–840.

22. Goldberg DP, Blackwell B. Psychiatric illness in general practice: a detailed study using a new method of case identification. *BMJ* 1970 May 23; **1**(5707): 439–443.

23. Goldberg DP, Gater R, Sartorius N, Ustun TB, Piccinelli M, Gureje O, et al. The validity of two versions of the GHQ in the WHO study of mental illness in general health care. *Psychol Med* 1997 Jan; **27**(1): 191–197.

24. Jackson A, Cooney C, Walsh JB, Coakley D. Caring for dementia sufferers in the community: the caregivers problems. *Ir Med J* 1991 Jun; **84**(2): 51–53.

25. Draper BM, Poulos CJ, Cole AM, Poulos RG, Ehrlich F. A comparison of caregivers for elderly stroke and dementia victims. *J Am Geriatr Soc* 1992 Sep; **40**(9): 896–901.

26. O'Reilly F, Finnan F, Allwright S, Smith GD, Ben-Shlomo Y. The effects of caring for a spouse with Parkinson's disease on social, psychological and physical well-being. *Br J Gen Pract* 1996 Sep; **46**(410): 507–512.

27. Donaldson C, Tarrier N, Burns A. Determinants of carer stress in Alzheimer's disease. *Int J Geriatr Psychiatry* 1998 Apr; **13**(4): 248–256.

28. Rosenvinge H, Jones D, Judge E, Martin A. Demented and chronic depressed patients attending a day hospital: stress experienced by carers. *Int J Geriatr Psychiatry* 1998 Jan; **13**(1): 8–11.

29. Matsuda O. Reliability and validity of the subjective burden scale in family caregivers of elderly relatives with dementia. *Int Psychogeriatrics* 1999; **11**(2): 159–170.

30. Nagatomo I, Akasaki Y, Uchida M, Tominaga M, Hashiguchi W, Takigawa M. Gender of demented patients and specific family relationship of caregiver to patients influence mental fatigue and burdens on relatives as caregivers. *Int J Geriatr Psychiatry* 1999 Aug; **14**(8): 618–625.

31. Groom MJ, Lincoln NB, Francis VM, Stephan TF. Assessing mood in patients with multiple sclerosis. *Clin Rehabil* 2003 Dec; **17**(8): 847–857.

32. Woods RT, Wills W, Higginson IJ, Hobbins J, Whitby M. Support in the community for people with dementia and their carers: a comparative outcome study of specialist mental health service interventions. *Int J Geriatr Psychiatry* 2003 Apr; **18**(4): 298–307.

33. Prince M. Care arrangements for people with dementia in developing countries. *Int J Geriatr Psychiatry* 2004 Feb; **19**(2): 170–177.

34. Secker DL, Brown RG. Cognitive behavioural therapy (CBT) for carers of patients with Parkinson's disease: a preliminary randomised controlled trial. *J Neurol Neurosurg Psychiatry* 2005 Apr; **76**(4): 491–497.

35. Love A, Street A, Harris R, Lowe R. Social aspects of caregiving for people living with motor neurone disease: their relationships to carer well-being. *Palliat Support Care* 2005 Mar; **3**(1): 33–38.

36. Roud H, Keeling S, Sainsbury R. Using the COPE assessment tool with informal carers of people with dementia in New Zealand. *N Z Med J* 2006; **119**(1237): U2053.

37. Elmstahl S, Malmberg B, Annerstedt L. Caregiver's burden of patients 3 years after stroke assessed by a novel caregiver burden scale. *Arch Phys Med Rehabil* 1996 Feb; **77**(2): 177–182.

38. Miyashita M, Yamaguchi A, Kayama M, Narita Y, Kawada N, Akiyama M, et al. Validation of the Burden Index of Caregivers (BIC), a multidimensional short care burden scale from Japan. *Health Qual Life Outcomes* 2006; **4**: 52.

39. Thomas P, Hazif-Thomas C, Delagnes V, Bonduelle P, Clement JP. [Vulnerability of caregivers for demented patients. The Pixel study]. *Psychol Neuropsychiatr Vieil* 2005 Sep; **3**(3): 207–220.

40. Thomas P, Lalloue F, Preux PM, Hazif-Thomas C, Pariel S, Inscale R, et al. Dementia patients caregivers quality of life: the PIXEL study. *Int J Geriatr Psychiatry* 2006 Jan; **21**(1): 50–56.

41. Elmstahl S, Ingvad B, Annerstedt L. Family caregiving in dementia: prediction of caregiver burden 12 months after relocation to group-living care. *Int Psychogeriatr* 1998 Jun; **10**(2): 127–146.

42. Andren S, Elmstahl S. Former family carers' subjective experiences of burden: a comparison between group living and nursing home environments in one municipality in Sweden. *Dementia* 2002; **1**(2): 241–254.

43. Andren S, Elmstahl S. Family caregivers' subjective experiences of satisfaction in dementia care: aspects of burden, subjective health and sense of coherence. *Scand J Caring Sci* 2005 Jun; **19**(2): 157–168.

44. Andren S, Elmstahl S. Relationships between income, subjective health and caregiver burden in caregivers of people with dementia in group living care: a cross-sectional community-based study. *Int J Nurs Stud* 2007 Mar; **44**(3): 435–446.

45. Glozman JM, Bicheva KG, Fedorova NV. Scale of Quality of Life of Caregivers/SQLC. *J Neurol* 1998 May; **245**(suppl1): S39–S41.

46. Zarit SH, Reever KE, Bach-Peterson J. Relatives of the impaired elderly: correlates of feelings of burden. *Gerontologist* 1980 Dec; **20**(6): 649–655.

47. Whitlatch CJ, Zarit SH, von Eye A. Efficacy of interventions with caregivers: a reanalysis. *Gerontologist* 1991 Feb; **31**(1): 9–14.

48. Schneider J, Murray J, Banerjee S, Mann A. EUROCARE: a cross-national study of co-resident spouse carers for people with Alzheimer's disease: I–Factors associated with carer burden. *Int J Geriatr Psychiatry* 1999 Aug; **14**(8): 651–661.

49. Spurlock WR. Spiritual well-being and caregiver burden in Alzheimer's caregivers. *Geriatr Nurs* 2005 May; **26**(3): 154–161.

50. Gort AM, Mingot M, Gomez X, Soler T, Torres G, Sacristan O, et al. Use of the Zarit scale for assessing caregiver burden and collapse in caregiving at home in dementias. *Int J Geriatr Psychiatry* 2007 Oct; **22**(10): 957–962.

51. Dias A, Dewey ME, D'Souza J, Dhume R, Motghare DD, Shaji KS, et al. The effectiveness of a home care program for supporting caregivers of persons with dementia in developing countries: a randomised controlled trial from Goa, India. *PLoS ONE* 2008; **3**(6): e2333.

52. Bachner YG, O'Rourke N. Reliability generalization of responses by care providers to the Zarit Burden Interview. *Aging Ment Health* 2007 Nov; **11**(6): 678–685.

53. Cifu DX, Carne W, Brown R, Pegg P, Ong J, Qutubuddin A, et al. Caregiver distress in Parkinsonism. *J Rehabil Res Dev* 2006 Jul; **43**(4): 499–508.

54. Rivera-Navarro J, Morales-Gonzalez JM, Benito-Leon J, Madrid Dymyelinating Diseases Group (GEDMA). Informal caregiving in multiple sclerosis patients: data from the Madrid Demyelinating Disease Group study. *Disabil Rehabil* 2003 Sep 5(18): 1057–1064.

55. Arai Y, Kudo K, Hosokawa T, Washio M, Miura H, Hisamichi S. Reliability and validity of the Japanese version of the Zarit Caregiver Burden interview. *Psychiatry Clin Neurosci* 1997 Oct; **51**(5): 281–287.

56. Boyer F, Drame M, Morrone I, Novella JL. Factors relating to carer burden for families of persons with muscular dystrophy. *J Rehabil Med* 2006 Sep; **38**(5): 309–315.

57. Schreiner AS, Morimoto T, Arai Y, Zarit S. Assessing family caregiver's mental health using a statistically derived cut-off score for the Zarit Burden Interview. *Aging Ment Health* 2006 Mar; **10**(2): 107–111.

58. Zarit SH, Todd PA, Zarit JM. Subjective burden of husbands and wives as caregivers: a longitudinal study. *Gerontologist* 1986 Jun; **26**(3): 260–266.

59. Zarit SH, Anthony CR, Boutselis M. Interventions with care givers of dementia patients: comparison of two approaches. *Psychol Aging* 1987 Sep; **2**(3): 225–232.

60. Anthony-Bergstone CR, Zarit SH, Gatz M. Symptoms of psychological distress among caregivers of dementia patients. *Psychol Aging* 1988 Sep; **3**(3): 245–248.

61. Hébert R, Bravo G, Girouard D. Fidélité de la traduction française de trois instruments d'évaluation des aidants naturels de malades déments. *Can J Aging* 1993; **12**(3): 324–337.

62. Mangone CA, Sanguinetti RM, Baumann PD, Gonzalez RC, Pereyra S, Bozzola FG, et al. Influence of feelings of burden on the caregiver's perception of the patient's functional status. *Dementia* 1993 Sep; **4**(5): 287–293.

63. Hadjistavropoulos T, Taylor S, Tuokko H, Beattie BL. Neuropsychological deficits, caregivers' perception of deficits and caregiver burden. *J Am Geriatr Soc* 1994 Mar; **42**(3): 308–314.

64. Rankin ED, Haut MW, Keefover RW, Franzen MD. The establishment of clinical cutoffs in measuring caregiver burden in dementia. *Gerontologist* 1994 Dec; **34**(6): 828–832.

65. Majerovitz SD. Role of family adaptability in the psychological adjustment of spouse caregivers to patients with dementia. *Psychol Aging* 1995 Sep; **10**(3): 447–457.

66. Molloy DW, Lever JA, Bedard M, Guyatt GH, Butt GML. Burden in care givers of older adults with impaired cognition: the relationship with dysfunctional behaviors, daily living and mood. *Ann RCPSC* 1996; **29**(3): 151–154.

67. Coen RF, Swanwick GRJ, O'Boyle CA, Coakley D. Behaviour disturbance and other predictors of carer burden in Alzheimer's disease. *Int J Geriatr Psychiatry* 1997 Mar; **12**(3): 331–336.

68. Coen RF, O'Boyle CA, Swanwick GRJ, Coakley D. Measuring the impact on relatives of caring for people with Alzheimer's disease: quality of life, burden and wellbeing. *Psychol Health* 1999; **14**(2): 253–261.

69. Hebert R, Bravo G, Preville M. Reliability, validity and reference values of the Zarit burden interview for assessing informal caregivers of community-dwelling older persons with dementia. *Can J Aging* 2000; **19**(4): 494–507.

70. Knight BG, Fox LS, Chou P. Factor structure of the burden Interview. *J Clin Geropsychology* 2000; **6**(4): 249–258.

71. Bedard M, Molloy DW, Squire L, Dubois S, Lever JA, O'Donnell M. The Zarit Burden Interview: a new short version and screening version. *Gerontologist* 2001 Oct; **41**(5): 652–657.

72. Colvez A, Joel ME, Ponton-Sanchez A, Royer AC. Health status and work burden of Alzheimer patients' informal caregivers: comparisons of five different care programs in the European Union. *Health Policy* 2002 Jun; **60**(3): 219–33.

73. Edwards NE, Ruettiger KM. The influence of caregiver burden on patients' management of Parkinson's disease: implications for rehabilitation nursing. *Rehabil Nurs* 2002 Sep; **27**(5): 182–86, 198.

74. Edwards NE, Scheetz PS. Predictors of burden for caregivers of patients with Parkinson's disease. *J Neurosci Nurs* 2002 Aug; **34**(4): 184–190.

75. Gallicchio L, Siddiqi N, Langenberg P, Baumgarten M. Gender differences in burden and depression among informal caregivers of demented elders in the community. *Int J Geriatr Psychiatry* 2002 Feb; **17**(2): 154–163.

76. Miyamoto Y, Ito H, Otsuka T, Kurita H. Caregiver burden in mobile and non-mobile demented patients: a comparative study. *Int J Geriatr Psychiatry* 2002 Aug; **17**(8): 765–773.

77. O'Rourke N, Tuokko HA. Psychometric properties of an abridged version of the Zarit Burden Interview within a representative Canadian caregiver sample. *Gerontologist* 2003 Feb; **43**(1): 121–127.

78. Dooley NR, Hinojosa J. Improving quality of life for persons with Alzheimer's disease and their family caregivers: brief occupational therapy intervention. *Am J Occup Ther* 2004 Sep; **58**(5): 561–569.

79. Taub A, Andreoli SB, Bertolucci PH. Dementia caregiver burden: reliability of the Brazilian version of the Zarit caregiver burden interview. *Cad Saude Publica* 2004 Mar; **20**(2): 372–376.

80. Ankri J, Andrieu S, Beaufils B, Grand A, Henrard JC. Beyond the global score of the Zarit Burden Interview: useful dimensions for clinicians. *Int J Geriatr Psychiatry* 2005 Mar; **20**(3): 254–260.

81. Serrano-Aguilar PG, Lopez-Bastida J, Yanes-Lopez V. Impact on health-related quality of life and perceived burden of informal caregivers of individuals with Alzheimer's disease. *Neuroepidemiology* 2006; **27**(3): 136–142.

82. Arai A, Matsumoto T, Ikeda M, Arai Y. Do family caregivers perceive more difficulty when they look after patients with early onset dementia compared to those with late onset dementia? *Int J Geriatr Psychiatry* 2007 Dec; **22**(12): 1255–1261.

83. Bridges-Webb C, Giles B, Speechly C, Zurynski Y, Hiramanek N. Patients with dementia and their carers. *Ann N Y Acad Sci* 2007 Oct; **1114**: 130–136.

84. Boutoleau-Bretonniere C, Vercelletto M, Volteau C, Renou P, Lamy E. Zarit burden inventory and activities of daily living in the behavioral variant of frontotemporal dementia. *Dement Geriatr Cogn Disord* 2008; **25**(3): 272–277.

85. Bruce JM, McQuiggan M, Williams V, Westervelt H, Tremont G. Burden among spousal and child caregivers of patients with mild cognitive impairment. *Dement Geriatr Cogn Disord* 2008; **25**(4): 385–390.

86. Gaugler JE, Roth DL, Haley WE, Mittelman MS. Can counseling and support reduce burden and depressive symptoms in caregivers of people with Alzheimer's

disease during the transition to institutionalization? Results from the New York University caregiver intervention study. *J Am Geriatr Soc* 2008 Mar; **56**(3): 421–428.

87. Ko KT, Yip PK, Liu SI, Huang CR. Chinese version of the Zarit caregiver Burden Interview: a validation study. *Am J Geriatr Psychiatry* 2008 Jun; **16**(6): 513–518.

88. Choo WY, Low WY, Karina R, Poi PJ, Ebenezer E, Prince MJ. Social support and burden among caregivers of patients with dementia in Malaysia. *Asia Pac J Public Health* 2003; **15**(1): 23–29.

89. Onishi J, Suzuki Y, Umegaki H, Nakamura A, Endo H, Iguchi A. Influence of behavioral and psychological symptoms of dementia (BPSD) and environment of care on caregivers' burden. *Arch Gerontol Geriatr* 2005 Sep; **41**(2): 159–168.

90. Goldstein LH, Atkins L, Landau S, Brown R, Leigh PN. Predictors of psychological distress in carers of people with amyotrophic lateral sclerosis: a longitudinal study. *Psychol Med* 2006 Jun; **36**(6): 865–875.

91. Kim SW, Kim JM, Stewart R, Bae KL, Yang SJ, Shin IS, et al. Correlates of caregiver burden for Korean elders according to cognitive and functional status. *Int J Geriatr Psychiatry* 2006 Sep; **21**(9): 853–861.

92. Zarit SH, Orr NK, Zarit JM. *The Hidden Victims of Alzheimer's Disease*. First edition. London and New York: New York University Press, 1985.

93. Kumamoto K, Arai Y. Validation of 'personal strain' and 'role strain': subscales of the short version of the Japanese version of the Zarit Burden Interview (J-ZBI_8). *Psychiatry Clin Neurosci* 2004 Dec; **58**(6): 606–610.

94. Coen RF, Swanwick GR, O'Boyle CA, Coakley D. Behaviour disturbance and other predictors of carer burden in Alzheimer's disease. *Int J Geriatr Psychiatry* 1997 Mar; **12**(3): 331–336.

95. Lee YR, Sung KT. Cultural influences on caregiving burden: cases of Koreans and Americans. *Int J Aging Hum Dev* 1998; **46**(2): 125–141.

96. Morales-Gonzales JM, Ito-Leon J, Rivera-Navarro J, Mitchell AJ. A systematic approach to analyse health-related quality of life in multiple sclerosis: the GEDMA study. *Mult Scler* 2004 Feb; **10**(1): 47–54.

97. Moniz-Cook E, Vernooij-Dassen M, Woods R, Verhey F, Chattat R, De VM, et al. A European consensus on outcome measures for psychosocial intervention research in dementia care. *Aging Ment Health* 2008 Jan; **12**(1): 14–29.

11

Translating patient-reported outcome measures (PROMs) for cross-cultural studies

Michele Peters

Introduction

An increasing number of multi-national studies are conducted within the field of health care. Because most instruments are originally developed in English (either U.K. or U.S.), an increasing number of instruments are translated to allow for cross-cultural comparisons. One example in neurodegenerative conditions is the PDQ-39 for Parkinson's disease, which was originally developed in U.K. English (1) and has been translated into more than 50 different languages. Patient-reported outcome measures (PROMs) are used in different countries to allow cross-national and cross-cultural comparisons of health outcomes. The importance of rigorous, high-quality translations is increasingly recognized, and a systematic review on translation methods has found that a rigorous and multi-step approach leads to a better translation (2). Internationally recognized translation guidelines were outlined by Guillemin and colleagues (3) more than 15 years ago. More recently, task forces such as the ISPOR (International Society for Pharmaeconomics and Outcomes Research) Translation and Cultural Adaptation group have outlined principles of good practice for translations and adaptations of PROMs (4).

To ensure that true cross-cultural comparisons are achieved, the process of translating needs to be rigorous and needs to include assessments of the quality of the translation. Thus, it is important to follow international guidelines to ensure the quality of the translation, to standardize the translation process within different countries, and to evaluate the validity of translated questionnaires. In some instances, specific guidelines, for example, SF-36 (5) or the EQ-5D (6), are related to the translation of a named PROM, and these must be adhered to if the translated instrument is to be recognized as an official version. Therefore, when translating an instrument, it is essential to first contact the original developers of the instrument to get their permission and to establish if any guidelines are available for translation of the instrument. Furthermore, it is important to meticulously describe the translation process in publications to allow readers to assess the rigor and quality of the translation process. This chapter focuses on the translation of existing instruments and outlines the different types of translations and current guidelines for the translation of instruments.

Translation

Many PROMs are initially developed for one study but are later translated to other languages, cultures, or both. Translating an existing instrument means a shorter developmental period and lower costs than required for developing a new

Quality of Life Measurement in Neurodegenerative and Related Conditions, eds., Crispin Jenkinson, Michele Peters, and Mark B. Bromberg. Published by Cambridge University Press. © Cambridge University Press 2011.

instrument cross-culturally (7), but this does not mean that no financial and time investment is necessary. Translations do cost money and require an investment of time, especially if they are carried out to a high standard. If the translation process is not successfully implemented, the validity of the research can be brought into question (8). The intent when translating a questionnaire is to develop another version of the instrument with equivalence to the original one (9).

For a limited number of PROMs, the initial process of development included concurrently developing multiple language versions (10, 11), which helped ensure that the instrument contains only items that are valid in a variety of cross-cultural settings. The concurrent development of several language versions is costly and highly time-consuming. Furthermore, even when several language versions are developed initially, there will be a limitation as to how many language versions are produced, and hence later translations of the instrument may still occur. The concurrent development of several language versions applies methods of translation similar to those used when an instrument is translated at a later stage.

In the literature, the terms "translation" and "adaptation" are used, and frequently these terms are used interchangeably. The Medical Outcomes Trust states that language adaptation might be differentiated from translation (12). If indeed translation and adaptation are different, translation of an instrument may be defined as the instrument's being translated from one language into another (e.g., English to French). Adaptation, on the other hand, may be defined as adapting questionnaires to country- or region-specific dialects (12) and to cultural context and lifestyle (3). According to that definition, an example of adaptation would be the development of a U.S. version of the PDQ-39 for Parkinson's from the original U.K. version (13) even though the authors refer to it as "translation" of the U.K. PDQ-39 to a U.S. PDQ-39. Adaptation can go as far as involving complete transformation of some items to capture the same concepts cross-culturally (14).

A more recent method that avoids having to adapt a PROM is to produce a "universal translation," meaning the development of a single translation that will be appropriate for use in different regions or countries where the same language is spoken (15, 16). The article by Wild et al. (16) gives useful and practical information on when and how to carry out a universal translation, as, for example, that translators should come from different countries. Universal translations still rely on traditional translation methods; the difference lies in the production of a single translated instrument that can be used in different regions or countries where the same language is spoken.

Types of translation

Two types of translation are used: symmetrical and asymmetrical. In symmetrical translation, the original and translated instruments need to be equally familiar and have loyalty of meaning and colloquialness (9) or, in other words, must be culturally relevant in the target population, have conceptual equivalence to the original, and employ language expressions that are commonly used in the target population. In asymmetrical translation, also called literal translation, emphasis is put on loyalty to one language, usually the original language (9). This means that items translated into another language maintain a one-to-one correspondence between words. Asymmetrical translation is therefore often unnatural in the translated version, and concerns arise for "functional equivalence" of words and concepts between the two languages; hence, international guidelines favor conceptual translation (3).

Translation methods

Three types of translation methods are used: 1) one-way translation, 2) the committee approach, and 3) forward and back translation. One-way translation is the fastest (and cheapest) method to translate a PROM; however, concerns arise about the quality of the translation, and it is generally not recommended. Views on whether forward and back translation or the committee approach is the preferred method of translation vary, but generally forward and back translation is recommended more frequently.

Forward and back translation is the most frequently recommended or used approach within translation guidelines (3, 4, 5, 9, 17). Forward and back translation requires at least two translators, who work independently. The first translator produces a translated version in the target language, and the second translator translates the translated version back to the original version (9). However, it is generally recommended that two translators produce a forward translation, and the two translated versions need to be reconciled before being back translated (2, 3, 4). Three methods of reconciliation have been described: 1) a translation panel with the key in-country person, all forward translators, and the project manager; 2) an independent native speaker of the target language who did not do the forward translation; or 3) an appointed in-country investigator, who may have prepared one of the forward translations and who will also conduct pilot testing and cognitive debriefing (4).

According to Wild et al. (4), guidelines vary as to how back translations should be carried out. Some guidelines recommend more than one back translation, whereas others recommend a back translation panel or a single back translation. Whichever option is chosen, once a PROM has been back translated, it will need to be reviewed (4). When discrepancies occur between the original and the back translated versions, researchers need to assess the significance of these discrepancies, and if necessary, modify the translated version to produce a more appropriate and adequate translation.

Another method of translation is panel translation (i.e., the committee approach); some authors believe this to be the best method to ensure high-quality translations (18). This approach involves two panels with five to seven members on each: one panel for the forward translation, and a second panel, including lay people who speak the target language only to assess the translation. A third panel, to include a backward translation, could also be involved. Thus, the panel approach may also involve forward and back translations, but the difference between the panel approach and forward and back translations lies in the fact that, in the panel approach, multiple translators translate the instrument simultaneously, whereas forward and back translation is carried out by one translator, or several translators who work independently.

Different translation techniques can be combined within one project and have been reported in the literature, such as forward and back translation, pilot-test techniques, and the committee approach (3), or back translation in combination with the committee approach (19). Ideally, a panel of bilingual experts compares the equivalence between forward and backward translation (19). Favorable results have been reported from using a combination of techniques; therefore, it is desirable to use multiple methods whenever possible (19).

After completion of the translation process, an instrument needs to be tested in its translated version and within the new target population. This should include pilot testing and cognitive debriefing (4). It is beyond the scope of this chapter to describe psychometric testing, but it is important to note that any translated instrument needs to be subjected to testing. Validating and testing a new language version of a PROM is important to verify the validity and reliability of the translated version. Equivalence will be supported further if the psychometric properties of the original and translated versions are found to be similar.

Quality of the translation

The quality of the translation is an important factor in producing an instrument that corresponds to the original. Quality of the translation is assessed by different types of equivalence between the original and target versions of the questionnaire. The more rigorous the translation process, the more likely the translation supports equivalence (9).

In back translation, when the original and the back translated version show no substantial differences, it suggests that the target version (from the middle of the process) is equivalent to the source language version (19). However, good back translation can *seemingly* create equivalence; therefore, researchers need to be careful. Problems may occur because translators may have a shared set of rules for translating certain nonequivalent words, and also, some back translators may be able to make sense out of a poorly written target language version (19). The bilingual translation from the source to the target may retain many of the grammatical forms of the source. This version would be easy to back translate but worthless for the purpose of asking questions of target-language monolinguals because its grammar is that of the source, not that of the target (19).

The Scientific Committee of the Medical Outcomes Trust described review criteria for the assessment of health status and quality of life instruments, including criteria for cultural and language adaptations and translations. Developers are recommended to describe the methods to achieve linguistic and conceptual equivalence, to identify and explain any significant differences between the original and translated versions, and to explain how inconsistencies were reconciled (12). When addressing equivalence, it is important to note the difference between semantic and conceptual equivalence, because items that are equivalent in meaning may not be equivalent conceptually (7). None of the translations of the Nottingham Health Profile (NHP) exactly mirrored the English version. Literal translations were limited to a few items, whereas other items were translated semantically or conceptually. For example, in Swedish, the use of the pronoun "I" posed problems because the preferred mode of expression is to distance the self from some experiences. Hence, the phrase "I am in pain when I walk" would translate more naturally as "it hurts when I walk" (7).

Other types of equivalence have been proposed to assess the quality of the translation. Examples of differences in the types and definitions of equiva-lence are shown in Table 11.1. The problem with the many different types of equivalence is that the definitions of the different types of equivalence are not always clear. A review focusing on "equivalence" (20) found 19 different types of equivalence. For some types of equivalence (e.g., semantic and operational equivalence), there is almost universal agreement on the definition, but for other types of equivalence (e.g., conceptual and functional equivalence), the study showed that consensus was notably lacking (20). In particular, a substantial amount of variation in the definition of conceptual equivalence was found.

Achieving equivalence between different language versions of a PROM can be challenging because not all concepts are equally applicable to different cultures. Herdman and colleagues (21) suggest that rather than using an "absolutist" approach to achieving equivalence, a "universalist" approach should be used. An "absolutist" approach assumes that there will be little or no change in the concept and organizations of a PROM across cultures, whereas a "universalist" approach does not make the assumption that constructs are the same across cultures. Six types of equivalence need to be taken into account when the universalist approach is used: 1) conceptual equivalence, 2) item equivalence, 3) semantic equivalence, 4) operational equivalence, 5) measurement equivalence, and 6) functional equivalence (21). Although the terminology used by Herdman and colleagues is the same or similar to other authors' terminology about equivalence, the definitions can differ (as shown in Table 11.1). The universalist approach is specific and may mean that some instruments will not be considered as suitable for translation because the different types of equivalence cannot be achieved between cultures.

Translators

Number of translators

Hilton and Skrutkowski (9) recommend at least two translators, one of whom will translate the

Table 11.1 Types of equivalence and definitions

Authors (year)	Type of equivalence	Definition
Guillemin et al. (1993) (3)	Semantic	Equivalence in the meaning of words. Achieving it may present problems with vocabulary and grammar.
	Idiomatic	Equivalent expressions have to be found for idioms and colloquialisms that are not translatable. This is more important for emotional and social dimensions.
	Experiential	Situations evoked or depicted in the original version should fit the target cultural context.
	Conceptual	Validity of the concept explored and the events experienced by people in the target culture.
Herdman et al. (1998) (21)	Conceptual	Questionnaire has the same relationship to the underlying concept in different cultures, primarily in terms of the domains included and the emphasis placed on domains.
	Item	Validity of items is the same in different cultures.
	Semantic	There is transfer of meaning across languages.
	Operational	Using a similar questionnaire format, instructions, mode of administration, and measurement methods.
	Measurement	Different language versions achieve acceptable levels in terms of psychometric properties (such as reliability, validity, responsiveness).
	Functional	The extent to which a measure does what it is supposed to do equally well in two or more cultures.
Hilton and Skrutkowski (2002) (9)	Content	Each item's content is relevant in each culture (some constructs cannot be insinuated into instruments for other cultures).
	Semantic	Similarity of meaning of each item in each culture after translation.
	Technical	Data collection method is comparable.
	Conceptual	Instrument measures the same theoretical construct in each culture.
	Criterion	Interpretation remains the same when compared with the norm for each culture.
Meadows (2003) (22)	Item or content	Each item describes a phenomenon for both cultures, or the situation described or experiences evoked in the original version are applicable to the target population.
	Semantic	The meaning of each item, word, or expression is retained after translation into the language of the target culture.
	Operational	The way in which data collection is carried out (self-completed versus structured interviews) may have differential effects on data collection.
	Conceptual	Existence and relevance of the concepts (ideas and experiences, etc.) in both cultures.
	Functional	The degree to which equivalence in the preceding stages has been achieved.

original version to the target language, and one of whom will back translate the translated version to the original language. Guillemin et al. (3) recommended producing several forward translations, with at least two independent translators and preferably a team of translators rather than individual translators. For panel translations, a translator panel of five to seven translators (18) is recommended.

Skills and background

Generally, there is consensus that the qualifications and skills of translators are important, and that competent translators should be used. However, the definition of a competent translator varies between authors. Competence may refer to the linguistic skills of the translator, and the use of linguistically competent translators who are conversant in the target language is recommended (22). Competence can also refer to the translator's area of expertise, and it is recommended that translators who are familiar with the content (i.e., subject area) involved in the source material be used (19). Brislin (19) showed that translators' familiarity with English contributed to translation quality and that translation quality was better for concepts with which the translators had greater familiarity. A systematic review of translations of quality of life instruments concluded that the people involved in translations are critical in determining a questionnaire's performance in a new country or culture (2).

For forward and back translations, it is always best to use translators who translate into their mother language (3, 4). Hilton and Srutkowski (9) believe that translators should include professional interpreters, lay people who are monolingual and representatives of the populations under study, people who are bilingual with the source language as their first language, and people who are bilingual with the target language as their first language. Furthermore, Wild et al. specify that translators should have prior experience in translating PROMs (4). However, it seems impossible to achieve this diversity, particularly when only two translators (one forward and one back) are involved in the research. Swaine-Verdier et al. (18), who are in favor of panel translations, recommend that translators should be as "ordinary" as possible (because the questionnaire is completed by "ordinary" people).

Instructions to translators

To ensure that translators use the same approach to their translations, they should be given instructions on how to proceed. Translators should be fully aware of their role and should ideally have prior experience in translations (22). Translators should be instructed to translate conceptually, rather than literally (5), and to refrain from using technical and difficult language (indication of reading age may be useful). Forward translators, but preferably not back translators, should be aware of the intent and concepts underlying the material (3). The use of dictionaries is not recommended because this might entice the translator to a literal, word-by-word translation rather than the conceptual translation of a whole sentence.

Assessors

Assessors, also called raters, are recommended as part of the translation process (3, 19, 22). Assessors are bilinguals who are concerned with assessing the quality and the equivalence between the original and the translated version. Ideally several assessors should examine the original and translated versions for errors (19), and a committee of assessors can be used to fulfill this role (3). Sperber (8) suggests that, prior to psychometric testing, a comparability and interpretability test should be carried out by at least 30 raters who rank the translated and back translated version in terms of comparability of language and similarity of interpretability. This gives the opportunity to revise items that score poorly or that are not thought to be equivalent to the original by the assessors, thus further increasing the likelihood of equivalence.

Reports about the translation process

It is important to carefully document the translation process, including consideration of format, administration, and translator selection; translation issues raised; and decisions made during the validation process (9, 23). Information on the translation procedure helps to assess the quality of the process and may give an indication of the quality of the translation, thus, increasing the credibility of the translation (2). A high-quality translation process is not a guarantee of a good translation, but a rigorous and inclusive translation process can increase the likelihood that the original and translated versions will be equivalent (9).

Conclusion

When translations are performed, it is important to use rigorous and well-documented methods. Forward and back translation is the preferred method, but it may be less important whether the translations (forward and back) are performed by individual and independent translators or a panel of translators. Because there is no scientific evidence on whether individual translations or panel translations produce higher-quality instruments, the decision of using individual translators or a panel may have to be based on the researchers' preference and practical issues such as the availability of suitable translators or other resources such as time and finances. A systematic review found no evidence in favor of one specific method of translation, but the authors concluded that a rigorous multi-step approach leads to better-quality translations and should therefore be used as a guarantee of quality (2). Furthermore, having standardized guidelines for translations can improve the quality of translations.

REFERENCES

1. Jenkinson C, Fitzpatrick R, Peto V, Greenhall R, Hyman N. The Parkinson's Disease Questionnaire (PDQ-39): development and validation of a Parkinson's disease summary index score. *Age Ageing* 1997 Sep; **26**(5): 353–357.

2. Acquadro C, Conway K, Hareendran A, Aaronson N. Literature review of methods to translate health-related quality of life questionnaires for use in multinational clinical trials. *Value Health* 2008 May; **11**(3): 509–521.

3. Guillemin F, Bombardier C, Beaton D. Cross-cultural adaptation of health-related quality of life measures: literature review and proposed guidelines. *J Clin Epidemiol* 1993 Dec; **46**(12): 1417–1432.

4. Wild D, Grove A, Martin M, Eremenco S, McElroy S, Verjee-Lorenz A, et al. Principles of good practice for the translation and cultural adaptation process for patient-reported outcomes (PRO) measures: report of the ISPOR Task Force for Translation and Cultural Adaptation. *Value Health* 2005 Mar; **8**(2): 94–104.

5. Bullinger M, Alonso J, Apolone G, Leplege A, Sullivan M, Wood-Dauphinee S, et al. Translating health status questionnaires and evaluating their quality: the IQOLA project approach. International Quality of Life Assessment. *J Clin Epidemiol* 1998 Nov; **51**(11): 913–923.

6. Rabin R, de Charro F. EQ-5D: a measure of health status from the EuroQol Group. *Ann Med* 2001 Jul; **33**(5): 337–343.

7. Hunt SM, Alonso J, Bucquet D, Niero M, Wiklund I, McKenna S. Cross-cultural adaptation of health measures. European Group for Health Management and Quality of Life Assessment. *Health Policy* 1991 Sep; **19**(1): 33–44.

8. Sperber AD. Translation and validation of study instruments for cross-cultural research. *Gastroenterology* 2004 Jan; **126**(1 suppl 1): S124–S128.

9. Hilton A, Skrutkowski M. Translating instruments into other languages: development and testing processes. *Cancer Nurs* 2002 Feb; **25**(1): 1–7.

10. WHOQOL group. The World Health Organization Quality of Life Assessment (WHOQOL): development and general psychometric properties. *Soc Sci Med* 1998 Jun; **46**(12): 1569–1585.

11. Niero M, Martin M, Finger T, Lucas R, Mear I, Wild D, et al. A new approach to multicultural item generation in the development of two obesity-specific measures: the Obesity and Weight Loss Quality of Life (OWLQOL) questionnaire and the Weight-Related Symptom Measure (WRSM). *Clin Ther* 2002 Apr; **24**(4): 690–700.

12. Scientific Advisory Committee of the Medical Outcomes Trust. Assessing health status and quality-of-life instruments: attributes and review criteria. *Qual Life Res* 2002 May; **11**(3): 193–205.

13. Bushnell DM, Martin ML. Quality of life and Parkinson's disease: translation and validation of the US Parkinson's Disease Questionnaire (PDQ-39). *Qual Life Res* 1999 Jun; **8**(4): 345–350.

14. Guillemin F. Cross-cultural adaptation and validation of health status measures. *Scand J Rheumatol* 1995; **24**(2): 61–63.

15. Eremenco SL, Cella D, Arnold BJ. A comprehensive method for the translation and cross-cultural validation of health status questionnaires. *Eval Health Prof* 2005 Jun; **28**(2): 212–232.

16. Wild D, Eremenco S, Mear I, Martin M, Houchin C, Gawlicki M, et al. Multinational trials: Recommendations on the translations required, approaches to using the same language in different countries, and

the approaches to support pooling the data: the ISPOR patient-reported outcomes translation and linguistic validation Good Research Practices Task Force report. *Value Health* 2008 Nov 12(4): 430–440.

17. Skevington SM, Sartorius N, Amir M. Developing methods for assessing quality of life in different cultural settings: the history of the WHOQOL instruments. *Soc Psychiatry Psychiatr Epidemiol* 2004 Jan; 39(1): 1–8.

18. Swaine-Verdier A, Doward LC, Hagell P, Thorsen H, McKenna SP. Adapting quality of life instruments. *Value Health* 2004 Sep; 7(suppl 1):S27–S30.

19. Brislin RW. Back-translation for cross-cultural research. *J Cross-Cultural Psychol* 1970; 1(3): 185–216.

20. Herdman M, Fox-Rushby J, Badia X. 'Equivalence' and the translation and adaptation of health-related quality of life questionnaires. *Qual Life Res* 1997 Apr; 6(3): 237–247.

21. Herdman M, Fox-Rushby J, Badia X. A model of equivalence in the cultural adaptation of HRQoL instruments: the universalist approach. *Qual Life Res* 1998 May; 7(4): 323–335.

22. Meadows KA. So you want to do research? 5: Questionnaire design. *Br J Community Nurs* 2003 Dec; 8(12): 562–570.

23. MAPI Institute. Linguistic Validation. Methodology. May 11, 2009. Available at: http://www.mapi-institute.com/linguistic-validation/methodology

12

Rasch analysis

Jeremy Hobart and Stefan Cano

Chapter overview

When rating scales are used as outcome measures, their core purpose is to measure people. We therefore require methods to ensure that they fulfill this purpose. Rasch analysis is a statistical method for analyzing rating scale data, constructing new rating scales, and evaluating and modifying existing scales. It is based on measurement principles and methods developed almost half a century ago by Georg Rasch, a Danish mathematician. The application of these principles and analyses has enormous potential to improve our ability to measure health outcomes and advance our clinical trials. This is because they enable us to construct rating scales that are high-quality measurement instruments and provide important information about the nature of the complex health constructs we are seeking to measure.

If this is the case, why is Rasch analysis not more widely used? There are many reasons. For instance, the literature is difficult to follow and is not accessible to clinical audiences. This is not helped because the field is often presented in a complex manner and, thus, misconceptions and misunderstandings are widespread. There is also a history of conflict between competing groups that has detracted from helping others get into the field. And there is reluctance of some to move outside of the comfort zone provided by standard (traditional) tests for

constructing scales and testing scale reliability and validity.

No doubt, much is involved with getting to grips with Rasch analysis. However, we believe it is much easier if the basic issues are followed before getting into the statistics. Therefore, the aim of this chapter is to set down, in nontechnical language, the basic principles related to, and underpinning, Rasch analysis to enable people to access the more difficult literature. First, we review some basics about rating scales and measurement. Second, we address the limitations of traditional psychometric methods and the history of the development of modern psychometric methods (Rasch measurement and item response theory). Third, we address the similarities and differences between Rasch measurement and item response theory. Last, we give an example of mechanics surrounding what happens when rating scale data are Rasch analyzed.

Rating scales as measurement instruments: basic principles

Rating scales are increasingly used as measurement instruments in clinical trials, clinical studies, clinical audit, and clinical practice. The results of these studies influence the care of individual people, the making of health policy, and the direction of future research. The inferences made from these studies

Quality of Life Measurement in Neurodegenerative and Related Conditions, eds., Crispin Jenkinson, Michele Peters, and Mark B. Bromberg. Published by Cambridge University Press. © Cambridge University Press 2011.

are based on the analysis of numbers generated by the rating scales used as outcome measures. If clinically meaningful interpretations are to be made from these studies, it is a requirement that the rating scales used are rigorous measures of the variables (aspects of health) they claim to quantify.

Psychometric methods are used in the development and evaluation of ratings scales and for analyzing their data. Three main types of psychometric methods are used for evaluating scales in health measurement: traditional psychometric methods, Rasch measurement, and item response theory (IRT). Each uses a different type of evidence to determine the extent to which a scale has achieved its goal of generating measurements. Before exploring these methods, we need to review the mechanics of rating scales.

How rating scales work

Some things that we wish to quantify can be measured directly using devices or machines. Examples include weight, height, and protein levels in the cerebrospinal fluid. Others cannot be measured directly. Examples include health variables such as disability, anxiety, fatigue, and quality of life. These must instead be measured indirectly through their observable manifestations. For example, we can measure the physical disability of a person only by engaging the person in physical tasks.

In fact, all measurements, whether direct or indirect, are of this nature. Thus, a person's weight can be determined only by engaging his/her weight with an instrument that reacts to it; the height of a person can be measured only by engaging it with an instrument against which we can read off its length; and so on. Likewise, we infer the extent to which a person is depressed by the symptoms of this health variable that the person manifests, either through observation or by formalizing some questions. So that this inferred aspect of health variables can be stressed, they are typically referred to in the rating scale literature as *latent traits*.

The Rivermead Mobility Index (RMI) is a clinician-scored rating scale purporting to measure mobility. It consists of 15 items. Each item concerns a mobility-related task that has two response options: "No" – I am unable to do this task; "Yes" – I am able to do this task. Typically, item scores are summed to give a total score that ranges from 0 (all "no" responses to items) to 15 (all "yes" responses to items).

Consider the aims of the RMI in greater detail. Mobility is being thought of (conceptualized) as a quantitative variable in the sense that it reflects a property that can have a range of values from "less" to "more." The RMI items attempt to map out this idea, and thus responses to its 15 items can be seen as indicators of the level of mobility. Essentially, the RMI seeks to map out mobility as a line varying from more to less on which people can be located. Thus, the 15 RMI items make operational (operationalize) the idea of a mobility variable. Because mobility is observed by a variety of manifestations, rather than directly, it is considered to be a latent (hidden) property. The words "trait" and "construct" are typically used instead of the word "property."

This conceptualization implies that each item represents a mark on the "ruler" of mobility mapped out by the RMI. More specifically, the mark defined by each item represents the transition point of the score from 0 to 1, that is, the point at which a person moves from scoring "0" (unable to do) to "1" (able to do). The aim of a psychometric analysis is to determine, using a range of evidence, the extent to which this conceptualization of a variable, in this instance, mobility by the RMI, has been achieved (1).

Traditional psychometric methods for evaluating scales and Classical Test Theory

Many different psychometric methods may be used. This chapter concerns three: traditional psychometric methods, Rasch analysis, and item response theory (IRT). Different methods use different types of evidence to determine the extent to which a quantitative conceptualization of a variable has been operationalized successfully. Traditional psychometric methods, the most widely used methods, use evidence predominantly from correlations and descriptive statistics.

Three main scale properties are examined by traditional psychometric methods: reliability, validity, and responsiveness. These properties are underpinned by a measurement theory called Classical Test Theory (CTT), which postulates the idea of an observed score, a true score, and an error score. The observed score (O) is the score that a person actually gets on a scale (sum of item scores). The true score (T) is the person's real score. This is the unobservable (theoretical) value we are trying to estimate. "E" represents the error associated with all measurements. CTT then postulates that the observed score (O) is the sum of the true score (T) and the error score (E). Thus,

$$O = T + E.$$

CTT assumes certain conditions to be true of the observed score, true score, and error, and the relationships between them. There are seven main assumptions. These include the following: the relationship between O, T, and E is additive; errors are uncorrelated with each other and with true scores; and observed, true, and error scores are linearly related (2). These assumptions enable a number of mathematical conclusions (proofs) to be derived from the seven assumptions of CTT and underpin methods of computing scale reliability and the error associated with scores (the standard error of measurement).

Despite the attractive simplicity of CTT, it has some critical limitations. Its two fundamental problems are 1) that "T" and "E" cannot be estimated in a way that enables us to verify if the theory is true; and 2) that the assumptions underpinning the theory cannot be tested, and we can only surmise when they would be appropriate (3). This means that most of its equations are unlikely to be contradicted by data (4) and demonstrated by Lord.[1] Thus, the lim-

---

[1] The other equations that arise from CTT arise or are related to the basic $O = T + E$. This means that they are subject to the same core limitation (i.e., assumptions underpinning the theory cannot be tested).

ited tautologic nature (4) of the equations of CTT have led it to be called weak true-score theory (2). Unfortunately, weak theories lead to weak conclusions, in this case, about the performance of scales and the measurement of people. It follows that traditional psychometric methods, based on CTT, also have major limitations. The most clinically important of these include the following:

- Item and total scores generated by rating scales are ordered counts with unequal intervals, not interval measurements.
- Results for scale reliability and validity tests are sample dependent.
- A person's measurement (e.g., physical impact of a condition) is scale dependent.
- There is no scientific strategy for dealing with missing item data (typically, we are encouraged to impute the mean score of the completed items).
- The standard error of measurement is considered to be the same whatever a person's measurement, implying that the measurement error for people at the floor and ceiling of a scale is the same as for those in the center.
- Traditional psychometric methods do not "scale" items, that is, they do not give items values that locate them on the measurement continuum. Thus, they neither map out the variable on which people can be measured nor mark out the continuum along which people can be located.

The limitations of CTT and traditional psychometric methods are significant. This fact, recognized in the psychometric literature for some time (5, 6), has opened the door to more sophisticated techniques.

Modern psychometric methods: Rasch measurement and item response theory

The term modern (or new) psychometric methods refers mainly to two methods: Rasch measurement and IRT. They represent a logical progression from CTT because they attempt to improve the scientific quality of the theory underpinning rating scales. Unlike CTT, modern psychometric methods focus on the relationship between a person's unobservable *measurement* on an underlying trait and his or her probability of responding to one of the response categories of a scale item. This approach has four key issues.

First, the term "person's unobservable measurement" is used because modern psychometric methods recognize the limitations of total scores (which are ordinal in nature) and instead locate people on a continuum. Second, a person's true interval-level location should govern his/her response to an item. This is logical. For example, if a person is very physically disabled, we expect him/her to answer "extremely" for most items on a "physical impact" scale. Thus, the response to any item *is a function of* someone's level of disability. Also logically, a person's response to an item is related to the difficulty of the tasks: physically demanding tasks (item 1) are more difficult than carrying things (item 3).

The third issue to note is use of the phrase "probability of responding to one of the categories of a scale item." This recognizes that it is unreasonable to try to predict exactly how someone will respond to an item. We can only say that one is likely to choose a specific response category. Thus, the relationship between true interval-level measurement and response to an item is best formalized in terms of probabilities. Finally, the focus shifts from the total score level in CTT to the item level in modern psychometric methods.

It seemed reasonable, therefore, to consider developing mathematical models that relate the probability of a response to an item to the person's location on the continuum measured by the item and some characteristics (parameters) of the items. The challenge then was to find, or derive, a mathematical model that links these variables together and to give the information required, using the responses of a sample of people to a set of items. Essentially, the mathematical model must use this information to allow us to determine if a set of items form a reliable and valid rating scale on which people can be located, preferably in interval-level units.

As pointed out earlier, two new psychometric methods are available. They have different origins and different directions and represent different perspectives. Thus, they are fundamentally different.

However, to complicate matters and ensure confusion, they also have important similarities.

Development of item response theory

Thurstone was the first person to attempt to bring strong theoretical and mathematical underpinnings to rating scales (7). This was followed by important contributions by Richardson (8), Ferguson (9, 10, 11) Lawley (12, 13), Tucker (14), Brogden (15), and Lazarsfeld (16). However, the work of Frederic Lord (17, 18) seems widely regarded to have been the birth of IRT. He is considered to be one of the first people to develop a mathematical model describing the relationship between a person's level of (dis)ability and his/her response to the items of a rating scale and to apply this model successfully to real data (19). Lord and Novick (20) went on to publish a landmark book on the topic in 1968.

Early work in IRT focused on trying to develop mathematical models that formalized CTT. Specifically, this work related a person's measurement on the construct to the features (parameters) of items that were seen to be important in traditional psychometric item analyses: item difficulty and item discrimination. In traditional psychometric methods, the "difficulty" of an item is indicated by its endorsement frequency, and the "discrimination" by the item-total correlation.

Mathematical models relating the probability of a response to an item to the person's location, the item's difficulty, and the item's discrimination are known as two-parameter (2PL) models. Examinations with these models did not necessarily account adequately for observed datasets (i.e., there was misfit). This led researchers to consider adding other item and person characteristics (parameters) to the basic 2PL model so the data might be better explained. In educational testing, where much of the early work was done, guessing responses to items was felt to be important; therefore, models including an item guessing parameter (21), a person guessing parameter (22), and a person discrimination parameter (23) were developed. Of these "multi-parameter" models, those mostly used are the basic 2PL model and the 3PL model, in which the third parameter is item guessing.

The general approach in the development of IRT was to try to develop mathematical models that *explained* the observed rating scale data. When the observed data were not adequately explained by the mathematical model, that is, when the data did not fit the chosen model closely enough, another model was tried. Thus, the justification for model selection was empirical evidence of its suitability (2). The purpose of choosing one model over another was that it accounted better for the data (24). The data were considered given. It is important to note that most circumstances of "modeling data" involve finding a model that fits the data. In addition, the finding that proposed models did not fit observed data meant that model development was also justified empirically.

Development of Rasch measurement

At the same time that Frederic Lord was developing his theories at the Educational Testing Service in the United States, Georg Rasch was developing his theories at the Danish Institute of Educational Research in Copenhagen (25). It is important to note that Rasch's work was independent of Lord's (and vice versa), although Lord discusses Rasch's work in his landmark text published 8 years later (20).

At the beginning, Rasch took a similar approach to Lord, in that he tried to model his data. He was studying students' ability to read texts of different difficulty and the distribution of errors. He chose to work with a Poisson model because this model is generally used as an error count model. However, to make the Poisson "work," he needed to have a parameter for each person's ability and each reading text difficulty. Thus, Rasch treated each student in his dataset as an individual. This contrasts with more conventional mathematical modeling, in which people tend to treat groups of individuals as random replications of each other, so that the error includes variation among individuals. He fixed those, and randomness was present only in the

response process of a person to an individual text (26, 27).

Over time, Rasch increasingly noticed that item locations and person locations could be estimated independently of each other. The implications of this are critical. It means that the measurement of people can be made independently of the *sampling distribution of the items used*, and the location of items on the continuum can be identified independently of the *sampling distribution of the people in whom they are derived*. Put another way, this means that the relative locations of any two people do not depend on the items they take and that the relative locations of any two items do not depend on the people from whom the estimates are made. This is Rasch's criterion of invariance – or stability (26).

Of course, there is one essential proviso: that the data fit the Rasch model. This is because the property of invariance is a consequence of the model, not of the data, or just the *application* of the model. Thus, for invariance to be a consequence of the data, the data must fit the Rasch model within statistical reason. But this means that when the data do fit the Rasch model, different subsets of items will give equivalent person estimates, and different subsets of persons will give equivalent item estimates. Rasch realized that this property was a fundamental one of a very important class of models. From there, he shifted his focus from describing datasets, to studying a class of models with a unique property. The implications are discussed below.

In the Rasch paradigm, the mathematical model is given primacy. When the data do not fit the Rasch model, another model is *not* chosen. Instead, the finding invokes an examination of the data to determine why, for example, a set of items hypothesized to be a measurement instrument is not performing as such. Thus, the justification for model selection is theoretical evidence of its suitability (2). The data are not considered given.

Rasch developed his model for dichotomous variables. His work was developed at the University of Chicago by Wright (28), with Stone (29) and Masters (30), and by Andrich, who generalized the Rasch

Rasch simple logistic model (SLM)

$$P_{ni} = \frac{e^{(B_n - D_i)}}{1 + e^{(B_n - D_i)}}$$

One-parameter logistic IRT model

$$P_{ni} = \frac{e^{(B_n - D_i)}}{1 + e^{(B_n - D_i)}}$$

Two-parameter logistic IRT model

$$P_{ni} = \frac{e^{[a_i(B_n - D_i)]}}{1 + e^{[a_i(B_n - D_i)]}}$$

Three-parameter logistic IRT model

$$P_{ni} = c_i + (1 + c_i) + \frac{e^{[a_i(B_n - D_i)]}}{1 + e^{[a_i(B_n - D_i)]}}$$

Figure 12.1 Formulas for Rasch's SLM, and the one-, two-, and three-parameter logistic models[2].
P_{ni} = probability that person "n" will respond "yes" to item I; B_n = the ability location of person "n"; D_i = the difficulty location of item "i"; α_i = the slope/discrimination of item "i"; c_i = the constant added for item "i" to take into account guessing.

Note that Rasch's SLM and the 1-PL have the same formula. This has led people to consider them to be the same thing and has resulted in considerable confusion. What is different about them is the paradigm in which they are used. In the Rasch paradigm, no other model is used, and when the data do not fit the model, an explanation for this "misfit" is sought. In the IRT paradigm, when the data do not fit the model, other models are tried to seek better fit.

model for use in rating scales with polytomous response categories (31).

Item response theory and Rasch measurement: similarities and differences

Similarities

Similarities between IRT and Rasch measurement have increased the potential for confusion. The first similarity is that both families are item response models for constructing and evaluating rating scales and for analyzing data. The second similarity is that both appeared at around the same time. The first written reports about both IRT and Rasch measurement were written in the 1950s (32), and landmark texts were published in the 1960s (20, 25).

Perhaps the greatest similarity between IRT and Rasch measurement is the structure of the mathematical models (33). Figure 12.1 shows the mathematical models of the Rasch model and the one-,

two-, and three-parameter models. All are "logistic" models. This simply means that central to them is the expression (e / 1+e). Rasch termed his model the simple logistic model (SLM), whereas the three IRT models are termed the one-, two-, and three-parameter logistic models (1-PL, 2-PL, 3-PL).[3] Second, the models are such that

- If C=0, then 3-PL becomes the 2-PL;
- If a=1, then 2-PL becomes the SLM;
- If a=1 and C=0, then 3-PL becomes the SLM.

This has led many people to consider the Rasch model as nothing more than a "special case" of the 2- and 3-PL models with convenient properties (34, 35) and to describe it as a one-parameter logistic model (1-PL). That perspective and terminology are reasonable if the aim is to find the model that best fits the data, but this view ignores the fundamental reasoning behind the development of the Rasch model and its value. This perspective is

---

[2,3] c = constant describing the lower asymptote due to guessing, a = discrimination.

not reasonable if the reasoning behind development of the Rasch model is taken into account. This is because the addition of parameters to the Rasch SLM prevents separate estimation of item and person parameters, and thus the property of invariance. Massof demonstrates this formally (33).

Differences

The fundamental difference between IRT and Rasch measurement is the approach to the problem, or the research agenda (26). IRT aims to find the item response model that best explains the data. Rasch measurement will use only the Rasch model, and if data do not fit this, researchers will seek to understand why and, if necessary, remove data, recollect data, or reconceptualize the construct. This is because proponents of IRT prioritize the data. In contrast, proponents of Rasch measurement prioritize the model.

Other differences between IRT and Rasch measurement arise from their different approaches, for example, how certain findings within the data are considered, interpreted, and managed. This particularly concerns features such as item discrimination and guessing. Both 2-PL and 3-PL item response models include an item discrimination parameter. This means that the discrimination of each item is estimated. The Rasch model does not have an item discrimination parameter. Thus, if items have empirically different discriminations, this is shown as misfit of the data to the Rasch model. More specifically, different item discrimination shows up as misfit for individual *items* that requires further qualitative exploration and explanation.

Similarly, the 3-PL model contains a guessing parameter for items. Thus, this is estimated in the analysis. The Rasch model does not contain a guessing parameter, and "guessing" shows up as a misfit for individual *people*. It is important to note that the analysis does not tell us that these individuals were guessing. It identifies their response pattern across items as inconsistent with expectations and hence misfitting. The cause of the misfit requires further qualitative exploration of the individuals.

Why proponents of item response theory favor their approach

Proponents of IRT give primacy to the data and to trying to best explain it. Thus, it is easy to understand why one might seek to find the item response model with the best fit. Another reason people favor the IRT approach is concern about using an item response model that does not include an estimate of item discrimination, given that empirical evidence demonstrates that items have different discriminate ability (36). A further reason supporting the IRT approach is concern about the concept of finding data to fit the model. This has been believed by some to disturb construct validity (36). However, giving primacy to the data does imply confidence that the data are not fallible. This might raise cause for concern given the ambiguities of items and the fact that many items could be placed in scales measuring a range of constructs.

Why proponents of Rasch measurement favor their approach

Rasch measurement proponents favor their approach because of the inherent properties of the model and because it offers the optimum criterion for fundamental measurement (26). It is appropriate to explore this statement further because it goes right back to the meaning of measurement itself.

Many psychometric textbooks quote the definition of measurement formalized by Stanley Smith Stevens (37). He defined measurement as "the assigning of number to things according to rules." Stevens proceeded not to define the rules for assigning numbers to things but rather to offer a four-level classification of scales (nominal; ordinal; interval; ratio) and the statistical tests that ought, or ought not, be applied to them. In general, these have been adopted as the basic scales of measurement and have had a major influence on psychometric theory and its development.

It is perhaps interesting to note that many standard psychometric texts over the years (3, 38, 39,

40, 41, 42, 43, 44, 45, 46) give little discussion to the topic of the nature of measurement despite the "tomes devoted to it" (38). In fact, measurement is a very important and advanced concept (26). It has been defined as the *sine qua non* of science (47). Helmhotz is reputed to have said all science is measurement (48), and it is widely acknowledged that advances in measurement methods have underpinned the progress of the physical sciences (26). Measurement in the physical sciences, which was called fundamental measurement by Campbell in the 1920s (49), has been studied and debated at length by mathematicians, philosophers, and social scientists to articulate the characteristics of measurement against which systems purporting to generate measurements (for example, rating scales) can be tested.

Underpinning most physical measurement systems, such as weight and height, is an empirical combining (concatenating) process. As Perline et al. state (50), (p. 238): "It is easy to show that two lumps of clay joined into one is equal to the sum of the weights of the individual lumps." Campbell (49), who deduced that the ability to concatenate is the fundamental property on which physical measurement (i.e., measurement in physics) is based, coined the term fundamental measurement and argued that there could be no fundamental measures in psychology because concatenation of psychological properties seemed impossible.

This challenge motivated the theory of conjoint measurement, which aimed to determine the conditions required for rating scales to achieve fundamental measurement. Luce and Tukey made an important contribution to the field in 1964 (51). Essentially, for an item response model to produce "fundamental measurements," it must satisfy the mathematical requirements of a noninteractive conjoint structure (52). These mathematical requirements concern relationships between the three key variables in the model: the person location and item location estimated by the model, and the observed responses to items. A noninteractive conjoint structure is one that exhibits additive relationships, double cancellation, solvability,

the Archimedean axiom, and independent effects that item locations and person locations have on observed responses.

The Rasch model satisfies these five conditions. Other item response models do not (26). This explains why the Rasch model offers the optimum potential for constructing fundamental measurements from rating scale data (26), why the status of other item response models as measurement models has been challenged (33), and why proponents of Rasch measurement favor their models and do not tend to use others.

Limitations of new psychometric methods

The main limitation of the new psychometric methods is that they require a complex, more advanced level of mathematical understanding, as well as investment in new training in the use of new software. Therefore, Rasch analysis appears complicated and is not widely used, and few clinicians and researchers are trained in its use and interpretation. Thus, the key question is, Do the clinical advantages of Rasch analysis outweigh the necessity for specialized knowledge and software? We believe that the new methods offer clinically meaningful scientific advantages that far outweigh concerns about the necessity for specialized knowledge and software. In particular, the benefits of Rasch analysis provide a substantial leap from traditional methods in measuring patient outcomes.

Worked example

The aim of this example is to compare and contrast scale evaluation using traditional and Rasch psychometric methods. We think this is a useful way to understand their similarities and differences. The example uses RMI data from 666 people in a large, U.K. multi-center clinical trial of cannabis in multiple sclerosis (CAMS). This scale has been chosen because each of the 15 items has only two response categories (yes/no).

Table 12.1 RMI summary of evaluation using traditional psychometric methods (n = 666)

Psychometric property	Values
Scaling assumptions	
Item mean scores – mean (SD); range	0.42 (0.44); 0.008–0.73
Item variances – range	0.18; 0.008–0.25
Corrected item-total correlations – range	0.10–0.76
Targeting	
RMI scale: midpoint; range	7.5; 0–15
RMI observed scores: mean (SD); range	6.3 (4.3); 0–15
Observed score range	0–15
Scale score range	0–15
Floor effect (% scoring 0)	11.9%
Ceiling effect (% scoring 15)	0.3%
Reliability	
Cronbach's alpha	0.91
Inter-item correlation; mean; range	0.38 (0.01–0.75)
SEM [SD × (1 – alpha)1/2]	1.29
95% CI around individual person scores	+/− 2.53
Validity (within-scale analyses)	
Corrected item-total correlations – range	0.10–0.76
Cronbach's alpha	0.91
Inter-item correlation; Mean; range	0.38 (0.01–0.75)

Evaluation of the RMI using traditional psychometric methods

Table 12.1 summarizes the results of traditional psychometric analyses. In brief, data quality was high, implying no problems using the RMI in this large sample. Scaling assumptions were largely satisfied. The 15 items had variable mean scores and standard deviations, implying that they were not parallel. Nevertheless, corrected item total correlations, with the exception of the "running" item, exceeded 0.30, implying that 14 of the items measured a common underlying construct and satisfying the criterion for summation without weighting. Scale-to-sample targeting was good, but the floor effect implied that a cohort of people with greater mobility problems were not measured well. Reliability was high. Evidence from within-scale analyses supports the validity of the RMI. Although the principal components analysis suggested that the one-component solution was the most satisfactory from a statistical perspective, this solution explained only 44% of the total variance.

Thus the RMI satisfies most traditional criteria for rigorous measurement. Some problems were demonstrated that suggest improvements could be made if the scale were considered for revision, specifically, consideration of removing the running item and extension of the measurement range into the more disabled range.

Evaluation of the RMI using Rasch analysis

Rasch analysis consists of gathering and integrating the evidence from a series of examinations. Typically, these analyses are not reported in the literature under the subheadings in the same way that we and others have used for traditional methods (reliability, validity, responsiveness). One reason for this is that these traditional terms do not allow evaluation of the scale to be considered separately from the measurement of people. Nor do they incorporate an indication of the suitability of the scale for measuring the sample, and the sample for evaluating the scale. With this in mind, we recommend considering reporting Rasch analyses under three main questions:

• Is the scale-to-sample targeting adequate for making judgments about the performance of the scale and the measurement of people?
• Has a measurement ruler been constructed successfully?
• Have the people been measured successfully?

The methods and different analyses underpinning each of these assessments are discussed fully elsewhere (5, 6). Two things are immediately noticeable: the extent of the information, and the graphics.

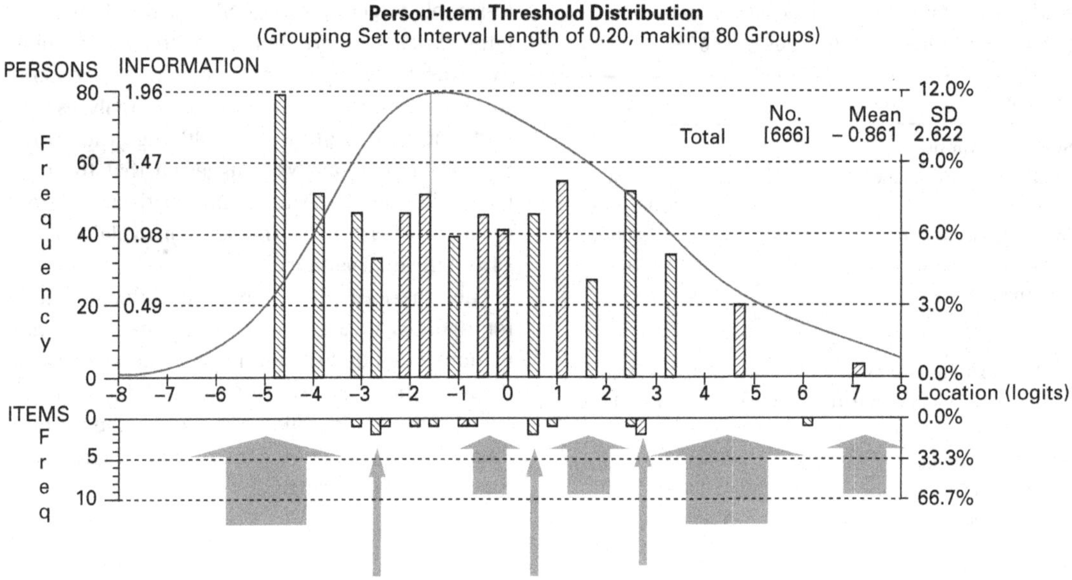

Figure 12.2 Targeting of the patient sample providing a representation of the measurement ruler mapped out by the 15 RMI items.

Is the RMI to CAMS sample targeting adequate for making judgments about performance of the RMI and measurement of people in the sample with MS?

Figure 12.2 shows targeting (match) of the patient sample (top histogram) to the items (bottom histogram). Item locations are covered by the people, but the person locations are not well covered by the items. Thus, this is a reasonable sample to examine the scale but a suboptimal scale for measuring the sample.

Has a measurement ruler been constructed successfully? Do the 15 RMI items map out a line on which people's mobility can be located?

The lower histogram in Figure 12.2 shows the relative difficulty of the 15 RMI items. They spread out and thus define a line (continuum) rather than just a point. Table 12.2 gives the location values and the associated standard errors. The 15 RMI items are bunched at three places on the continuum: "sitting

balance" (−2.781) and "lying to sitting" (−2.707); "walking outside on even ground" (+0.444) and "stairs" (+0.515); and "walking outside on uneven ground" (+2.641) and "up and down four steps" (+2.715). This raises the possibility that one of each pair of items may be redundant. Notable gaps are apparent in the continuum they map out (marked with thick arrows). Gaps imply limited measurement at those areas on the continuum. Thus, Figure 12.2 provides a clear representation of the mobility measurement ruler mapped out by the 15 RMI items, with its adequacy and limitations explicit. It is clear to see how such a figure could be invaluable during scale construction.

Do the 15 RMI items work together to define a single variable?

A central theme of a Rasch analysis is examination of the "fit" of the observed data to the expectations of the mathematical model. By fit, we mean the extent to which observed responses of persons to items are

Table 12.2 RMI items, item locations, SE, fit, and chi-square probability (n = 585; 666, with 81 extremes excluded)

RMI Item	Item location	Location SE	Fit residual	Chi-square value	Chi-square probability
1. Turning over in bed	−3.032	0.13	−0.031	4.557	0.4722
2. Lying to sitting	−2.707	0.125	−0.803	31.761	0
3. Sitting balance	−2.781	0.126	1.626	51.566	0
4. Sitting to standing	−1.863	0.117	2.188	17.23	0.0041
5. Standing supported	−0.619	0.115	−2.85	13.742	0.0173
6. Transfer	−2.423	0.122	−1.514	29.498	0
7. Stairs	0.515	0.119	−1.143	11.585	0.0409
8. Walking inside, with aid if needed	−1.568	0.116	−2.729	28.581	0
9. Walking outside (even ground)	0.444	0.119	−2.75	11.453	0.0431
10. Walking inside, no aid	2.566	0.144	0.088	7.322	0.1978
11. Picking off the floor	0.94	0.122	−3.775	25.877	0.0001
12. Walking outside (uneven ground)	2.641	0.146	−0.503	4.76	0.4459
13. Bathing	−0.872	0.115	1.217	8.77	0.1186
14. Up and down four steps	2.715	0.148	−0.759	3.971	0.5536
15. Running	6.042	0.356	−0.202	10.973	0.0519

SE = standard error.

predicted by, or recovered from, the mathematical model.

Table 12.2 includes fit residuals and chi square values for the 15 RMI items. Fit residuals range from −3.775 to +2.188. Four items (items 11, 5, 9, 8) have fit residuals outside the range of −2.5 to +2.5, indicating that the observed responses to these four items are not consistent with those predicted by the Rasch model. It is noteworthy that fit residuals for three of these four items (items 5, 9, 8) lie within the range +/−3.0 and thus only a small amount outside the recommended range. Therefore, only item 11 (picking off the floor) notably fails this one criterion of fit. This indicates that some misfit of the observed data with the Rasch model needs to be explored and explained.

Chi-square values range from 3.971 (item 14; "up and down four steps") to 51.566 (item 3; "sitting balance"). Although chi-square probabilities are significant at the 0.01 level, for the last six items Andrich (31) recommends examination of the values themselves and how they change sequentially across items, rather than a binary interpretation of

their associated probabilities. For the RMI, a gradual increase is seen for 10 items from chi square = 3.971 up to chi square = 17.230; then a larger step (item 11 = 25.877) is followed by a fairly gradual increase for the next three items (chi square = 28.581 to 31.761) before a large step can be taken to the final item (item 3; chi square = 51.566).

A third indicator of observed data-to-Rasch–model fit is the item characteristic curve (ICC). This is a graphic rather than numeric indicator of fit. It brings perspective to, and aids the interpretation of, the two fit statistics detailed above, which are sample-size dependent. ICC's plot the expected response (predicted from the model) to an item at each and every level of the measurement continuum. Figure 12.3 shows the ICC for the worst-fitting item (3 = sitting balance), indicating that the fit is less of a concern than the statistical values might imply.

What do the fit statistics mean for the 15 RMI items? The implication of misfit is that it undermines the inferences made from the data. Essentially, for the total score to be a sufficient statistic,

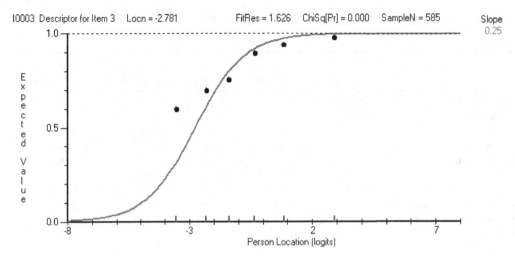

Figure 12.3 Item characteristic curve for item 3, including class intervals.

and for the estimates of items and persons generated to be invariant, and on an equal interval scale, the data need to fit the Rasch model. The question then becomes to what extend does the misfit associated with a specific analysis disrupt this process.

One common approach to the problem of misfitting items is to remove them to create a modified RMI with better fit statistics. A better approach is to try to diagnose why misfit has occurred in some items, given that the 15 items of the RMI are conceptually related to mobility – the construct the RMI seeks to measure.

Item 11 ("picking off the floor") failed all three item fit criteria. One explanation of the misfit is that this item involves more than mobility and is less related to mobility than the other items. Another explanation is that there may have been some ambiguity, or that the items may not be a common task for people to do. So, there may be some estimating by people as to their ability to do the task – or the interviewers set different standards for success and failure.

Item 7 ("stairs") also failed all three item fit criteria and demonstrated a similar pattern of fit results to item 11. As it stands, item 7 is ambiguous in that the number of stairs constituting a flight varies widely. Some people might not do their flight of stairs

because there are many. Accordingly, they would report "unable" when they are able to do a few stairs – which for others might constitute a flight. In addition, there is no clarification of "help," which can be seen in many forms (hand rail, verbal encouragement, hands on help from another person). Thus, many explanations are available for misfit, and were one to modify the RMI, it would be appropriate to address these issues before removing items. It is perhaps surprising to note that managing a flight of stairs (location = −1.568) appears considerably easier than going up and down four steps (location = +2.715).

Items 3, 7, and 11 came out worst. All three items have some degree of ambiguity. Item 3 involves a judgment of time and is not a regular task. It is uncertain why 10 seconds was used as the criterion. Item 7 does not define what constitutes a "flight of stairs" or "help." But it seems interesting that Item 3 (sitting balance) failed two item fit criteria. It had the largest chi-square values and therefore chi-square probability. The ICC shows that the slope of the observed responses is flatter than the ICC. Thus, the item is less discriminating than the model requirements. This explains the positive fit residual. Therefore, at the more disabled end of the continuum, more people are able to do this task than predicted; furthermore, people in four successive class intervals and, by definition, at different levels of disability, tend to get the same mean score on the item. One explanation is that item 3 may be difficult to interpret. It is uncertain why 10 seconds was used as the criterion for sitting on the edge of the bed without help.

Does the response to one item directly influence the response to another?

For the RMI, in this sample none of the residual correlations exceeded 0.30. This implies that responses on items are independent of each other and that the items are locally independent.

Are locations of the items stable across clinically important groups?

We examined item functioning across the three treatment arms of the study (placebo, cannador, marinol). No evidence suggested that the three groups handled any of the items differently. Thus we have evidence that item performance across the three treatment groups is stable and that the three groups can be measured on a common ruler.

Have the people in the sample been measured successfully?

Are persons in the sample separated along the line defined by the items?

Figure 12.2 shows the distribution of person measurements (locations) relative to item locations. The sample is well spread, with values ranging from around −4.75 to +7 logits. The mean is −0.861 (SD 2.622), indicating that the sample is off center of the items (because the mean of the item locations is always zero).

One numeric indicator of the degree to which a scale has been successful in separating this sample of people with MS is the Person Separation Index (PSI (53)). This is computed from the person location estimates as the variation among person locations relative to the error of estimate for each person. Thus, it is consistent with the traditional definition of reliability of a scale: how reliably the scale distinguishes between responders. The PSI tells us how much of the variation in person estimates is error variance, that is, the extent to which scores are associated with random error. Thus, the PSI is a reliability indicator, and like most reliability indicators, it goes from 0 (all error) to 1.0 (no error). The fact that it focuses (in both name and computation) on the separation of persons indicates that the PSI is not a property of the scale but a property of the scale in relation to the specific sample of persons measured. In contrast, the analogous reliability statistic of traditional psychometric analysis, Cronbach's alpha, has the same formulaic structure as the PSI but relates the variance among persons to the variance among items. A number of other advantages of the PSI over Cronbach's alpha are known.

The distribution of people in the sample has some notable features. The sample is not normally distributed. This is neither expected, nor wanted, because the distribution of the sample is an empirical finding rather than a requirement. However, it does have implications by suggesting that it would be advantageous not to make assumptions of the distribution of samples and traits in populations. The largest frequency of patients (n ≈ 80, ≈12%) is at the floor of the scale range, and about 50% are within the lower third of the scale range. This provides further evidence of suboptimal targeting of the RMI to the study sample, especially in the context of a clinical trial, where the ability to detect change is paramount.

Figure 12.4 shows the plot of RMI total scores against the intervalized measurements they imply. The curve is S-shaped, although not substantially so. Nevertheless, these vary 4.7-fold across the range of the scale.

Figure 12.5 plots the SE against each RMI location. The curve is U-shaped and indicates that standard errors vary 3-fold across the range of the scale, are greatest at the extremes, and are smallest at the center of the scale range. This is logical. People who

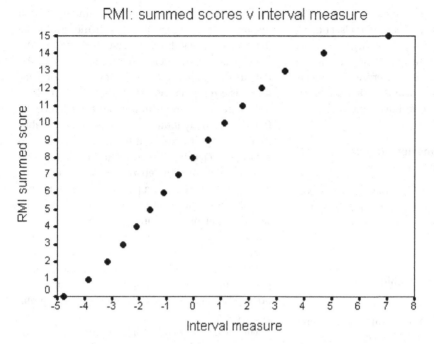

Figure 12.4 Plot of RMI total scores against the intervalized measurements they imply.

score at the floor and the ceiling are those for whom we have the least confidence about their estimate – we do not know how far above or below the ceiling or floor they really lie. There are two implications of the U-shaped curve. First, the most precise measurement occurs in the center of the range covered by a scale. Second, statistical significance of change is influenced by a person's location at each measurement time point (e.g., pretreatment and posttreatment), as well as by the size of the change score.

How valid is each person's measurement?

The item fit residual, as discussed above, summarizes the extent to which responses to each individual item are consistent with those expected by the Rasch model. This value is achieved for each of the 15 RMI items by summarizing the residuals arising from 585 patients' responses to that item. Similarly, we can achieve a value for each of the 667 patients by summarizing the residuals from each person's responses to the 15 RMI items. This is called the person fit residual; it summarizes the extent to which responses by each person are consistent with those expected by the Rasch model and is used to identify misfitting individuals. In this sample, no person fit residuals were outside the range $-/+2.5$.

Comparison of results from the two analytic methods

This analysis of RMI data using both traditional and Rasch psychometric analyses offers the opportunity to compare and contrast the two approaches and to highlight some of the similarities and differences between them.

In Rasch analysis, the 15 items of the RMI have been located, relative to each other, on an interval-level continuum. Moreover, these estimates are independent of the distributional properties of the sample from which the estimates were made, and

Plot of standard error against location

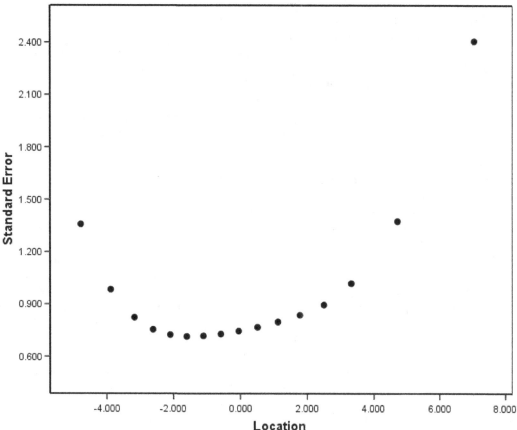

Figure 12.5 Plot of standard error against location.

we have an associated estimate of the error associated with the location. The fact that these estimates are freed up from the sample distributional properties is a fundamental requirement if we are to determine the stability of these locations, and thus the stability of the ruler they imply, across clinically different samples. Traditional psychometric methods do not generate estimates of item locations. This does not mean we cannot get an idea of their potential locations – this can be achieved by examining the item mean scores. However, these values are not on an interval-level scale and are dependent on the distribution of the sample from which they were derived. Thus, inferences about the potential stability of items (even if they could be made) could not be understood meaningfully.

In Rasch analysis, the extent to which a set of items works together to define a single variable – their internal consistency – is determined rigorously: the fit of the observed responses to a mathematical model. In traditional methods, the internal consistency of a set of items is determined by correlational analyses: corrected item total correlations, Cronbach's alpha, homogeneity coefficients. Rasch analysis and traditional methods came to different conclusions about the extent to which the 15 RMI items make up a conformable set. The latter implied that the items were a cohesive set but identified item 15 ("running") as poorly related to the others. Rasch analysis identified problems with a number of items that warranted further explanation. Certainly, attention needs to be paid to the wording of some items and their descriptions. Item 15 was fine, and the reasons for its poor item total correlation are its distant location from the other items and its relative targeting to the sample. This highlights a poorly understood limitation of correlations (54).

Finally, in terms of examining items, Rasch analysis enabled a formal examination of dependency among items and differential performance of items. This is not possible with traditional methods.

The change in mobility measurement implied by a 1-point change in RMI raw score varies 4.7-fold across the scale range. This has critical implications for clinical trials, where accurate measurement of change underpins the inferences made. It also has implications for performing basic statistical tests on RMI raw scores. It questions the legitimacy of adding (which underpins means and SDs), subtracting (which underpins change score analysis), dividing, and multiplying, and of all the statistical tests that handle data in this way. In contrast, it is legitimate to undertake these statistical analyses on Rasch-derived measurements because they are on an interval scale.

Another advantage of Rasch analysis is that it generates a standard error for each person location. In contrast, traditional analyses generate a single estimate of the standard error that is considered applicable across the whole range of the scale. The problem with a single estimate of error is that it is illogical – it is clear that the people for whom we have the least confidence about their measurement are those at the extremes of the scale range. The availability of individualized standard errors makes measurement at the individual person level a legitimate process. This means that rating scale data from clinical trials and other studies could be analyzed for individual person clinical decision making as well as a group comparisons study. In contrast,

raw scores are not considered suitable for individual person level analysis (55).

The demonstration that variable standard errors are associated with different person location estimates is important for another reason. It demonstrates that significant change for any one individual is not simply a function of the magnitude of his/her change. It also depends on the location of the individual on the continuum at the measurement time points. This important fact is not accounted for in group-based analyses of change.

Summing up

From the preceding discussion, it seems clear that Rasch analysis offers substantial clinical and scientific advantages over traditional psychometric methods in the development and evaluation of rating scales, and in the analysis of rating scale data. Nevertheless, few publications have concluded that the benefits are modest (56, 57). This has led a number of people to argue that traditional psychometric methods are just as good as new psychometric methods. However, these studies simply examined the impact of inferences on a single study, using Rasch-transformed summed scores versus summed scores; therefore the findings are not surprising for a number of reasons. First, summed scores are monotonically related to the interval measurements they imply. Second, group-based and individual person-based analyses can come to different conclusions. Third, neither of these studies examined differences at the individual person level. Fourth, the impact of inferences will be study dependent (thus findings from a single study will not generalize), and it will be impossible to determine in advance the situations in which a difference might be found.

More important, we think the main problem with these studies comparing Rasch analysis with traditional scoring is that they have missed the point. As we have seen, the ability to construct interval measurements from ordinal rating scale data is one of a series of advantages that Rasch analysis offers over traditional psychometric methods. Their major role will be in developing newer scales (58), making recommended modifications of scales developed using traditional psychometric approaches, and providing information about the constructs being measured (26). Because rating scales are increasingly the central dependent variables on which treatment decisions are made about patients we treat, we feel there can be no compromise in the efforts made to achieve rigorous measurements in clinical studies.

REFERENCES

1. Andrich D, Styles IM. *Report on the Psychometric Analysis of the Early Development instrument (EDI) Using the Rasch Model*. Perth, WA: Murdoch University, 2004.
2. Novick MR. The axioms and principal results of classical test theory. *J Math Psychol* 1966; **3**: 1–18.
3. Allen MJ, Yen WM. *Introduction to Measurement Theory*. Monterey, CA: Brooks/Cole, 1979.
4. Lord FM. *Applications of Item Response Theory to Practical Testing Problems*. Hillsdale, NJ: Lawrence Erlbaum Associates, 1980.
5. Hobart J, Cano S. Improving the evaluation of therapeutic intervention in MS: the role of new psychometric methods. *Monogr UK Health Technol Assess Prog* 2009; **13**(12): 1–200.
6. Hobart J, Cano S, Zajicek J, Thompson A. Rating scales as outcome measures for clinical trials in neurology: problems, solutions, and recommendations. *Lancet Neurol* 2007; **6**: 1094–1105.
7. Thurstone LL. Theory of attitude measurement. *Psychol Rev* 1929; **36**: 222–241.
8. Richardson M. The relationship between item difficulty and the differential validity of a test. *Psychometrika* 1936; **1**: 33–49.
9. Ferguson GA. Item selection by the constant process. *Psychometrika* 1942; **7**: 19–29.
10. Ferguson GA. On the theory of test development. *Psychometrika* 1949; **14**: 61–68.
11. Ferguson L. A study of the Likert technique of attitude scale construct. *J Soc Psychol* 1941; **13**: 51–57.
12. Lawley DN. The factorial analysis of multiple item tests. *Proc Roy Soc Edinburgh* 1944; **62-A**: 74–82.
13. Lawley DN. On problems corrected with item selection and test construction. *Proc Roy Soc Edinburgh* 1943; **6**: 273–287.
14. Tucker LR. Maximum validity of a test with equivalent items. *Psychometrika* 1946; **11**: 1–13.
15. Brogden H. Variation in test validity with variation in the distribution of item difficulties, number of items, and degree of their intercorrelations. *Psychometrika* 1946; **11**: 197–214.
16. Lazarsfeld PF. The logical and mathematical foundation of latent structure analysis. In: Stouffer SA et al., eds. *Measurement and Prediction*. Princeton: Princeton University Press, 1950.
17. Lord F. A theory of test scores. *Psychometric Monogr* 1952; No. **7**.
18. Lord FM. The relation of the reliability of multiple-choice tests to the distribution of item difficulties. *Psychometrika* 1952; **17**(2): 181–194.
19. Hambleton RK, Swaminathan H. Item response theory: principles and applications. Boston: Kluwer-Nijhoff, 1985.
20. Lord FM, Novick MR. *Statistical Theories of Mental Test Scores*. Reading, MA: Addison-Wesley, 1968.
21. Birnbaum A. Some latent trait models and their use in inferring an examinee's ability. In: Lord FM, ed. *Statistical Theories of Mental Test Scores*. Reading, MA: Addison-Wesley, 1968.
22. Waller M. Estimating parameters in the Rasch model: removing the effects of random guessing. Princeton, NJ: Educational Testing Service, 1976.
23. Lumsden J. Person reliability. *Appl Psychol Meas* 1977; **1**: 477–482.
24. Thissen D, Steinberg L. A taxonomy of item response models. *Psychometrika* 1986; **51**(4): 567–577.
25. Rasch G. Probabilistic models for some intelligence and attainment tests. Copenhagen, Chicago: Danish Institute for Education Research, 1960.
26. Andrich D. Controversy and the Rasch model: a characteristic of incompatible paradigms? *Med Care* 2004; **42**(1): I7–I16.
27. Andrich D, personal communication, 2006.
28. Wright BD. Solving measurement problems with the Rasch model. *J Educ Meas* 1977; **14**(2): 97–116.
29. Wright BD, Stone MH. Best Test Design: Rasch Measurement. Chicago: MESA, 1979.
30. Wright BD, Masters G. *Rating Scale Analysis: Rasch Measurement*. Chicago: MESA, 1982.
31. Andrich D. A rating formulation for ordered response categories. *Psychometrika* 1978; **43**: 561–573.

32. Wright BD. IRT in the 1990's: which models work best? *Rasch Meas Trans* 1992; **6**(1): 196–200.

33. Massof R. The measurement of vision disability. *Optometry Vision Sci* 2002; **79**: 516–552.

34. Divgi D. Does the Rasch model really work for multiple choice items? Not if you look closely. *J Educ Meas* 1986; **23**(4): 283–298.

35. Suen HK. *Principles of Test Theories*. Hillsdale, NJ: Lawrence Erlbaum Associates, 1990.

36. Cook K, Monahan P, McHorney C. Delicate balance between theory and practice. *Med Care* 2003; **41**(5): 571–574.

37. Stevens SS. On the theory of scales of measurement. *Science* 1946; **103**(2684): 677–680.

38. Nunnally JC. *Psychometric Theory*. 1st ed. New York: McGraw-Hill, 1967.

39. Cronbach LJ. *Essentials of Psychological Testing*. 5th ed. New York: Harper Collins, 1990.

40. Anastasi A, Urbina S. *Psychological Testing*. 7th ed. Upper Saddle River, NJ: Prentice-Hall, 1997.

41. Ghiselli E. *Theory of Psychological Measurement*. New York: McGraw-Hill, 1964.

42. Helmstadter G. *Principles of Psychological Measurement*. New York: Appleton-Century-Crofts, 1964.

43. Horst P. *Psychological Measurement and Prediction*. Belmont, CA: Wadsworth, 1966.

44. Kaplan RM, Saccuzzo DP. *Psychological Testing: Principles, Applications, and Issues*. 3rd ed. Pacific Grove, CA: Brooks/Cole, 1993.

45. Torgerson WS. *Theory and Methods of Scaling*. New York: John Wiley and Sons, 1958.

46. Brown FG. *Principles of Educational and Psychological Testing*. Hinsdale, IL: Dryden Press, 1970.

47. Bohrnstedt GW. Measurement. In: Rossi PH, Wright JD, Anderson AB, eds. *Handbook of Survey Research*. New York: Academic Press, 1983; 69–121.

48. Von Helmholtz H. All science is measurement. Unreferenced citation. In: Hill AB. *Principles of Medical Statistics*. New York: Oxford University Press, 6.

49. Campbell N. *Physics: The Elements*. London: Cambridge University Press, 1920.

50. Perline R, Wright BD, Wainer H. The Rasch model as additive conjoint measurement. *Appl Psychol Meas* 1979; **3**(2): 237–255.

51. Luce RD, Tukey JW. Simultaneous conjoint measurement: a new type of fundamental measurement. *J Math Psychol* 1964; **1**: 1–27.

52. Michell J. *An Introduction to the Logic of Psychological Measurement*. Hillsdale, NJ: Lawrence Erlbaum Associates, 1990.

53. Andrich D. An index of person separation in latent trait theory, the traditional KR20 index, and the Guttman scale response pattern. *Educ Psychol Res* 1982; **9**(1): 95–104.

54. Duncan OD. Probability, disposition and the inconsistency of attitudes and behaviours. *Synthese* 1985; **42**: 21–34.

55. McHorney CA, Tarlov AR. Individual-patient monitoring in clinical practice: are available health status surveys adequate? *Qual Life Res* 1995; **4**: 293–307.

56. McHorney CA, Haley SM, Ware JEJ. Evaluation of the MOS SF-36 Physical Functioning Scale (PF-10): II. comparison of relative precision using Likert and Rasch scoring methods. *J Clin Epidemiol* 1997; **50**(4): 451–461.

57. Prieto L, Alonso J, Lamarca R. Classical test theory versus Rasch analysis for quality of life questionnaire reduction. *Health Qual Life Outcomes* 2003; **1**: 27.

58. Hobart JC, Riazi A, Thompson AJ, et al. Getting the measure of spasticity in multiple sclerosis: the Multiple Sclerosis Spasticity Scale (MSSS-88). *Brain* 2006; **129**(1): 224–234.

13

A method for imputing missing questionnaire data

Crispin Jenkinson, Robert Harris, and Ray Fitzpatrick

Introduction

When conducting research with questionnaire-based outcome instruments, it is inevitable that some data will be missing. Rigorous analyses of the data quality of patient-completed questionnaires are becoming more common (1, 2, 3, 4), but an area that can cause concern in surveys using health status measures, and especially in clinical trials, is that of missing data (5, 6). Increasingly, trials use results from self-reported health status instruments as primary endpoints, and missing data from such measurements can potentially reduce analytic power and be a source of bias (7). The purpose of this chapter is to evaluate a simple missing data algorithm for the imputation of missing dimension scores on the 39-item Parkinson's Disease Questionnaire (PDQ-39).

The Parkinson's Disease Questionnaire (PDQ-39) (8, 9) is the most widely used disease-specific measure of health status in Parkinson's disease and has been recommended as the most comprehensively validated for competing PD-specific outcome measures (10, 11). The instrument was developed in the United Kingdom but has been translated into more than 30 languages, including Spanish, American English, French, German, Polish, and Japanese (12, 13, 14, 15, 16, 17), and has been used in both single-country (18) and cross-cultural trials (19). Typically, the instrument has been shown to have rela-

tively low levels of missing data, but inevitably with questionnaire-based outcome instruments, some data will be missing.

Data Imputation

One of the most widely used techniques for data imputation currently used within the social sciences is the "expectation maximization" (EM) computational algorithm for multiple imputation (20). The EM approach is an iterative procedure with two discrete steps. First, the "expectation" step computes the expected value of the complete data log likelihood based on complete data cases and the algorithm's "best guess" as to what the sufficient statistical functions are for the missing data based on existing data points. The "maximization" step procedure substitutes the expected values (typically, means and covariances) for the missing data obtained from the expectation step and then maximizes the likelihood function as if no data were missing to obtain new parameter estimates. The new parameter estimates are substituted back into the expectation step, and a new maximization step is performed. The procedure iterates through these two steps until convergence is obtained. Convergence occurs when the change in parameter estimates from iteration to iteration becomes negligible (21). EM has a number of advantages over rival imputation methods based on multiple

Quality of Life Measurement in Neurodegenerative and Related Conditions, eds., Crispin Jenkinson, Michele Peters, and Mark B. Bromberg. Published by Cambridge University Press. © Cambridge University Press 2011.

regression, not least that it is an established method that makes fewer demands of data in terms of statistical assumptions, and it appears, in general, to be more accurate (7). Furthermore, EM is implemented in a wide variety of computer packages, including popular statistical software such as the Statistical Package for the Social Sciences (SPSS).

Methods

Analysis plan

Data from a survey of patients registered with the Parkinson's Disease Society were analyzed to determine whether EM could accurately estimate mean scores and distributions on the eight dimensions of the 39-item Parkinson's Disease Questionnaire (PDQ-39). This was achieved through a six-stage process:

1) Any case from the dataset that contained any missing PDQ-39 dimension scores was deleted. This led to a dataset that had a complete set of scores for all respondents on all eight dimensions of the PDQ.

2) Dimension scores were deleted from this newly created subset of the original dataset, reflecting the manner in which data had been missing in the original complete dataset (i.e., the pattern of missing data was identical to the original data, although the cases from which deletions were made were selected randomly).

3) The data that had been deliberately removed were then imputed using EM, assuming a normal multivariate distribution, and mean scores, standard deviations, median, and 25th and 75th percentiles for each dimension were calculated: these results were compared with the original scores before deletion of data. Both parametric (t-test) and nonparametric (Wilcoxon) tests were used to determine whether data were statistically significantly different. This procedure was then repeated, with random selection of another set of cases for data deletion to check the results of the first analysis.

4) Ten percent of responses to each PDQ-39 dimension were randomly deleted and then data imputed as before, and results were compared with the original dataset. Once again, this procedure was repeated with another random selection of data deleted and imputed.

5) It has been suggested that quality of life data are most likely to be missing among the most severely ill of respondents (22, 23). Consequently, another analysis was undertaken, restricting the 10% of deletions and imputations to those cases in the bottom third of scores on the PDQ-39 Index (24), which is a summary score calculated on the basis of all eight dimensions. Once again, this procedure was repeated.

6) The purpose of this sixth step was to ascertain whether EM is an appropriate algorithm for use in smaller datasets. Consequently, a subset of 200 cases of the respondents who had complete data in the original dataset was selected. Ten percent of data for each dimension was deleted and then imputed using EM as before. This step was then repeated.

The original dataset is referred to here as DATA_ORIGINAL.

The dataset derived from DATA_ORIGINAL, which contains only cases with complete data for all eight dimensions of the PDQ-39, is called DATA_FULL.

The dataset created from DATA_FULL, where PDQ-39 values have been deliberately removed, is called DATA_VR.

The dataset created from DATA_FULL, where deletions are restricted to the most severely ill respondents, is called DATA_ILL.

The dataset that contains a small subset of DATA_FULL is called DATA_FULL-SMALL.

Survey design

The data analyzed here were gained from a postal survey of randomly selected members of 13 local branches of the Parkinson's Disease Society (PDS). The survey contained the PDQ-39 and demographic questions. A thank you/reminder letter was sent out to all members after 3 weeks. Full details of the survey can be found elsewhere (25).

Table 13.1 Descriptive statistics for all respondents on the eight dimensions of the PDQ-39 (n = 715)

PDQ Dimension	Mean	(SD)	Min-Max	Percentiles		
				25	50	75
Mobility	59.13	(29.95)	0–100	35.00	62.50	85.00
ADL	51.66	(27.52)	0–100	29.17	50.00	75.00
Emotional well-being	38.04	(23.47)	0–100	20.83	37.50	54.17
Stigma	30.74	(26.23)	0–100	6.25	25.00	50.00
Social support	24.98	(24.24)	0–100	0	16.67	41.67
Cognitions	43.34	(23.95)	0–100	25.00	43.75	62.50
Communication	33.50	(25.37)	0–100	8.33	33.33	50.00
Bodily discomfort	48.93	(25.46)	0–100	25.00	50.00	66.67

The Questionnaire

The PDQ-39 comprises 39 questions measuring eight dimensions of health: mobility, activities of daily living (ADL), emotional well-being, stigma, social support, cognition, communication, and bodily pain. Dimension scores are coded on a scale of 0 (perfect health as assessed by the measure) to 100 (worst health as assessed by the measure). The contents of the instrument were developed on the basis of exploratory in-depth interviews with patients with Parkinson's disease. These interviews generated a large number of candidate questionnaire items. Items were scrutinized for ambiguity or repetition, and a long-form questionnaire was developed and piloted to test basic acceptability and comprehension. A postal survey was conducted using this initial version of the questionnaire to produce a more usable questionnaire with a smaller number of items and to identify scales in the instrument to address different dimensions of Parkinson's disease. Data from this survey were factor analyzed and the eight domains identified, containing a total of 39 items. Additional studies have tested and confirmed the reliability and validity of the instrument. (26)

Results

A total of 1,372 PDS members were surveyed; of these, 851 (62.03%) questionnaires were returned.

Of these, 839 (61.15%) had been completed or partially completed. Twelve (0.87%) were returned blank with notice that the person was unable to participate in the survey. The first stage in testing EM on the PDQ-39 was creating a dataset with complete data for every case. Of the 839 questionnaires returned, complete data on the PDQ were available in 715 (85.22%) cases, and it is this subset of the data that is analyzed here (called DATA_FULL). The average age of respondents was 70.48 years (SD 90.57; min = 32.89, max = 90.57, n = 713). Four hundred thirty-two (60.42%) of the respondents were male, and 283 (39.58%) female. Descriptive statistics for the eight dimensions of the PDQ-39 are reported in Table 13.1.

The second stage in testing EM on the PDQ-39 involved removing data from the DATA_FULL dataset. The distribution of missing data in the subsequent dataset, DATA_VR, replicated the pattern of missing data in the original dataset (DATA_ORIGINAL). In the original dataset, 125 cases were missing a score on at least one dimension as the result of missing data. Consequently, data in DATA_FULL were deleted in 125 cases; cases for deletion were chosen randomly, but the deletion of data exactly mirrored that in the original dataset. The distribution of dimensions with complete data is shown in Table 13.2. Because the number of cases with missing data in DATA_VR is exactly the same as in DATA_ORIGINAL, the proportion of cases with missing data is somewhat higher. Consequently, DATA_VR contains a higher proportion of missing

Table 13.2 Descriptive statistics for DATA_VR (and number of cases with complete data for each dimension) before imputation of data

PDQ Dimension	Mean	(SD)	n	Percentiles		
				25	50	75
Mobility	59.37	(30.12)	664	35.00	62.50	85.00
ADL	51.80	(27.67)	694	29.17	50.00	75.00
Emotional well-being	38.01	(23.61)	674	20.83	37.50	54.17
Stigma	30.67	(26.25)	681	6.25	25.00	50.00
Social support	24.99	(24.13)	680	0	16.67	41.67
Cognitions	43.67	(24.00)	691	25.00	43.75	62.50
Communication	33.56	(25.42)	697	8.33	33.33	50.00
Bodily discomfort	49.11	(25.27)	701	25.00	50.00	66.67

Table 13.3 Descriptive statistics after imputation of data (n = 715)

PDQ Dimension	Mean	(SD)	Min-Max	Percentiles		
				25	50	75
Mobility	59.42	(30.06)	0–100	37.50	62.50	85.00
ADL	51.76	(27.69)	0–100	29.17	50.00	75.00
Emotional well-being	37.99	(23.59)	0–100	20.83	37.50	54.17
Stigma	30.72	(26.25)	0–100	6.25	25.00	43.75
Social support	25.11	(24.18)	0–100	0	25.00	41.67
Cognitions	43.62	(24.00)	0–100	25.00	43.75	62.50
Communication	33.60	(25.41)	0–100	16.67	33.33	50.00
Bodily discomfort	49.10	(25.27)	0–100	33.33	50.00	66.67

data than is typical of PDQ-39 datasets: this strategy was deliberately chosen to test the data imputation algorithm in datasets with higher than typical amounts of missing data. Descriptive statistics for this dataset prior to imputation of data is shown in Table 13.2.

The third stage in testing EM on the PDQ-39 involved applying the EM algorithm to the dataset. Descriptive statistics are reported in Table 13.3. Mean differences between original and imputed scores for all eight dimensions were very small (see Table 13.4). Correlations between the two datasets were high (ICC [intraclass correlation coefficient] = 0.95, or higher, p < 0.001).

The procedures outlined above were then repeated, but missing data were created for another random sample from DATA_FULL to create a new

DATA_VR. Data reflected the results gained above with very small differences for all PDQ-39 dimensions between the original dataset and the dataset containing imputations (less than +/− 0.4). Correlations between the original data and the imputed data for each dimension were high (ICC = 0.97, or higher, p < 0.001).

The fourth step in testing the EM procedure on the PDQ-39 involved removing 10% of data per dimension (from DATA_FULL) and then imputing values for this missing data. This led to 297 (41.54%) cases with complete data, with the remainder requiring at least one dimension score to be imputed. Descriptive statistics and mean differences between the original data and the imputed dataset, are shown in Table 13.5, as are descriptive statistics for the dataset, including the imputations.

Table 13.4 Mean differences (NS) and intraclass correlations (p < 0.001) between original and imputed datasets

PDQ Dimension	Mean difference (SD)	95% CI	Paired sample correlations
Mobility	0.30 (6.79)	−0.20–0.80	0.97
ADL	0.10 (3.08)	−0.13–0.32	0.96
Emotional well-being	−0.05 (4.64)	−0.39–0.29	0.96
Stigma	−0.02 (5.23)	−0.41–0.36	0.96
Social support	0.15 (5.27)	−0.24–0.53	0.95
Cognitions	0.28 (4.03)	−0.02–0.57	0.95
Communication	0.10 (3.34)	−0.14–0.35	0.95
Bodily discomfort	0.17 (4.65)	−0.17–0.51	0.95

Table 13.5 Descriptive statistics and mean differences between the original data and those imputed when 10% of data per dimension was removed

	Mean	SD	Min-Max	Mean difference (SD) from original dataset	Mean 95% lower	Difference CI higher
Mobility	59.02	(28.71)	0–100	−0.11 (8.72)	−.75	.53
ADL	51.44	(26.18)	0–100	−0.22 (8.05)	−.81	.37
Emotional well-being	38.37	(22.72)	0–100	0.33 (6.18)	−.12	.79
Stigma	30.69	(24.84)	0–100	−0.05 (7.92)	−.63	.53
Social support	24.87	(23.05)	0–100	−0.09 (7.47)	−.64	.45
Cognitions	43.22	(22.91)	0–100	−0.11 (7.00)	−.63	.40
Communications	33.43	(24.19)	0–100	−0.07 (7.35)	−.61	.47
Bodily discomfort	48.97	(24.40)	0–100	0.04 (8.10)	−.55	.64

Mean differences between original and imputed scores for all eight dimensions were very small. Correlations between the two datasets were high (ICC = 0.95, or higher, p < 0.001). The procedures outlined above were then repeated, but missing data were created for another 10% random sample for each dimension from DATA_FULL: only 307 (42.94%) cases had complete data across all dimensions of the PDQ-39. Data reflected the results gained above with mean differences for all PDQ-39 dimensions between the original dataset and the dataset containing imputations being very small (less than +/− 0.35). Similarly, results for all eight dimensions were highly correlated (ICC = 0.95, or higher, p < 0.001).

The fifth stage in testing the EM algorithm was similar to that just described, but 10% of cases were all removed from respondents who scored in the bottom third of scores on the PDQ-39 Index, creating a dataset called DATA_ILL. This led to 492 (68.81%) cases with complete data and the remainder requiring at least one dimension score to be imputed. Results in this analysis were similar to those from the random deletions undertaken previously. Mean differences between original and imputed scores for all of the eight dimensions were very small (see Table 13.6). Correlations between the two datasets were high (ICC = 0.97, or higher, p < 0.001). Results are reported in Table 13.6. The procedures outlined above were then repeated, but missing data were created for another 10% random sample from the bottom third of scores on the PDQ-Index for each

Table 13.6 Descriptive statistics and mean differences between original data and those imputed when 10% of data, restricted to the most severely ill, was removed

	Mean	SD	Min-Max	Mean difference (SD) from original dataset	Mean 95% lower	Difference CI higher
Mobility	59.89	(28.47)	0–100.00	−0.77 (7.64)	−1.33	0.21
ADL	52.18	(26.84)	0–100.00	−0.52 (5.59)	−0.93	−0.1
Emotional well-being	38.18	(23.08)	0–100.00	−0.14 (4.68)	−.043	0.20
Stigma	31.18	(25.70)	0–100.00	−0.44 (4.96)	−0.80	0.80
Social support	25.72	(23.34)	0–100.00	−0.74 (6.17)	−1.19	−0.29
Cognitions	43.83	(23.25)	0–100.00	−.049 (5.06)	−0.86	−0.12
Communications	33.92	(24.76)	0–100.00	−0.43 (7.64)	−0.99	0.13
Bodily discomfort	49.02	(24.51)	0–100.00	−0.01 (6.68)	−0.50	0.48

Table 13.7 Results of data imputation on a random subset (n = 200)

	Mean (SD) original sample, n = 200		Mean (SD) imputed sample, n = 200		Mean difference (SD)	95% confidence interval of the difference	
						Lower	Upper
Mobility	59.73	(30.16)	58.72	(28.47)	−1.00 (9.36)	−2.31	0.30
ADL	53.29	(27.44)	52.40	(25.85)	−0.90 (8.54)	−2.09	0.29
Emotional well-being	37.83	(24.39)	38.16	(23.81)	0.33 (5.44)	−.429	1.09
Stigma	33.31	(27.61)	32.98	(26.42)	−0.34 (8.23)	−1.48	0.81
Social support	25.00	(24.98)	24.86	(23.95)	−0.15 (7.01)	−1.12	0.83
Cognitions	44.00	(24.29)	44.63	(22.96)	0.63 (7.80)	−0.45	1.72
Communications	35.00	(26.07)	35.41	(23.99)	0.41 (9.44)	−0.90	1.73
Bodily discomfort	50.46	(26.57)	50.72	(28.47)	−0.35 (7.48)	−1.39	0.70

dimension from DATA_FULL: only 489 (68.39%) cases had complete data across all dimensions of the PDQ-39. Data reflected results gained above with mean differences for all PDQ-39 dimensions, with the original dataset and the dataset containing imputations being very small (less than +/−0.88). Similarly, results for all eight dimensions were highly correlated (ICC = 0.97, or higher, p < 0.001).

In the sixth stage in testing the EM algorithm on the PDQ-39, 200 cases from the original dataset were randomly selected, and 10% of responses to each dimension randomly removed from this subset were then imputed. This dataset is called DATA_FULLSMALL. The purpose of this procedure was to see if data imputation works on datasets smaller than those previously analyzed here. The results of this procedure are reported in Table 13.6. Only 88 respondents (44.0%) had complete data after random deletion of data. All PDQ-39 dimensions had ranges of 0 to 100 both for the original 200-case dataset and for the dataset containing imputations. Results for all eight dimensions were highly correlated (ICC = 0.93, or higher, p < 0.001). The procedures outlined above were then repeated, but missing data were created for another 10% random sample for each dimension from the 200 cases of the sample: only 82 (41%) respondents had complete data for the PDQ-39. Data reflected the results gained above with mean differences for all PDQ-39 dimensions between the original dataset and the dataset containing imputations being small (less than +/7−0.70). Similarly, results for all eight dimensions were highly correlated (ICC = 0.95, or higher, p < 0.001).

CONCLUSION

This chapter has evaluated a widely used missing data algorithm (expectation maximization – EM) for use with the Parkinson's Disease Questionnaire (PDQ-39). It has also been tested on the ALSAQ-40, an Amyotrophic Lateral Sclerosis/Motor Neuron Disease questionnaire (23). Missing data can lead to problems in analyses of data and, in treatment trials, can cause loss of power and are potentially a source of bias. Furthermore, the common use of listwise deletion (i.e., completely omitting cases with missing data) not only can lead to bias but could be viewed as unethical because patients have given time to complete the survey; however, it is possible that imputation of values may severely skew results and hence be inappropriate (27). This informed the decision to undertake the analyses that have been reported in this chapter.

The procedure used here imputes dimension scores and not individual item responses. This approach was adopted because previous analyses have shown that the eight dimensions of the PDQ-39 are tapping aspects of a broad, general underlying phenomenon (overall health). Indeed, the concept of unidimensionality underlies the PDQ-39 Single Index Score, which is calculated by summing scores for the eight dimensions (28). Consequently, one would expect there to be a pattern to dimension scores, and the results gained here would support this hypothesis. Indeed, differences between the original full dataset and the consequent datasets in which data have been deleted and then imputed are very small and are unlikely to be meaningful.

It is not advisable to use this, or any other data imputation algorithm, on smaller (n < 200/(100 for ALSAQ-40)) datasets than that presented here. Indeed, the use of EM on small datasets can produce misleading variance to the distribution of data (28). Furthermore, datasets with very large amounts of missing data (in excess of 10%) must be viewed with caution, because this is a high rate of missing data atypical of the PDQ-39 or ALSAQ-40 and is likely to reflect some aspect of the sample surveyed or the method of data collection. Indeed the PDQ-39 and ALSAQ-40 exhibit low levels of missing data compared with generic instruments that have been used in elderly samples (29). However, in the analyses undertaken here, we have adopted conservative estimates (i.e., large) for missing data, and the success in imputing the data scores suggests that the imputation method will work in more typical datasets from which fewer data are likely to be missing. Results reported here provide encouraging evidence of a method of imputation for data on health-related quality of life. Furthermore, we have explored the possibility that missing data are systematically related to the overall health status of individuals, and the algorithm performs well.

In conclusion, EM is recommended as a method for imputing PDQ data in surveys and trials. However, this should not be done at the expense of trying to determine what the reasons for such missing data may be and whether strategies may exist for improving data collection.

REFERENCES

1. Berzon RA. Understanding and using health-related quality of life instruments within clinical research studies. In: MJ Staquet, RD Hays, PM Fayers, eds. *Quality of Life Assessment in Clinical Trials: Methods and Practice.* Oxford: Oxford University Press, 1998.
2. Jenkinson C, Fitzpatrick R, Norquist J, Findley L, Hughes K. Cross cultural validation of the Parkinson's Disease Questionnaire: tests of data quality, score reliability, response rate and scaling assumptions in

America, Canada, Japan, Italy and Spain. *J Clin Epidemiol* 2003; **56**: 843–847.

3. Friedman LM, Furberg CD, DeMets DL. *Fundamentals of Clinical Trials*. New York: Springer, 1998.

4. Jenkinson C, Levvy G, Fitzpatrick R, Garratt A. The Amyotrophic Lateral Sclerosis Assessment Questionnaire (ALSAQ-40): tests of data quality, score reliability and response rate in a survey of patients. *J Neurol Sci* 2000; **180**: 94–100.

5. Efficace F, Bottomley A, Vanvoorden V, Blazeby J. Methodological issues in assessing health-related quality of life of colorectal cancer patients in randomised controlled trials. *Eur J Cancer* 2004; **40**: 187–197.

6. Vercherin P, Gutknecht C, Guillemin F, Ecochard R, Mennen L-I, Mercier M. Non-reponses aux questionnaires de qualite de vie SF-36 dans un echantillon de l'etude SU.VI.MAX. *Rev Epidemiol Sante Publique* 2003; **51**: 513–525.

7. Fairclough D, Peterson H, Chang V. Why are missing quality of life data a problem in clinical trials of cancer therapy? *Stat Med* 1998; **17**: 667–677.

8. Peto V, Jenkinson C, Fitzpatrick R, Greenhall R. The development and validation of a short measure of functioning and well-being for individuals with Parkinson's disease. *Qual Life Res* 1995; **4**: 241–248.

9. Jenkinson C, Fitzpatrick R, Peto V. *The Parkinson's Disease Questionnaire: User Manual for the PDQ-39, PDQ-8 and the PDQ Summary Index*. Oxford: University of Oxford Health Services Research Unit, 1998.

10. Marinus J, Ramaker C, van-Hilten JJ, Stiggelbout AM. Health related quality of life in Parkinson's disease: a systematic review. *J Neurol Neurosurg Psychiatry* 2002; **72**: 241–248.

11. Damiano AM, Snyder C, Strausser B, Willian MK. A review of health related quality-of-life concepts and measures for Parkinson's disease. *Qual Life Res* 1999; **8**: 235–243.

12. Katsarou Z, Bostantjopoulou S, Peto V, Alevriadou A, Kiosseoglou G. Quality of life in Parkinson's disease: Greek translation and validation of the Parkinson's disease questionnaire (PDQ-39). *Qual Life Res* 2001; **10**: 159–163.

13. Martinez-Martin P, Frades-Payo B, Fontan-Tirado C, Martinez-Sarries F, Guerrero M, del-Ser-Quijano T. Valoracion de la calidad de vida en la enfermedad de Parkinson mediante el PDQ-39. *Estudio Piloto Neurologia* 1997; **12**: 56–60.

14. Martinez-Martin P, Frades B, Jimenez-Jimenez F, Pondal M, Lopez-Lozano JJ, Vela L, Vazquez A, del-Val-Fernandez J, Divi M, Fabregat N, Tuldra A, Crespo-Maraver MC, Molinero LM. The PDQ-39 Spanish version: reliability and correlation with the short-form health survey (SF-36). *Neurologia* 1999; **14**: 159–163.

15. Bushnell DM, Martin ML. Quality of life and Parkinson's disease: translation and validation of the US Parkinson's Disease Questionnaire (PDQ-39). *Qual Life Res* 1999; **8**: 345–350.

16. Sobstyl M, Zabek M, Koziara H, Kadziolka B. Evaluation of quality of life in Parkinson's disease treatment. *Neurol Neurochir Polska* 2003; **37**(suppl 5): 221–230.

17. Jenkinson C, Fitzpatrick R, Norquist J, Findley L, Hughes K. Cross cultural validation of the Parkinson's Disease Questionnaire: tests of data quality, score reliability, response rate and scaling assumptions in America, Canada, Japan, Italy and Spain. *J Clin Epidemiol* 2003; **56**: 843–847.

18. Wade DT, Gage H, Owen C, Trend P, Grossmith C, Kaye J. Multidisciplinary rehabilitation for people with Parkinson's disease: a randomised controlled trial. *J Neurol Neurosurg Psychiatry* 2003; **74**: 158–162.

19. Gershanik O, Emre M, Bernhard G, Sauer D. Efficacy and safety of levodopa with entacapone in Parkinson's disease patients suboptimally controlled with levodopa alone, in daily clinical practice: an international, multicentre, open label study. *Prog Neuropsychopharmacol Biol Psychiatry* 2003; **27**: 963–971.

20. Schafer JL. *Analysis of Incomplete Multivariate Data*. London: Chapman and Hall, 1997.

21. Little RJA, Rubin DB. The analysis of social science data with missing values. In: Fox S, Long JS, eds. *Modern Methods of Data Analysis*. Newbury Park, CA: Sage, 1990.

22. Fayers PM, Machin D. *Quality of Life: Assessment, Analysis and Interpretation*. Chichester: John Wiley and Sons, 2000.

23. Kopp I, Lorenz W, Rothmund M, Koller M. Relation between severe illness and non-completion of quality-of-life questionnaires by patients with rectal cancer. *J R Soc Med*. 2003 Sep; **96**(9): 442–448.

24. Jenkinson C, Fitzpatrick R, Peto V, Greenhall R, Hyman N. The PDQ-39: development of a Parkinson's disease summary index score. *Age Ageing* 1997; **26**: 353–357.

25. Peto V, Jenkinson C, Fitzpatrick R. Determining minimally important differences for the Parkinson's Disease Questionnaire (PDQ-39). *Age Ageing* 2001; **30**: 299–302.

26. Peto V, Jenkinson C, Fitzpatrick R. PDQ-39: A review of the development, validation and application of a Parkinson's disease quality of life questionnaire and its associated measures. *J Neurol* 1998: **245**(suppl 1): S10–S14.

27. VonHippel PT. Biases in SPSS 12.00 missing value analysis. *Am Statistician* 2004; **58**: 160–164.

28. Gelman A, King G, Lin C. Not asked and not answered: multiple imputation for multiple surveys. *J Am Stat Assoc* 1999; **93**: 846–857.

29. Kosinski M, Bayliss M, Bjorner JB, Ware JE. Improving estimates of SF-36 Health Survey scores for respondents with missing data. *Monitor* 2000; Fall Edition: 8–10.

14

Individualized quality of life measurement in neurodegenerative disorders

Mark B. Bromberg

Introduction

Quality of life (QoL) is an important element in the overall management of patients. It is a unique and complex concept whose elements are expressed in a variety of definitions. The various definitions emphasize different aspects and factors that have, in turn, spawned a large number of QoL measurement instruments. Most assessments of QoL focus on the impact of impaired health on the "quality" of the patient's life. Among the spectrum of health conditions and diseases, neurodegenerative disorders have special and distinguishing clinical features that affect QoL in unique ways because the negative impact of the disorders on health cannot be reversed.

The field of QoL can be approached from many directions, including philosophical, clinical, procedural, and statistical. By early 2009, more than 128,000 articles appear in PubMed under the heading "quality of life." A lesser number appear for amyotrophic lateral sclerosis (ALS), 337; Parkinson's disease (PD), 922; and Alzheimer's disease (AD), 795. Although all approaches are important and contribute to the field, this chapter considers QoL from the clinical perspective. Specifically, what clinically useful information can a health care provider derive from studies of QoL in patients with neurodegenerative disorders? How can this information be used to understand QoL issues and help patients cope with their disease? The chapter emphasizes the different philosophical approaches to QoL and resultant instruments, and less emphasis is placed on the procedural and statistical aspects of assessing QOL instruments.

It will be argued that QoL definitions that allow subjects to define what is important to them and QoL instruments that include existential questions are the most appropriate for patients with neurodegenerative disorders. In contrast, instruments that assess general health, although appropriate for a broad range of health-related issues, miss important factors and issues of QoL in patients with these disorders. This chapter focuses on efforts to measure QoL in the more common neurodegenerative disorders: ALS, PD, and AD.

Unique features of neurodegenerative disorders

An important feature of neurodegenerative disorders is that they are slowly and inexorably progressive. Currently, no means are known to reverse nerve damage and restore lost function. Most neurodegenerative disorders have no clinically effective treatment for the degenerative process, and nerve cells continue to lose function and die. Available treatments show statistical efficacy, but the magnitude of the effect is small and is not likely to

Quality of Life Measurement in Neurodegenerative and Related Conditions, eds., Crispin Jenkinson, Michele Peters, and Mark B. Bromberg. Published by Cambridge University Press. © Cambridge University Press 2011.

be noticed by the patient. Treatments for symptom management are helpful but tend to become less effective with disease progression. Accordingly, neurodegenerative disorders result in progressive loss of function over time and are associated with shortened life span. Median survival from diagnosis ranges from 2 to 4 years for ALS (1), 11.8 years for PD (2), and 9.3 years for AD when diagnosed at age 60 years, and 2.7 years when diagnosed at age 95 years (3). ALS is unique in that the disease process itself leads uniformly to death from respiratory failure, whereas the shortened life spans in PD and AD are due to secondary issues or are associated with comorbidities.

Clinical features of amyotrophic lateral sclerosis

A number of clinical issues associated with neurodegenerative disorders can influence QoL and its measurement. ALS involves degeneration of nerves subserving muscle strength and the smooth execution of movements. Patients differ in the initial site of weakness, but with progression, many patients experience disturbed speech, and oral communication becomes problematic. Most patients also experience weakness of hand muscles, and both writing and typing become challenging. Computer-based communication devices are available, but a minority of patients use such devices. Leg strength is affected, leading to impaired mobility, and activities of daily living require greater assistance.

Another issue in ALS is the recognition of a high incidence of frontal-temporal lobe dementia (FTLD), with 30% to 50% of patients showing some symptoms or signs on neuropsychometric testing (4). FTLD involves difficulties with word finding, decision making, and behavior. The degree of FTLD varies among patients, and at the extreme, some patients who present with symptoms of dementia will be found at the time of diagnosis of FTLD to also have ALS. More commonly, from the perspective of the patient presenting with symptoms of ALS, symptoms of FTLD will be evident by reduced speech output and difficulty making decisions. The overall impact of FTLD on patient well-being and how it affects the completion of QoL instruments remain unknown.

Clinical features of Parkinson's disease

PD involves degeneration of neurons in the basal ganglia leading to difficulties controlling movement, but muscle strength remains normal. Major clinical features include tremor, bradykinesia, and rigidity, and lesser features include dysarthria, dysphagia, shuffling gait, gait freezing, neurobehavioral abnormalities, and dementia (5). PD can affect mental function. Dementia has been reported in 48% of patients after 15 years of parkinsonian symptoms, and the dementia includes memory and executive functioning (6). A similar percentage of patients display depression, apathy, anxiety, and hallucinations, and a lesser percentage obsessive-compulsive behavior. Many of these clinical features can affect completion of QoL instruments.

Clinical features of Alzheimer's disease

AD involves degeneration of neurons in the temporal lobes affecting memory and other areas of the brain that interferes with social function or activities of daily living. A spectrum of cognitive changes is recognized, including mild cognitive impairment, preclinical AD, prodromal AD, and full AD dementia (7). These stages are associated with short-term memory impairment at early stages and loss of well-remembered information at later stages. Early word-finding difficulties can progress to anomia. Executive function is impaired to varying degrees. There is frequently a lack of awareness of any dysfunction (8). There will be different challenges in completing QoL instruments at different stages of AD, and it is unlikely that objective and full evaluation will be possible at late stages.

Challenges measuring quality of life in neurodegenerative disorders

Each neurodegenerative disorder imposes unique challenges in measuring QoL. Three issues relate to

ALS: (1) progressive loss of physical function and independence in all patients; (2) progressive loss of the ability to communicate in most patients; and (3) the effects of FTLD on language, judgment, and affect in up to one third of patients. QoL instruments that include questions related to physical function will yield scores that are uniformly low and that will progressively fall over time. Communication issues can likely be overcome by giving additional time and attention and letting the subject use the most effective means of communication. At this time, it is not clear how FTLD might affect answers to specific QoL questions.

The main issue in PD and AD is progression of dementia that may reach an extreme degree in late AD. This may affect the subject's ability to read, comprehend, and respond to questions. Some questions in QoL instruments refer to historical or demographic issues, and others address personal or internal issues that rely on memory and judgment. One approach is to ask a caregiver (family member or professional provider) to serve as a proxy in assessing QoL of a demented subject. However, responses may not be congruent between the caregiver and patient, and caregivers tend to rate the patient's QoL lower than does the subject (9). Other potentially significant issues in assessing QoL in demented subjects are difficulties with executive function and indifference (apathy), but it is not clear how these might affect answers to specific questions.

Another factor in assessing QoL in a disease setting is that the overall or ideal medical goal is to return patients to better or normal health. Because no cures or markedly effective treatments are known for any neurodegenerative disorder, answers to QoL questions that address expected or actual treatment outcome will result in low ratings.

Uses of quality of life instruments

QoL instruments may be used for a variety of purposes. When deciding which instruments to use to assess QoL in patients with neurodegenerative disorders, the overall goals and evaluation of resultant data should be considered. QoL assessments can be performed on an individual to help identify specific issues affecting his or her QoL or can be performed on groups of subjects, such as healthy subjects or those with a specific disease. QoL can be assessed at a single point in time (cross-sectional study) or serially over time (longitudinal studies), such as healthy subjects as they age or patients at early and late stages of a disease. Comparisons can be made between groups, such as healthy subjects compared with age-matched subjects with a disease. Within a disease, QoL comparisons can be made before and after a treatment or intervention, which is an important issue because regulatory agencies wish to determine not only if a drug has an impact on the course of the disease but also whether it has a positive effect on patient QoL. QoL is frequently assessed directly with a single instrument, but it is also common to give a battery of instruments at the same time to validate or further define certain issues related to QoL.

A number of issues need to be considered when evaluating QoL data in the literature. When multiple instruments are given at the same time, conclusions may be reached from statistical associations that may have little clinical validity. Similarly, many QoL instruments have a number of subcomponents or domains, and subcomponent or domain analysis may yield statistical associations that are challenging to relate to clinical features. Distinctions between types of QoL instruments are not always made when results are reported in the literature. For example, although an instrument may be designed and designated correctly as being of the health-related type, subsequent discussions frequently revert to the term "QoL," and conclusions are reported as such. When multiple instruments are compared to validate a health-related instrument, the test instrument is frequently declared to "be a valid QoL instrument" for the disease when this is true only in a statistical sense and it is left open as to whether it has clinical validity.

A separate but important factor in the setting of degenerative diseases is consideration of the QoL of the caregiver, for with disease progression, there are greater needs for patient care in terms of time and effort. The growing burden can affect many aspects of a caregiver's QoL, but only infrequently does it directly affect his or her physical health. As a result, health-related instruments are unlikely to yield an accurate picture of how providing care affects QoL. This means that the same health-related instruments cannot be applied to patient and caregiver for valid comparisons. Although caregiver QoL is an important issue, it will not be considered further in this chapter.

Quality of life definitions and measurement instruments

It would be ideal if QoL could be unambiguously defined before a QoL assessment instrument is designed. It is unlikely that any one definition will satisfy all perspectives. Accordingly, a large number of instruments have been developed on the basis of different definitions and perspectives of QoL. This, in turn, has led to different results in the same study population. The World Health Organization (WHO) has suggested that quality of life is defined as individuals' perceptions of their position in life in the context of the culture and value system in which they live and in relation to their goals, expectations, standards, and concerns. It is a broad-ranging concept affected in a complex way by the person's physical health, psychological state, level of independence, social relationships, and relationships to salient features of the environment.

Working from this definition, QoL can be divided into two broad categories: those that relate to general health, including "physical health, psychological state, level of independence," and those that include individuals' subjective perceptions of "goals, expectations, standards and concerns, social relations, [and] their relationships to salient features of environment." The importance of health is based on empirical evidence that health (having good health or absence of ill health) is mentioned frequently when subjects are queried about elements that make up QoL. The individual's sub-

jective perceptions are intuitively important. QoL instruments may include objective and subjective elements. Objective elements are usually assessed by a series of direct questions, but subjective elements are harder to assess by direct questions but can be approached using visual analogue scales or open questions.

QoL instruments can be divided into several broad types: 1) instruments may assess health-related QoL focus or many of the factors expressed in the WHO definition; 2) instruments or sections of instruments that focus on the individual's perceptions include existential questions; 3) disease-specific instruments focus on unique issues related to a particular disease; 4) open or individualized instruments allow individuals to determine what is important for their QoL; and 5) single-topic instruments address specific areas in the physical, social, and psychological areas. They are usually used to validate subsections of larger instruments, and because they are highly focused and do not purport to assess QoL, they will not be discussed further.

Health-related quality of life instruments

Health-related QoL has been defined as "the value assigned to the duration of life as modified by the social opportunities, perceptions, functional states and impairments that are influenced by disease, injuries, treatment or policy" (10). Health-related QoL instruments include a number of domains, where a domain is defined as an area of life that can be differentiated from other areas. A number of health-related QoL instruments have been devised to assess various aspects of physical health. They usually evolve from interviews with subjects to define domains, and questions are written to evaluate the domains. Domains commonly include physical health, mental health, social functioning, role limitations due to physical problems, role limitations due to emotional problems, energy and vitality, pain, and general health perception. Instruments are assessed for validity and reliability by statistical means, and attempts are made to reduce the number of questions to a minimum without losing information. Through this process, the statistical distributions of domain scores (subscores) and total scores are determined for a healthy population, and then comparisons with test populations are made.

The Short-Form 36 (SF-36) Health Survey (11) is probably the most well-used health-related QoL instrument and will serve as an example, because it has been applied in each of the neurodegenerative disorders and can serve as a comparison with other QoL instruments. It consists of 36 questions (*Items*) distributed across eight domains (*Scales*) and two Summary Measures (Physical Health and Mental Health). The summary measure of "Physical Health" includes domains of Physical Functioning, Role-Physical, Bodily Pain, and General Health. The summary measure of "Mental Health" includes domains of Vitality, Social Function, Role-Emotional, and Mental Health. A review of the 36 individual questions indicates that some of the questions can address more than one general category. Up to 11 questions query the effects of general health, and 19 query issues related to physical function, energy, or fatigue. The overall effect is that for neurodegenerative disorders, half to two-thirds of the questions in the SF-36 reflect the negative burden of disease. With no chance of improvement for neurodegenerative disorders, QoL will necessarily deteriorate regardless of the patient's subjective views. One can dissect health-related QoL results by subscale analysis, but from the clinical perspective, this leads away from a global view of QoL.

Existential quality of life instruments

Existential instruments are based on a simple definition of QoL as "subjective well-being" (12). It has been recognized that certain elements that make up QoL may be missed when instruments focus on health-related domains. Existential questions represent a wide variety of general issues, including perception of purpose, meaning of life, capacity for personal growth and transcendence, and specific issues such as religiosity, intimacy, loneliness, rela-

tionships, environment, social interactions, values, coping, interests, desires, and goals.

The McGill Quality of Life (MQoL) instrument was developed with the notion that the existential domain is important in an individual's QoL, especially among patients with advanced illness (it was originally developed for patients with cancer), and that reliance on the physical domain makes it difficult to assess positive contributions to QoL (13). Thus, the MQoL incorporates existential questions and is less heavily weighted toward physical function. It also includes a single question on quality of life (MQoL-SIS). The importance of existential issues has been investigated, and the existential questions have been shown to correlate well with the single QoL question (12).

Disease-specific and domain-specific quality of life instruments

When it is believed that unique issues are related to a particular disease, disease-specific instruments are developed to include questions that address the unique aspects of the disease. Disease-specific instruments attempt to be more sensitive to changes related to the particular disease compared with instruments that are applicable to a wide variety of subjects. These instruments include a focus on specific areas, such as functional abilities, psychological well-being, social well-being, memory, and other items. The elements expanded upon are frequently derived from interviews with subjects who have the disease.

Many disease-specific QoL tools are designed to be health-related instruments with special emphasis on issues related to the specific disease. Accordingly, they are generally affected by the same limitations as general health-related QoL instruments. A number of these instruments include existential questions, and thus there is overlap between disease-specific or domain-specific instruments and existential instruments. In particular, the ALS-Specific Quality of Life Instrument (ALSSQoL) is singled out as an attempt to move away from weighting toward health-related domains and to include existential items and an individualized or open scale (14).

Individualized quality of life instruments

A different approach is based on allowing the individual to define QoL. This has led to a number of instruments that do not impose predefinitions but rely upon the subject's unique perspective. It is argued that such instruments do not focus on health, or any other domain, and therefore are less likely to bias subjects to their illness or lack of effective therapy and allow other potentially positive factors to be included. Individualized instruments may take several forms, from a single visual analogue or Likert global scale to multi-question or multi-step instruments. Individualized instruments have been designed that vary in their approach, but most rely on responses to a set number of open questions (15). Many have not gone beyond the early development stage, and clinical experience is limited (16).

The Schedule for the Evaluation of Individual Quality of Life (SEIQoL) is based on the definition of QoL that states "it is what the individual says it is" (17). The SEIQoL is a three-step "open" instrument. The first step is a semistructured interview during which subjects are asked to consider their life and to designate or nominate five areas or domains of life they consider important in their overall QoL at the current time. If five areas are not forthcoming, a list is offered of suggestions based on past experience. The second step involves rating how each of the five areas is going for them using their own criteria applied to a 100-mm visual analogue scale between the extremes of 0 = "worst possible" and 100 = "best possible." The third step is to quantify the relative importance or weight of each area based on judgment analysis. The judgment analysis step was a formal and time-consuming process that was recognized as a limitation for older subjects, those with reduced cognitive function, or those with other physical infirmities. This led to the development of a more simple third step that directly weights each domain by the use of an apparatus and is referred to as the Schedule for the Evaluation of Individ-

ual Quality of Life-Direct Weighting (SEIQoL-DW) (18). The direct weighting apparatus is a five-sector pie chart in which each sector represents one of the five nominated areas and each sector can be adjusted with respect to the other sectors to set a relative degree of importance for each (each sector represents a chosen number of degrees of the 360-degree pie). A computer version of the SEIQoL-DW has been developed and has been shown in a small sample to yield similar results compared with the written version (19).

Another definition of QoL states that it is "the extent of which our hopes and ambitions are matched by experience" (20). This approach has led to the Patient-Generated Index instrument (PGI), which has three steps (21). In the first, subjects are asked to select the five most important areas of their lives affected by their condition (or to select five from a list of 20 items if subjects have difficulty generating five on their own). The second step is to rate how badly each area is affected on a scale of 0 (worst they can imagine) to 100 (exactly as they would like to be). The third step is to imagine that they can improve some or all of their chosen areas, and "points" are given to spend across one or more of the areas that the subject would most like to improve (thus representing relative importance of potential improvements). ·

Although the SEIQoL-DW and the PGI are similar in some aspects, especially with respect to the first two steps, they differ in several ways. First, the SEIQoL-DW is completely open and is not linked to ill health, whereas the PGI focuses on the subject's underlying health-related issues. Second, the PGI asks about possible improvement in health, but improvements in health are unrealistic goals for neurodegenerative disorders.

Qualty of life investigations in neurodegenerative disorders

Much effort has been expended to study QoL in neurodegenerative disorders, and most reports are based on health-related instruments, but a limited number of studies, particularly in ALS, have used existential and individualized instruments. This section focuses on comparisons between health-related instruments (using the SF-36) such as disease-specific and individualized instruments and those with existential elements for ALS, PD, and AD.

Amyotrophic lateral sclerosis

The inexorable progression of weakness in ALS has influenced the development of QoL instruments and has affected the results of health-related QoL instruments. Progression in ALS can be measured directly by quantitative isometric muscle strength testing (22) and indirectly by a functional rating scale. The ALS Functional Rating Scale (ALS-FRS) (23) and a later revised version that includes more detailed questions about respiratory function (ALSFRS-R) (24) are commonly used measures of disease progression. These scales have very high correlations with muscle strength and can be used as a proxy for strength (23). Not unexpectedly, when either quantitative strength or the ALS-FRS or ALSFRS-R is used as a comparison, high correlations are seen with functional domains in health-related instruments. For the SF-36, there are high correlates between the Physical Function scale (particularly for leg strength) and isometric limb strength and between the perceptions of physical health and strength (25). High correlations are also seen between the Physical Function scale and the ALSFRS-R (26). It was also noted that there are floor and ceiling effects for a number of domains in the SF-36 when applied to ALS patients, emphasizing a limitation of the instrument (27). The Sickness Impact Profile (SIP) instrument (28) correlates well with quantitative strength measurements in both cross-sectional and serial studies (29). The SIP consists of 132 questions, and a subset of 19 questions was selected that address function (ALS/SIP-19) (30); this short instrument correlates highly with quantitative strength and the ALSFRS (31). Thus, the 19 questions account for the overall high correlations of the full SIP with patient function.

In contrast to the correlations between disease progression and health-related instruments is the lack of correlations between progression and QoL when instruments with existential elements or those with individualized formats are used. Despite the inexorable progression of ALS, neither the disease itself nor the disability it causes is foremost on the minds of ALS patients as assessed by these instruments. When patients were asked, as part of the SEIQoL-DW instrument, to name five areas they consider important in making up their QoL, the area of "health" was mentioned with low frequency (by 15% in one study and by ~50% in other studies). The areas most frequently nominated from three studies are family, finances, activities (recreational), dependency, friends-friends/social life, health, and profession (32, 33, 34).

The MGQoL instrument, which includes existential items, has been administered serially to ALS patients and compared with the ALSFRS and ALS/SIP-19 scales (35). Although clear loss of function is seen over 5 to 9 months of assessment by the ALSFRS and ALS/SIP-19, no significant change is seen in the MGQoL. A similar pattern has been observed in serial studies using the SEIQoL-DW, with little change in overall index score over time (32, 33, 34). The ALSSQoL has been compared with the ALSFRS-R, and despite low functional scores, there are high scores on the ALSSQoL (14). There are also high correlations between the ALSSQoL and the SEIQoL-DW. It has been pointed out that patients feel that the SEIQoL-DW has greater validity for them and that the SIP imparts significantly more emotional distress because of its length and the general negativity of the questions. Thus, with instruments that include existential items or allow the subject to nominate important areas, patients report the preservation of a relatively good QoL despite the progressive loss of strength and function.

A structured review of the literature on QoL instruments in ALS focused on data related to validity, reliability, and responsiveness (36). Instruments for which there were sufficient data included the SF-36, SIP, MQoL, SIP/ALS-19, ALSAQ-40, ALSSQoL-46,

SEIQoL-DW, EuroQoL, and EQ-5D. The report concluded that SF-36 and ALSAQ-40 were well tested for validity and reliability but acknowledged that there was a need for questionnaires to include areas on religious and spiritual beliefs and that the ALSSQoL may bridge the gap between traditional health status instruments (SF-36, SIP, ALSAQ-40) and individual instruments (MQoL) or open instruments (SEIQoL-DW). It was also acknowledged that the effects of cognitive impairment have not been addressed in QoL instruments.

Parkinson's disease

The SF-36 has been compared with the PDQ-39, and there were good correlations between matching scales (37). There were also good correlations between patient perceptions of clinical features of PD and the PDQ-39 and with physician assessment scales. These correlations relate to the physical aspects of PD and are consistent with the high proportion of questions in the PDQ-39 related to physical function. However, other areas not included in the SF-36 were found to be important to PD patients.

A comparison has been made between the SEIQoL-DW and the PDQ-39 (38). The most common domains designated in the SEIQoL-DW were family (87.7%) and health (52.8%), with lower percentages for leisure activities, marriage, and friends. When correlated with the PDQ-39, only the domains of social support, cognitive impairment, and emotional issues in the PDQ-36 correlated with the SEIQoL-DW. Predictors of QoL differed between the two instruments: for the PDQ-39, predictive negative elements were the number of symptoms, disease stage, and depression (measured by the Beck Depression Inventory), whereas for the SEIQoL-DW, the predictive negative element was depression. The conclusion was that psychosocial issues rather than physical issues and the stage of the disease are important elements in QoL in PD.

The motor symptoms of PD frequently respond to medication, at least early in the course of the disease, and this might be expected to improve QoL. However, health-related QoL instruments have not always been found to correlate with objective improvement on motor function scales (39).

Alzheimer's Disease

The SF-36 has been assessed in patients with AD and has revealed challenges, making it largely unsuitable, especially when dementia is severe (40). Thirteen percent of patients refused to complete the questions, and help from the interviewer was required in 73%, whereas data were incomplete in patients with Mini-Mental State Examination (MMSE) scores of <10 (30 is normal state).

An important question for assessing QoL in AD is the ability of patients with more severe dementia, which can include lack of insight, to meaningfully complete an instrument (41). When the QoL-AD instrument was assessed in patients with MMSE scores <12, those with scores from 3 to 11 could complete the 13-item instrument with a degree of validity and reliability, but those with scores <3 could not complete any of the items (42, 43). Highest correlations on the QoL-AD were seen with mood state, as assessed by a 12-question health-related instrument derived from the SF-36, with lesser correlations seen with physical health and activities of daily living.

In a study that used the SEIQoL-DW in 20 patients with dementia, the majority displayed poor understanding of the domain rating concept, and only six who were less cognitively impaired completed the instrument (44). Thus, the SEIQoL-DW may be limited to patients who are early in the course of their dementia. Another study queried AD patients with mild dementia (MMSE scores 2 to 25; mean, 13.5) (45). Patients were asked a set of questions that are similar to the first step in the SEIQoL-DW: 1) How do you describe your QoL? 2) What things give you your QoL? 3) What things take away from your QoL? 4) What things make your QoL better? 5) What things make your QoL worse? From patient responses, the following themes emerged: social interaction, physiologic well-being, religion and spirituality, independence, financial security, and health. It is noted that subjects did not focus on activities of daily living, cognitive difficulties, or other disease-related issues.

Another study assessed nine QoL instruments, including the QoL-AD, DQoL, and SEIQoL-DW (46). No instrument was found to be appropriate for all stages of AD: the SEIQoL-DW was found to be useful for mildly to moderately affected subjects, and the QoL-AD was useful for subjects with MMSE scores >3.

Healthy subjects

It is reasonable to compare QoL instruments and data from patients with neurodegenerative disorders to data from healthy subjects, and in particular from healthy elderly, because neurodegenerative disorders occur more commonly with advancing age. Most QoL instruments given to healthy subjects are health-related instruments. Data in the literature on other instruments have focused more on individualized instruments than on those with existential elements. In a study using the original SEIQoL, among 60 subjects >65 years in age and with no medical problems, the areas nominated as important domains by 75% to 95% of subjects were family, social and leisure activities, health, living conditions, and religion (47). A comparison was made with 42 healthy young subjects (mean age, 28.8 years; range, 19 to 51 years) who also nominated family (60%), happiness (48%), and work (38%), but other domains were not included by the elderly. The index scores were statistically significantly higher for the elderly (82.0) compared with the younger group (77.5).

Impact of the response shift

Given the progressive decline in function in neurodegenerative disorders, the data showing a relatively preserved assessment of QoL using instruments focusing on existential elements or individualized instruments must be explained. The factor that allows a reasonable QoL in the setting of incurable diseases can be explained by the "response shift." The response shift represents internal reconceptualization and recalibration of an individual's internal framework for judging QoL (48, 49). It includes a catalyst (such as the underlying disease) modified by a variety of factors and preexisting components (including sociodemographics, personality, expectations, spirituality) and the influence of adaptive components (including coping mechanisms, social support, and goal reformatting), leading to a response shift and the perceived QoL. A striking example of a response shift in ALS comes from a German patient completing the SEIQoL-DW (33). He listed football (soccer) as one of the five important elements in his quality of life. Over time, as he became weaker, he shifted from actively playing football to watching football. Despite this shift in type of involvement, football remained high as a source of satisfaction, and its relative contribution to quality of life remained unchanged. In the extreme, patients have been known to state that a progressive disease has given more meaning to their lives than before the disease was diagnosed.

It can be argued that response shifts are normal adaptive, psychological homeostatic mechanisms for coping with a wide range of life's disturbances, including normal aging and unfulfilled hopes and plans. Although the response shift can be viewed as a natural process with aging, it may not go well with everyone, especially when faced with a severe disease. When shifts do not go well, an individual may experience variable degrees of stress and a lower QoL (49).

The effect of the response shift is being studied using individualized QoL instruments. One example is from a group of patients receiving an intervention (receipt of dentures) who were given the SEIQoL-DW before and after the intervention (50). It is interesting to note that the index score did not change after dentures were received; however, when patients were asked to retrospectively evaluate their QoL before the intervention (then-test), the reevaluation scores were lower. The rationale is that by retrospectively evaluating their QoL, they will be using the same internal criteria as they are using after the intervention. Differences in weighting between the original and the reevaluation represent the response shift. Further evaluation revealed that 80% of patients nominated at least one different cue or domain after the intervention, and this was felt to represent reconceptualization as an adaptation to changing circumstances. When patients were asked to reevaluate their weightings for the cues, they frequently rated them lower, and this was interpreted to represent recalibration.

In another study, patients who received a diagnosis of metastatic cancer and who were enrolled in a palliative care program completed the SEIQoL-DW within 3 months of the time of diagnosis and at two later times 3 months apart (51). The index score improved over time. An interesting pattern in nominating cues was observed: at the first testing only 9% of patients were able to nominate five domains despite prompting, at the second testing 21% nominated five domains, and by the third testing 57% nominated five domains. The explanation offered is that at the time of diagnosis, patients had scaled back some of their goals, and that with passage of time, some patients were able to expand the number of goals (representing a positive change). Among the patients who could not nominate five domains, it was hypothesized that this likely represented a lesser degree of positive change, or a negative change.

How well these findings in other diseases can be generalized to neurodegenerative diseases is not clear. However, it is the author's experience with ALS that, at the time of diagnosis, many patients immediately look ahead and express the opinion that they do not want to be "bed bound and paralyzed and dependent upon others," but they infrequently return to these concerns over the course of progression (52). This change in expectations in ALS is interpreted as being similar to that in patients in the study of metastatic cancer who have a very focused outlook early on, manifested by the inability to name five domains, but who later are able to expand their outlook and are more likely to name five domains.

Discussion

It is argued in this chapter that the unique features of neurodegenerative disorders have a marked impact on the selection of QoL instruments and interpretation of the data. The primary issue with health-related and disease-specific instruments is that they include domains related to physical disabilities that in turn do not relate to factors that patients feel are important for their QoL. It should be noted that, although health-related and disease-specific instruments are frequently compiled after discussions with patients to determine what is important to them, the same factors appear not to be mentioned when subjects are asked to nominate domains important in their QoL with individualized instruments. This is likely due to the fact that health-related and disease-specific instruments do not take into consideration the effects of response shifts. The reason for this is not entirely clear but likely includes the fact that health-related and disease-specific instruments (as well as other QoL instruments) ask fixed questions that do not easily allow for how the subject shifts responses to underlying conditions.

Much effort has been expended to assess construct and face validity of QoL instruments for both health-related and disease-specific instruments. This is a statistical exercise that, if successful, leads to the statement that the instrument has been "validated" for general health-related use or for a particular disease. When an instrument is found to be valid, it is likely reliably tracking some state or domain in the test population. However, that state or domain may not actually be important for the patient in the assessment of QoL or for the clinician in trying to use the information. This is particularly true for neurodegenerative disorders, where most instruments are validly tracking the degenerative aspects of the disease but are missing elements that are important clinically. Thus, it is argued that physical function and dysfunction are not necessarily key determinants in the patient's QoL.

It is recognized among groups interested in QoL that the effects of the response shift are important for patients with progressive disease. For example, the SEIQoL-DW has been administered to patients with cancer (metastatic cancers, Hodgkin's lymphoma, leukemia, prostrate, small-cell lung, mesothelioma, gastrointestinal cancers, treatment with stem cell transplantation), congenital heart disease, type 1 diabetes mellitus, cystic fibrosis, multiple sclerosis, HIV, mental illness, poststroke, in a palliative care program, and to the healthy elderly. The general results of these studies, many of which include comparisons with other QoL instruments, support the differences between instruments and indicate that individualized instruments assess what appear to be important issues to patients that are not captured by health-related instruments. Many of these reports recognize and discuss the element of the response shift that is not captured by health-related instruments.

The SEIQoL-DW is the most individualized or open QoL instrument currently available. However, it is not without issues. The optimum number of domains to inquire about is not clear, and although more than five may more fully reflect factors in a patient's QoL, not all subjects can give five. Further, it may be that, although the first five are readily offered, more important ones may be apparent to the patient only upon deeper reflection. When subjects cannot nominate five domains important for their QoL, the SEIQoL-DW manual gives a list of suggestions to offer subjects. It has been pointed out that there may be a potential bias when patients cannot nominate five domains and suggestions are offered (53). There can be a cognition element, and patients with an MMSE <20 may have problems comprehending and completing the SEIQoL-DW (47). In a large sample of patients (120 with ALS) completing the SEIQoL-DW, 90% of the selected domains reflected family or significant others, and only 15% reflected health or physical function (54). There is a concern that the administration manual requires verbatim instruction when asking about domains: "...the things that make your life a relatively happy or sad one at the moment...", and thus the SEIQoL-DW may be focusing

on happiness rather than on other aspects of QoL (53).

Another issue is whether the index score derived from the SEQoL-DW is a valid measure of aggregate QoL among groups, and its use in comparing groups is questioned (53). Among ALS patients, there are poor correlations between the SEIQoL-DW index score and the MQoL-SIS. The SEIQoL-DW manual recommends caution in using and comparing index scores among subjects, because the sum of products of individual domain levels by their weights may vary independently.

Another use of the SEIQoL-DW or similar open instruments that allow patients to nominate important areas affecting their QoL is the ability to detect and address areas of concern. In one study of oncology patients, the SEIQoL-DW appeared to empower the patient and allow for a broader approach to patient care (55).

At the end of this evaluation, it is clear that health-related QoL instruments do not address certain important areas that affect QoL in patients with neurodegenerative disorders and do not address the effects of the response shift. On the other hand, relatively few fully developed QoL instruments include existential elements or are individualized. The two most promising instruments are the SEIQoL-DW and the MQoL. The SEIQoL-DW has been used in a number of disorders, including ALS and PD, but there are issues with its usability with marked dementia and whether it in fact focuses on happiness rather than on QoL. The MQoL has been used in a large variety of disorders but in few neurodegenerative disorders other than ALS. A modification of the MQoL for ALS has been developed (ALSSQoL), but has not been extended to other neurodegenerative disorders. Of note, the MQoL-SIS has high correlations with the MGQoL full-scale score and the SEIQoL-DW and also with other instruments, and perhaps its directness and simplicity offer a lot of information (56, 53). It remains unclear how to assess QoL in neurodegenerative diseases that affect cognition.

What information do QoL instruments provide to the clinician? Most clinicians would agree that, despite the progressive nature of degenerative disorders, patients remain, in general, relatively positive in their outlook. Thus, any QoL scale that shows a decline is not congruent with clinical experience. Detailed assessment of health-related domains within an instrument, such as the various domains available in the SF-36, is generally a research exercise that is inefficient to apply in the clinic. It is important when counseling patients early on with their diseases to give them a realistic outlook of how they will feel at different stages, and instruments with existential elements or individualized instruments appear to provide reliable data to give to patients. An attraction of open instruments, particularly the SEIQoL-DW, is the ability to determine what domains in their life are going well or are not going well, and this information provides the chance to compliment, address, or intervene as needed. Without effective therapy, one goal of a clinician is to help the patient with a neurodegenerative disease work through the response shift.

Conclusion

Measuring QoL is a very challenging exercise as evidenced by the various QoL definitions and constructs that have led to large number of assessment instruments. Assessing QoL of patients with progressive disorders is most important while searches are made for effective interventions. It is also essential to include the effects of response shifts. It is unlikely that a single QoL instrument can cover all neurodegenerative disorders. It may be that a single-item QoL question will serve to adequately assess a complex and individual situation and allow for comparisons between and among groups of patients. An open instrument (SEIQoL-DW) may provide unique insights into individual issues. A multi-domain instrument with existential questions (MGoL or ALSSQoL) may provide a broader view of the many factors that contribute to QoL. Finally, a variety of instruments may be necessary in disorders that include a major element of dementia.

REFERENCES

1. Traynor B, Codd M, Corr B, Forde C, Frost E, Hardiman O. Clinical features of amyotrophic lateral sclerosis according to the El Escorial and Airlie House diagnostic criteria: a population-based study. *Arch Neurol* 2000; **57**: 1171–1176.

2. Driver JA, Kurth T, Buring JE, Gaziano JM, Logroscino G. Parkinson disease and risk of mortality: a prospective comorbidity-matched cohort study. *Neurology* 2008; **70**: 1423–1430.

3. Brookmeyer R, Corrada MM, Curriero FC, Kawas C. Survival following a diagnosis of Alzheimer disease. *Arch Neurol* 2002; **59**: 1764–1767.

4. Lomen-Hoerth C, Anderson T, Miller B. The overlap of amyotrophic lateral sclerosis and frontotemporal dementia. *Neurology* 2002; **59**: 1077–1079.

5. Jankovic J. Parkinson's disease: clinical features and diagnosis. *J Neurol Neurosurg Psychiatry* 2008; **79**: 368–376.

6. Verbaan D, Marinus J, Visser M, van Rooden SM, Stiggelbout AM, Middelkoop HA, et al. Cognitive impairment in Parkinson's disease. *J Neurol Neurosurg Psychiatry* 2007; **78**: 1182–1187.

7. Dubois B, Feldman HH, Jacova C, Dekosky ST, Barberger-Gateau P, Cummings J, et al. Research criteria for the diagnosis of Alzheimer's disease: revising the NINCDS-ADRDA criteria. *Lancet Neurol* 2007; **6**: 734–746.

8. Talwalker S, Overall JE, Srirama MK, Gracon SI. Cardinal features of cognitive dysfunction in Alzheimer's disease: a factor-analytic study of the Alzheimer's Disease Assessment Scale. *J Geriatr Psychiatry Neurol* 1996; **9**: 39–46.

9. Sands LP, Ferreira P, Stewart AL, Brod M, Yaffe K. What explains differences between dementia patients' and their caregivers' ratings of patients' quality of life? *Am J Geriatr Psychiatry* 2004; **12**: 272–280.

10. Patrick DL, Erikson P. *Health Status and Health Policy. Allocating Resources to Health Care.* New York: Oxford University Press; 1993.

11. Ware J, Sherbourne C. The MOS 36-item short-form survey (SF-36). I. Conceptual framework and item selection. *Med Care* 1992; **30**: 473–483.

12. Cohen SR, Mount BM, Tomas JJ, Mount LF. Existential well-being is an important determinant of quality of life. Evidence from the McGill Quality of Life Questionnaire. *Cancer* 1996; **77**: 576–586.

13. Cohen S, Mount B, Strobel M, Bui F. The McGill Quality of Life Questionnaire: a measure of quality of life appropriate for people with advanced disease: a preliminary study of validity and acceptability. *Palliat Med* 1995; **9**: 207–219.

14. Simmons Z, Felgoise S, Bremer B, Walsh S, Hufford D, Bromberg M, et al. The ALSSQOL: balancing physical and nonophysical factors in assessing quality of life in ALS. *Neurology* 2006; **67**: 1659–1664.

15. Dijkers MP. Individualization in quality of life measurement: instruments and approaches. *Arch Phys Med Rehabil* 2003; **84**: S3–S14.

16. Patel KK, Veenstra DL, Patrick DL. A review of selected patient-generated outcome measures and their application in clinical trials. *Value Health* 2003; **6**: 595–603.

17. O'Boyle C, McGee H, Joyce C. Quality of life: assessing the individual. In: Albrecht G and Fitzpatrick R, eds. *Quality of Life in Health Care. Advances in Medical Sociology*. Vol **5**. Greenwich, CT: JAI Press, Inc., 1994; 159–180.

18. Hickey A, Bury G, O'Boyle C, Bradley F, O'Kelly F, Shannon W. A new short form individual quality of life measure (SEIQoL-DW): application in a cohort of individuals with HIV (AIDS). *BMJ* 1996; **313**: 29–33.

19. Ring L, Hofer S, Heuston F, Harris D, O'Boyle CA. Response shift masks the treatment impact on patient reported outcomes (PROs): the example of individual quality of life in edentulous patients. *Health Qual Life Outcomes* 2005; **3**: 55.

20. Calman KC. Quality of life in cancer patients – an hypothesis. *J Med Ethics* 1984; **10**: 124–127.

21. Ruta DA, Garratt AM, Leng M, Russell IT, MacDonald LM. A new approach to the measurement of quality of life: The patient-generated index. *Med Care* 1994; **32**: 1109–1126.

22. Andres P, Hedlund W, Finison L, Conlon T, Felmus M, Munsat T. Quantitative motor assessment in amyotrophic lateral sclerosis. *Neurology* 1986; **36**: 937–941.

23. ALS-CNTF Treatment Study (ACTS) phase I-II Study Group. The amyotrophic lateral sclerosis functional rating scale. *Arch Neurol* 1996; **53**: 141–147.

24. Cedarbaum J, Stambler N, Malta E., Fuller C, Hilt D, Thurmond B, et al. The ALSFRS-R: a revised ALS functional rating scale that incorporates assessments of respiratory function. *J Neurol Sci* 1999; **169**: 13–21.

25. Shields RK, Ruhland JL, Ross MA, Saehler MM, Smith KB, Heffner ML. Analysis of health-related quality of life and muscle impairment in individuals with amyotrophic lateral sclerosis using the medical out-come survey and the Tufts Quantitative Neuromuscular Exam. *Arch Phys Med Rehabil* 1998; **79**: 855–862.

26. De Groot IJ, Post MW, van Heuveln T, Van Den Berg LH, Lindeman E. Cross-sectional and longitudinal correlations between disease progression and different health-related quality of life domains in persons with amyotrophic lateral sclerosis. *Amyotroph Lateral Scler* 2007; **8**: 356–361.

27. Bourke SC, McColl E, Shaw PJ, Gibson GJ. Validation of quality of life instruments in ALS. *Amyotroph Lateral Scler Other Motor Neuron Disord* 2004; **5**: 55–60.

28. Bergner M, Bobbitt R, Carter R, Gilson B. The Sickness Impact Profile: development and final revision of a health status measure. *Med Care* 1981; **19**: 787–805.

29. McGuire D, Garrison L, Armon C, Barohn R, Bryan W, Miller R, et al. Relationship of the Tufts Quantitative Neuromuscular Exam (TQNE) and the Sickness Impact Profile (SIP) in measuring progression of ALS. *Neurology* 1996; **46**: 1442–1444.

30. McGuire D, Garrison L, Armon C, Barohn R, Bryan W, Miller R, et al. A brief quality-of-life measure for ALS clinical trials based on a subset of items from the Sickness Impact Profile. *J Neurol Sci* 1997; **152**: S18–S22.

31. Bromberg M, Anderson F, Davidson M, Miller R, Group ACS. Assessing health status quality of life in ALS: comparison of the SIP ALS-19 with the ALS Functional Rating Scale and the Short Form-12 Health Survey. *Amyotroph Lateral Scler* 2001; **58**: 320–322.

32. Bromberg M, Forshew D. Comparison of instruments addressing quality of life in patients with ALS and their caregivers. *Neurology* 2002; **58**: 320–322.

33. Neudert C, Wasner M, Borasio GD. Patients' assessment of quality of life instruments: a randomised study of SIP, SF-36 and SEIQoL-DW in patients with amyotrophic lateral sclerosis. *J Neurol Sci* 2001; **191**: 103–109.

34. Neudert C, Wasner M, Borasio GD. Individual quality of life is not correlated with health-related quality of life or physical function in patients with amyotrophic lateral sclerosis. *J Palliat Med* 2004; **7**: 551–557.

35. Robbins R, Simmons Z, Bremer B, Walsh S, Fischer S. Quality of life in ALS is maintained as physical function declines. *Neurology* 2001; **56**: 442–444.

36. Epton J, Harris R, Jenkinson C. Quality of life in amyotrophic lateral sclerosis (motor neuron disease): a structured review. *Amyotroph Lateral Scler* 2008; 1–12.

37. Jenkinson C, Peto V, Fitzpatrick R, Greenhall R, Hyman N. Self-reported functioning and well-being in patients

with Parkinson's disease: comparison of the short-form health survey (SF-36) and the Parkinson's Disease Questionnaire (PDQ-39). *Age Ageing* 1995; **24**: 505–509.

38. Lee MA, Walker RW, Hildreth AJ, Prentice WM. Individualized assessment of quality of life in idiopathic Parkinson's disease. *Mov Disord* 2006; **21**: 1929–1234.

39. Gallagher DA, Schrag A. Impact of newer pharmacological treatments on quality of life in patients with Parkinson's disease. *CNS Drugs* 2008; **22**: 563–586.

40. Novella JL, Jochum C, Ankri J, Morrone I, Jolly D, Blanchard F. Measuring general health status in dementia: practical and methodological issues in using the SF-36. *Aging (Milano)* 2001; **13**: 362–369.

41. Walker MD, Salek SS, Bayer AJ. A review of quality of life in Alzheimer's disease. Part 1: Issues in assessing disease impact. *Pharmacoeconomics* 1998; **14**: 499–530.

42. Hoe J, Katona C, Roch B, Livingston G. Use of the QOL-AD for measuring quality of life in people with severe dementia – the LASER-AD study. *Age Ageing* 2005; **34**: 130–135.

43. Logsdon RG, Gibbons LE, McCurry SM, Teri L. Assessing quality of life in older adults with cognitive impairment. *Psychosom Med* 2002; **64**: 510–519.

44. Coen R, O'Mahoney D, O'Boyle CA, Joyce CRB, Hiltbrunner B, Walsh JB, et al. Measuring the quality of life of patients with dementia using the Schedule for the Evaluation of Individual Quality of Life. *Irish J Psychiatry* 1993; **14**: 154–163.

45. Byrne-Davis LM, Bennett PD, Wilcock GK. How are quality of life ratings made? Toward a model of quality of life in people with dementia. *Qual Life Res* 2006; **15**: 855–865.

46. Scholzel-Dorenbos CJ, Ettema TP, Bos J, Boelens-van der Knoop E, Gerritsen DL, Hoogeveen F, et al. Evaluating the outcome of interventions on quality of life in

dementia: selection of the appropriate scale. *Int J Geriatr Psychiatry* 2007; **22**: 511–519.

47. Browne JP, O'Boyle CA, McGee HM, Joyce CR, McDonald NJ, O'Malley K, et al. Individual quality of life in the healthy elderly. *Qual Life Res* 1994; **3**: 235–244.

48. Sprangers MA, Schwartz CE. Integrating response shift into health-related quality of life research: a theoretical model. *Soc Sci Med* 1999; **48**: 1507–1515.

49. Wilson I. Clinical understanding and clinical implications of response shift. *Soc Sci Med* 1999; **45**: 1577–1588.

50. Ring L, Lindblad AK, Bendtsen P, Viklund E, Jansson R, Glimelius B. Feasibility and validity of a computer administered version of SEIQoL-DW. *Qual Life Res* 2006; **15**: 1173–1177.

51. Sharpe L, Butow P, Smith C, McConnell D, Clarke S. Changes in quality of life in patients with advanced cancer: evidence of response shift and response restriction. *J Psychosom Res* 2005; **58**: 497–504.

52. Bromberg MB. Asssessing Quality of Life in ALS. *J Clin Neuromusc Dis* 2007; **9**: 318–325.

53. Westerman M, Hak T, The AM, Groen H, Van Der Wal G. Problems eliciting cues in SEIQoL-DW: quality of life areas in small-cell lung cancer patients. *Qual Life Res* 2006; **15**: 441–449.

54. Felgoise SH, Stewart JL, Bremer BA, Walsh SM, Bromberg MB, Simmons Z. The SEIQoL-DW for assessing quality of life in ALS: strength and limitations. *Amyotroph Lateral Scler* 2009; **10**: 456–462.

55. Kettis-Lindblad A, Ring L, Widmark E, Bendtsen P, Glimelius B. Patients'and doctors' views of using the schedule for individual quality of life in clinical practice. *J Support Oncol* 2007; **5**: 281–287.

56. Chio A, Gauthier A, Montuschi A, Calvo A, Di Vito N, Ghiglione P, et al. A cross sectional study on determinants of quality of life in ALS. *J Neurol Neurosurg Psychiatry* 2004; **75**: 1597–1601.

Index